# Here's what readers are saying about
## The Body Sculpting Bible for Men

I'm in week three of your advanced program. What a great program! At 46 years old, I've led a healthy lifestyle for many years and have been working out for 25-plus years...The first two weeks on your programs, I've seen distinct changes in my body. More muscle definition and greater muscle size.

—*David D.*

I just wanted to send a big thank you for your fantastic book. I have been on this program for just a few weeks now, and I've already seen big differences! Thank you so much for putting out such a COMPLETE and thorough book. I do not know of any other one source that puts together so much great and necessary detail.

Keep up the great work. You've already made a big difference in my life. I also recently bought the Power Block dumbbells on your recommendation, and I love them, too!

—*Rob V. (Lake Forest, Calif.)*

I started your program six weeks ago, and I am in the best shape of my life. I used the 14-day Body Sculpting Workout #2 and it has given me incredible results! You guys have done a great job of informing and motivating the reader for a great routine. Again, this book was a revelation to me in many ways. I feel like this book cuts straight to the point in a fresh, straightforward way.

—*Michael F.*

This is one of the most informative fitness books I have ever laid my eyes on. I have used this book to change my entire workout. The photographs are amazing. Detail, detail, detail. This is a must BUY...

—*Richard B.*

I have been following this book for two months and I have never felt better. I have learned a lot and turned my wife on to the womens edition, and she follows it and loves it. Thanks!

—*A reader from Ft. Myers, Fla.*

This book addressed exactly what I was looking for. All the exercises are thoroughly detailed and they explain the mistakes that you should avoid while performing them. The majority of the exercises described in the book are done with free weights, so machines are not required. Almost all of the workouts can be done at home with a basic dumbbell set. I found the book's coverage of nutrition and fat burning extremely helpful. Workout charts and sample diets are also included, so you know exactly how to start. The book also covers all levels of body sculpting. I have already begun to see my body take shape and am very satisfied with this book.

*—A reader from Connecticut*

Great book! Easy to read, covers the entire subject...workouts, nutrition, supplements, etc. I've been doing it for six weeks and have seen great results. The concept of the 14-day workout makes sense and allows for a schedule that can last a lifetime. I highly recommend this book!

*—A reader from Bordentown, N.J.*

I've been a personal trainer in New York City for the last eight years and have read countless books on the subject of fitness.

For the last two months I have implemented *The Body Sculpting Bible* techniques into my personal training programs and have seen truly impressive results with all of my clients.

No other book has provided me with such effective and useful tools that have helped me help my clients achieve great progress in such a short amount of time.

Because of this book, my personal training business has absolutely increased. If you're looking for a straightforward, realistic, and effective fitness book for men, this is a must read!

*—A reader from New York City*

These guys did an excellent job. The book is easy to understand, and rich in information and routines that anyone can follow. I've already read many books, but none of them compares to *The Body Sculpting Bible*....If you were looking for a great fitness book, you've found it. Most importantly, this 14-day program WORKS!

*—Norberto F. (Sao Paulo, Brazil)*

I wanted to start a weight-training program to finally get the body I wanted. I tend to try and research what I need to do before starting anything and this book was amazing. The mind to body connection helps with focusing on what muscles need to be exercised and keeping proper form in the movements. The nutrition information is excellent for the beginner. With all the supplements out there it gives a wonderful easy to understand guide to what you should take to help get the body you're looking for. The programs are easy to follow and detailed. The thing I like most about the book though is that it doesn't offer a quick fix—it gives you the foundation to start building a strong muscular body. So if you are looking to start a new workout routine and to pack on muscle and take off the fat, I highly recommend this book.

*—Lenny (Glendale, Ariz.)*

# THE BODY SCULPTING BIBLE FOR MEN

## THIRD EDITION

### FEATURING THE 14-DAY BODY SCULPTING WORKOUT

## JAMES VILLEPIGUE
## HUGO A. RIVERA

### PHOTOGRAPHY BY
### PETER FIELD PECK

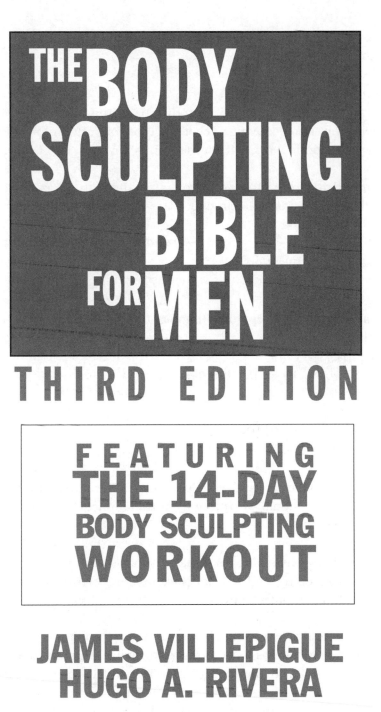

hatherleigh

The Body Sculpting Bible For Men, Third Edition

Hatherleigh Press is committed to preserving and protecting the natural resources of the Earth. Environmentally responsible and sustainable practices are embraced within the company's mission statement.

Library of Congress Cataloging-in-Publication Data

Villepigue, James C.
  Body sculpting bible for men / James Villepigue, Hugo Rivera. -- 3rd ed.
      p. cm. --  (Body sculpting bible)
  ISBN 978-1-57826-400-1 (pbk.)
1.  Bodybuilding.  I. Rivera, Hugo A., 1974- II. Title.
  GV546.5.V54 2011
  613.7'13--dc23
                          2011043138

*The Body Sculpting Bible For Men* is available for bulk purchase, special promotions and premiums. For more information on reselling and special purchase opportunities, please call us at 1-800-528-2550 and ask for the Special Sales Manager.

Cover Design by Deborah Miller  and Heather Daugherty
Interior Design by Deborah Miller, Allison Furrer, Jasmine Cordoza, and Nick Macagnone

10 9 8 7 6 5 4 3 2 1
Printed in the United States

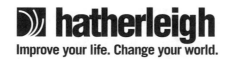

hatherleigh
Improve your life. Change your world.

# Dedications

This book is dedicated to my beautiful wife Lina who always loves and supports me uncondition-ally throughout any project, to my son Chad who is my pride and joy, to my parents and grandpar-ents for always believing in me and who always ensured that I would get the best education possi-ble as I was growing up, to my brother Raul whose computer knowledge made it possible for me to go online, to my in-laws who are always there to help me and provide me with support in times of need, and finally to God for giving me the talent to put this work together.

**Hugo A. Rivera**

I would like to begin by dedicating this landmark Revised Edition to the most important people in my life. To my, as always, remarkable mom, Nancy: I am so blessed by God to be your son and I thank you for all of your limitless love and support. You are an inspiration to so many mothers!

To my incredibly successful sister, Deborah: I am so proud of your strong will and your drive to succeed. You have become such a remarkable businesswoman and I am so psyched to see how far you can take it!

To my beloved dad, Jim, my best pal and navigator: I love you and miss you so much. Thank you for instilling in me your boundless love, deep emotions, and adventurous spirit. I honor you absolutely every moment of my life.

To God, again and as always, thank you, thank you, thank you!

To the newest edition of my family: my very beautiful, incredibly sweet, and extraordinarily tal-ented wife, Heather Villepigue, I love you, my baby, and I am so blessed to have you by my side. Thank you!

**James Villepigue**

# Special Thanks from James Villepigue

I would like to thank my partner and dear friend Hugo Rivera: We have come such a long way together bro; here's to many more years of wonderful success and friendship!

To my great friend Andrew Flach: Life has thrown us some curve balls but we continue to hit them out of the park.  You are truly one of my greatest friends and mentors.

To my consigliore, Kevin Moran, thank you for your great talent, your warm nature and your awesome friendship.

As always, thank you to the greatest photographer in all of health and fitness, Peter Field Peck. You're the greatest!

A huge thanks to Alyssa, Andrea, and Debbie.  You are all so talented and always manage to bring our work to its highest level.

To my amazing family, my grandparents, Charles and Gloria Hopf: You are two of my biggest fans. I am so honored to be your grandson!

To my aunt Joyce, uncle Tony, and my cousin Joey: All I can say is thank you! I love you all much more than you could ever know!

To my aunt Kathy, I am so lucky to have such a beautiful godmother like you. I love you.

To my newest business partner, Edward Abel: You have been a great friend! Here's to the future of TKO Business Coaching, Inc.

A huge thank you to the PowerHouse Gym in Syosset, New York.  You made this Revised Edition possible!

Additionally, I would like to thank all of my wonderful friends and all of the amazingly dedicated readers of our *Body Sculpting Bible* books. Recently I have met many of you while on the road speaking and I feel so lucky to have met you. I wish everyone continued success and look forward to meeting you all and helping you make your fitness, business, and life dreams a reality! All my love!

# Foreword to the Original Edition

If you decided you wanted to build a house the first thing you would do after acquiring the land would be to hire an architect to make the blueprints for your future dream home. I also imagine that you would do your homework to find someone you really trust to design the biggest purchase of your lifetime. That process can be quite confusing and a bit frustrating because of the different styles and many options available in a market where there are so many qualified parties.

Once you have made your decision, you are "off to the races" as they say. The first thing you will receive from your architect (next to a whopping bill!) will be your own set of blueprints for your dream home. From there on in it is simply a matter of following those blueprints exactly, step by step, until the process is done. As hard as it is along the way, the end result will hopefully be one of joy and excitement as you enter your new home for the first time.

Let's imagine for a moment that you begin to doubt the process half way through the building process. You panic and get additional blueprints from the architect that was second on your list or your spouse says, "I told you this guy was better". The last thing you would do would be to abandon the original plan and start with the new ones. You would have a complete mess. Everything would fall apart and you would have wasted precious time and money along the way.

That is a simple analogy of what most people do when attempting to get in the best shape of their lives. I have competed for years and helped many others do the same. I have learned over the years that there are many good ways to get in shape. I would run if I heard someone touting that their system is "the best" or "the only way." We know in this industry that many people claim to be experts in the attempt to collect on innocent people looking for the so coveted "magic bullet." Guess what my friends? There is no such thing as a "magic bullet."

I am going to give you the bottom line; it takes work to get in shape. It also takes a plan. James Villepigue and Hugo Rivera have worked hard to layout a time-tested plan of proper exercise, nutrition and supplementation coupled with consistency. They don't claim they have any new revelation or secret snake oil. They have done some homework and presented quality, time honored information in an easy to understand format.

Another thing I have learned along the way is that people want results today. They become impatient so they abandon their original blueprint. If results don't come when they want, they automatically move to the next set of plans. When you combine systems and pick and choose what you like you dilute the plans all together. The one thing I advocate is to find a program you trust and stick it out until the end. The program laid out in this book will work. It will work if you apply the principles and follow through until the end. Don't abandon the plan halfway through. Don't let friends, experts, critics or anyone confuse your desire to attain better health through fitness.

Anyone involved in the fitness industry wants to help people; as health professionals we should collaborate in that single purpose. I might have a book someday and I would expect that others would advocate the use of the principles I choose to teach. By agreeing to write this foreword, I am acknowledging that I see James and Hugo desiring to help people get healthier and I am all for it.

Read the book; decide if the information is right for you and your goals. If it is, then by all means go for it! Take action today, make some positive changes and share the book with everyone you care about.

—Clark Bartram
Host of *American Health & Fitness*

# Preface

**Hi Folks! Welcome to the 3rd Edition of our *Body Sculpting Bibles*!**

If you have already purchased our previous *Body Sculpting Bible* editions in the past, then we want to extend to you our most sincere gratitude for giving us the support you have since the beginning. If you are a new reader, then we want to personally congratulate you for taking your first step towards achieving the leaner, firmer, and stronger body that you are looking for.

*The Body Sculpting Bible* series has been around for over 11 years now. That's an extraordinary length of time for a fitness book series. Most fitness books only last a year or two in the marketplace, if they even last that long.

So why have our books survived the test of time, and even flourished, when others seem to just disappear? Here are a few reasons why the *Body Sculpting Bible* series has differed from other fitness books:

## THE WHO, WHAT, WHEN, WHERE, WHY & HOW

- **Who are the Creators:** James Villepigue and Hugo Rivera have been in the fitness industry and lifted in the trenches for a combined amount of over 40 years. They walk the talk and play the part.
- **What are They Most Recognized For:** The essence of the *Body Sculpting Bible* books is the underlying original 14-Day Body Sculpting Program—one of the very first periodized weight training programs for the mainstream fitness enthusiast. These systems utilize a logically arranged `muscle confusion' approach that yields the fastest and most consistent long-term body composition results possible.
- **When Were the Books First Created:** Back in 1998, the authors just happened to meet in Florida while working out separately. They started talking and two years later, they had developed this best-selling fitness book series.
- **Where:** James and Hugo spent over one year writing the books and accomplished the collaborative work by way of phone and Internet.
- **Why:** The authors had discovered that average people needed top-tier fitness information and more guidance to help them achieve their dream physiques.
- **How:** James and Hugo created step-by-step guidelines and a direct plan of action that anyone could follow, all based on scientific analysis. Much like a business plan, where everything is laid out for success, the Body Sculpting Bible books equip people with the means to achieve body sculpting perfection.

Why is it that the *Body Sculpting Bibles* have sold well over one million copies and are revered as one of the most successful fitness book franchises in history? Well, they're solid books and provide a comprehensive, yet solid, plan of specific action steps to help you on your way. When we first set out, we offered one of the very first mainstream periodization programs called "The 14 Day Body Sculpting Program". Many of our innovative training principles were initially considered radical, but they were quickly embraced by our readers and fans because they worked (and worked very well).

So, yes, the *Body Sculpting Bible* books have had wild success, but we are not sitting pretty. Yes, we've managed to help hundreds of thousands of average people just like you to shape up, gain confidence, preserve their youth, and improve many areas of their lives. But still, there are millions of people we still need to help.

We came to the realization that we needed to come back and refresh some of the material within the book. As time passes, things naturally change as new research is conducted and new science comes about. It is up to us, as fitness experts, to take the science, decipher it, and pass it on in a way that makes sense and is easy for you to understand.

So, with that said, we're on a mission to help millions more people get up and get out of their own way. Get up off that couch, rid yourself of the fast food, do what most people won't take the time to do, and let's get you to a place of total body transformation and life empowerment.

Over the years, we have had to rely mostly on the books and e-mail to stay in communication with our fans. No longer do we each exist in a place where we are isolated in our home-land or limited to our own cities and close surroundings. The internet has allowed us to reach out and digitally shake hands with our global friends.

The new global approach of this latest edition was developed for two reasons. First, we want you to be an ambassador for fitness in your hometown. We want you to stand proud and represent where you're from. Gather your local friends, family, co-workers, and anyone else and create a fitness force. With this book, we want you to lead your clan and build them up to extraordinary health and fitness levels. Together, we can combat fat, obliterate obesity, do-in diabetes, kill many cardiac problems, and take more control over our lives than ever before.

The second reason for this global approach is that, even though we have greater reach to the world than ever before, many of us still hide behind our computers. It's time to reach out and tell the world who you are. We know the world is facing a lot of difficulties right now, and there is no better time to take a stand and refuse to give in to adversity. Today we are battling wars, a bullied economy, and the fight against obesity. The grim reality is that most people have not gotten healthier over the last decade. In fact, they have gotten even unhealthier! Perhaps this is partly a result of the negative things that are going on in the world at this time. Maybe the stress from everything that is happening has affected people and thus, they take comfort in food.

However, here is our advice to you: there is too much going on in the world that we have little or absolutely no control over. But here's the great news: there are some things that we can control. We can control our ability to do our very best in building ourselves up, both inside and out, so that we create better outcomes for ourselves and for the people around us. When we build ourselves up both physically and emotionally, we empower ourselves and we place ourselves in a rare position that allows us to have more control over many different things in our lives.

It is our hope that you will take advantage of this powerful opportunity by following our lead, and we promise to help you achieve many truly remarkable and life-altering changes.

## WHAT'S NEW?

In this new edition we have updated our supplements section in order to make it current. We have also added new Body Sculpting Workouts to offer more variety and provide you with a workout that best fits your needs. In addition, we have added more sample diet plans to give you more concrete ideas of what you should be eating on a daily basis.

Since the beginning of the series, over 10 years ago, our goal has been to help people achieve the physique that they desire without having to deal with the pitfalls and the challenges that we experienced ourselves. A decade later, our commitment to help others is larger than ever! And thanks to the internet and to social networks like Facebook, we can now reach millions of people with just one click!

Before you put this book down today, go to your computer and visit us here: www.facebook.com/bodysculptingbibles. This will now become the new *Body Sculpting Bible* home base and it's a place where you will find accountability from us and your fellow readers, where you will maintain motivation to keep going, and where you can communicate with us directly.

By frequenting our Facebook Fan Page, you will always be on top of your game and you can count on it. Whether you have questions, need support, motivation, or information on training, nutrition, or supplementations, we are here to help you succeed in achieving your physique goals. We want to turn this page into a massive community of like-minded people whose goal is to not only improve their physiques but also their lives and the lives of many others!

Over the years, we have been blessed with the great opportunity to touch the lives of well over 1 million people and now that we have Facebook, we feel that we can reach more people than we ever thought possible. And now, we are not alone, since we have you to help us spread the word and finally get people off the couch and into shape!

With that said, we're calling on you to help us make great change. We need you to help us touch the lives of many other people. The way to do this is simple:

1.  **Become a fan of our Facebook Fan Page:** www.facebook.com/bodysculptingbibles.
2.  **Share this page with your friends:** In this manner, you can help us reach out to others who are looking to get in shape but may not know how to do it.
3.  **Share your expertise:** Don't be shy. Many of you are very talented and can help others by sharing your expertise. If you have read the books and used the information to transform your own life, this puts you in a position of power to help others achieve the same.

In fact, we have thousands of readers who, after reading the *Body Sculpting Bible*, decided to make a career out of fitness! While that may not be your goal, definitely don't be shy in sharing your expertise as just a simple word of encouragement can make a huge difference in the life of someone who could use a helping hand.

We look forward to working with all of you as we continue to improve our bodies (and lives). We are so excited to be connecting with new people throughout the world and together we can have a huge impact on global health!

See you soon on Facebook!

Best Always,
**James & Hugo**

# Quick Start

To get started with the *14-Day Body Sculpting Workout* as quickly as possible, follow the reading outline below. It will take you approximately 60 minutes at the most to go through this outline. We feel you'll need this basic understanding of the *14-Day Body Sculpting Workout* principles in order to harness the maximum benefits of the program.

## CHAPTER 2

| | |
|---|---|
| The Zone-Tone Concept | 33 |
| The First Component: | 42 |
| Determination | |

## CHAPTER 3

| | |
|---|---|
| Putting It All Together | 57 |
| How Does the 14-Day Body | |
| Sculpting Workout Work? | 60 |
| Choosing the Best Time to Work Out | 61 |
| Workout Clothing | 62 |
| How Fast Should You Lift The Weight? | 62 |
| Muscle Soreness | 63 |
| Breathing While Performing an Exercise | 65 |
| Warming Up Before Training and Stretching | 65 |
| Selecting the Weight for Each Exercise | 66 |

## CHAPTER 4

| | |
|---|---|
| Nutrition Basics | 72 |
| Characteristics of a Good | 77 |
| Nutrition Program | |
| Designing Your Diet | 81 |
| Tips for Choosing Food | 92 |
| Beverage Tips | 93 |
| Cooking Tips | 94 |
| Supplementation Recommendations | |
| Summary | 100 |

## CHAPTER 13

| | |
|---|---|
| Choose between: The Break-In Routine | 312 |
| The 14-Day Body Sculpting Workout | 316 |
| The 14-Day Rapid Body Sculpting Workout | 334 |
| The Advanced 14-Day Body Sculpting Workout | 346 |
| The 14-Day Body Sculpting Mass Workout | 370 |
| The 14-Day Bodyweight | |
| Body Sculpting Workout | 376 |

Depending on your knowledge of how to perform the exercises, read the exercise descriptions that pertain to the routine that you choose.

We do recommend that you read through the entire book progressively to obtain the full benefits that the program has to offer. There is more than just training information in this book. This book will not only teach you how to change your physique, it will also teach you how to change your life!

# Table of Contents

**INTRODUCTION**   **1**

The Weight Loss Obsession   2

A Book Designed Only for Men   5

The 14-Day Body Sculpting Workout   5

More on the 14-Day Body Sculpting Workout   6

**PART 1:**
**THE FOUNDATIONS OF PHYSICAL PERFECTION**   **9**

**CHAPTER 1: COMMON MYTHS & MISCONCEPTIONS**   **11**

Common Myths Debunked   12

Unnecessary Gadgets   14

Fat Burning Creams   15

Weight Loss Clinics   15

Drugs for Weight Loss   15

The Most Common & Fatal
Dieters' Mistake: Thinking
that Eating Less is Better   16

Bulimia   17

Low Carb/High Protein/High Fat Diets   18

Steroids; The Good, the Bad and the Ugly   19

Conclusion   22

**CHAPTER 2: THE POWER OF THE MIND:**
**POWERFUL METHODS FOR ACHIEVING**
**SUCCESS**   **25**

Things Don't Always Have to Be
As Complicated As They Might Seem   26

Different Routines: Some Work, Most Don't!   26

Expectations and Desire;
Expect and You Shall Receive   27

Mind Sculpting: Visualization
and Mental Imagery
(Think and Become!)   27

Applying the Visualization
Technique: An Introduction
to Self-Hypnosis for
Unprecedented Results   30

The Zone-Tone Concept   33

The 10 Commandments of
Body Sculpting Perfection   35

Life's Dilemmas, Simple Solutions;
Some People Make Excuses,
Others Find Solutions   37

The Blueprint for a Perfect Body   38

The Many Benefits of Exercise
and Correct Eating: You Will Get
Much More Than You Hoped For!   39

Turn Off the Stress Light!   41

The Formula for Success   42

The First Component:
Determination   42

The Other Components of the
Formula for Success   43

**PART 2: THE BUILDING BLOCKS OF**
**BODY SCULPTING**   **45**

**CHAPTER 3: TRAINING**   **51**

Weight Training   52

Characteristics of a Good
Weight-Training Program   52

Aerobic Training   56

Putting It All Together 57
How Does the 14-Day Body
Sculpting Workout Work? 60
Choosing the Best Time
to Work Out 61
Workout Clothing 62
How Fast Should You
Lift the Weight? 62
Muscle Soreness 63
Breathing While Performing
an Exercise 65
Warming Up Before Training
and Stretching 65
Selecting the Weight for
Each Exercise 66
Overtraining 68
Skipping Workouts 68

## CHAPTER 4: NUTRITION 71

Nutrition Basics 72
Glycemic Index 73
Characteristics of a
Good Nutrition Program 77
Designing Your Body Sculpting Diet 81
Break-In Body Sculpting Diet Plan 82
The 14-Day Body Sculpting Diet Plan 83
Advanced Body Sculpting Diet Plan 85
Designing Your Diet 89
Dieting to Add Muscle Mass 89
Tips for Choosing Foods 92
Beverage Tips 93
Quick and Easy Recipes 93
Cooking Tips 94
Eating on the Run: Fast Foods 96
Supplementation 98
Supplementation Recommendations
Summary 100
All About Protein and Biological Values 101

Creatine Monohydrate 104
Glutamine 107
Conclusion 108

## CHAPTER 5: REST & RECOVERY 109

The Sleep Cycle 110
Maladies Caused by
Sleep Deprivation 111
Are You Sleep Deprived? 112
Sleeping Pills 112
Conclusion 113

## PART 3: BODY SCULPTING EXERCISES 115

## CHAPTER 6: LEGS 117

Foot Stances and Quadriceps
and Hamstring Development 118

## CHAPTER 7: BACK 163

A Word about Exercises that Utilize
Various Hand Positions and How
Variation can Affect Different
Muscle Groups 164

## CHAPTER 8: CHEST 191

Proper Alignment 192

## CHAPTER 9: SHOULDERS 215

## CHAPTER 10: TRICEPS 239

## CHAPTER 11: BICEPS 261

## CHAPTER 12: ABDOMINALS 283

Every time we turn on the TV or read the latest muscle magazine we are bombarded with the latest way to lose fat, gain muscle and achieve the body of our dreams in only five minutes a day. We are constantly exposed to empty promises telling us that all we have to do to build a buff body is buy some fancy new machine (that may be as cheap as three small credit card installments of $75.99), take some new hyped up "magic" pill or go on a "new" diet, and that dream body will miraculously appear.

If you've ever bought one of those "body in a box" gadgets or machines, recall the process that took place when you received it. You used it for a few weeks, if at all, right? Eventually it ends up becoming a great place to lay your clothes. The only thing that ends up losing weight in this case is our wallet.

With so many diets, gadgets and magic potions available to us, it is no wonder that we become confused about how to properly get in shape. This is one of the major reasons why we decided to write this book. We are sick and tired of seeing and hearing about how people are ripped off by these "get fit quick" schemes and hokey solutions that provide nothing more than a healthy pile of junk. In addition, having dealt with weight problems throughout our youth, we naturally relate to people who want desperately to change the way they look and don't know how to go about doing so. We will show you that you can lose fat very easily without starving yourself. In fact, you may end up eating much more than you ever have in your life and still achieve the perfectly shaped physique you've been hoping for! We will also show you how to create lean muscle without having to exercise for hours a day. You don't even need to join a health club if you don't want to. Our goal is to share with you all of the

knowledge that we have accumulated in our combined 20 years of bodybuilding experience. With this newfound knowledge you will soon be in total control of how you look and feel. No longer will it be a dreadful experience to step on the scale, try on those old jeans, put on that favorite suit that stopped fitting long ago. No longer will you be at the mercy of an infomercial because you'll know exactly what to do in order to look the way you want.

Now that we've laid out our goals, let's go and learn about how you can reach yours.

## THE WEIGHT LOSS OBSESSION

Have you noticed how many people are obsessed with losing weight? It is truly unbelievable how this obsession can play into all other aspects of our lives. When we feel fat and out of shape, it can bring on very strong feelings of insecurity and depression. Is it hard for you to believe that not looking good can go hand in hand with not feeling good about yourself? I think not! I respect someone who might not be in the best shape but still feels very confident about himself and how he looks and feels. However, I do see that the majority of people who are out of shape are very unhappy about their appearance, and this usually transfers into most aspects of their lives.

There is increasing evidence that the American fixation with diet and weight loss is hazardous. Concerns about weight many times lead to obsessions about diet and weight control, dysfunctional lifestyles, abnormally high patterns of exercise, disordered eating patterns, metabolic depression and inadequate nutrition. Study after study has proven the ineffectiveness of dieting. Many of these studies were done on the commercial weight loss industry, including the companies who promote "losing weight." There exists a misconception that losing "weight" is the best way to feel and look good, which weight-loss companies would love you to believe. What exactly does losing weight entail? Losing weight in the traditional sense includes losing muscle, bone density, water and even organ tissue. Don't think for a second that these vital components of your body aren't being cannibalized upon during the losing "weight" stages. Is this healthy? Certainly not! But the diet and weight-loss industry will have you believe it is. Could this be a reason why people are not optimally healthy and even worse, are becoming sick? Indeed it is.

Conventional weight loss programs focus on caloric reduction, often without providing proper nutrition. These programs are not concerned with how you feel, exercise, or the reasons why you are losing weight. Reducing your caloric intake to a point where you burn many more calories than you are consuming is fine. But without exercise to help build and sustain lean muscle tissue, your body will be forced to cannibalize itself. Commercial weight loss programs can help you lose "weight," but along with that, there is a good chance that you'll also feel terrible, weaken your immune system risking sickness as a result, and in most cases gain all of your weight back plus more. In contrast, exercising will build muscle which in turn will help neutralize your fat loss. Your body will keep what you need for healthy maintenance, and burn off the rest for energy expenditures. In addition, the nutrients that you consume must be in balanced ratios that provide sufficient protein, carbohydrate and fat intake for optimal health. Do you think that these diet companies provide you with all of this? Their end result might cause you to lose weight, but not the kind you want to lose.

First we ask you to stop obsessing about your body weight. Instead, focus on bodily measurements, fat composition and the way that you look in the mirror. Why? Because weight cannot give you a true indication of how much fat you are carrying. Remember, body weight is a combination of the weight of all of your bone structure, organs, muscles, water and fat. Therefore, if you lose five pounds in one week, how can you be assured that those five pounds were from fat? Think about it. It could have been two pounds of muscle, two pounds of water and one pound of fat. If this is the case, you are now in a worse situation than you were before the five-pound loss. Why? Because your metabolism will end up being slower and you will have lost body shape (muscle increases your metabolism and also gives shape to your body). This is why crash diets don't work. They cause you to lose mostly muscle and water, while simultaneously creating fat storage. These diets trick the body into thinking that it is starving. When the body thinks this is the case, it begins storing fat for future use and eating away at valuable muscle. So while you may achieve your ideal weight, you'll look very different than you envisioned.

Therefore, in order to achieve the look that you desire, forget about reaching your so-called ideal body weight. Humans are made up of simply too many varying frames and sizes, making it impossible to determine universal weight standards. Such a thing just isn't realistic (at least not since the 1960's). Just follow the guidelines prescribed in the Nutrition chapter and let the fat calipers, tape measure and the mirror tell you when you have arrived at your destination.

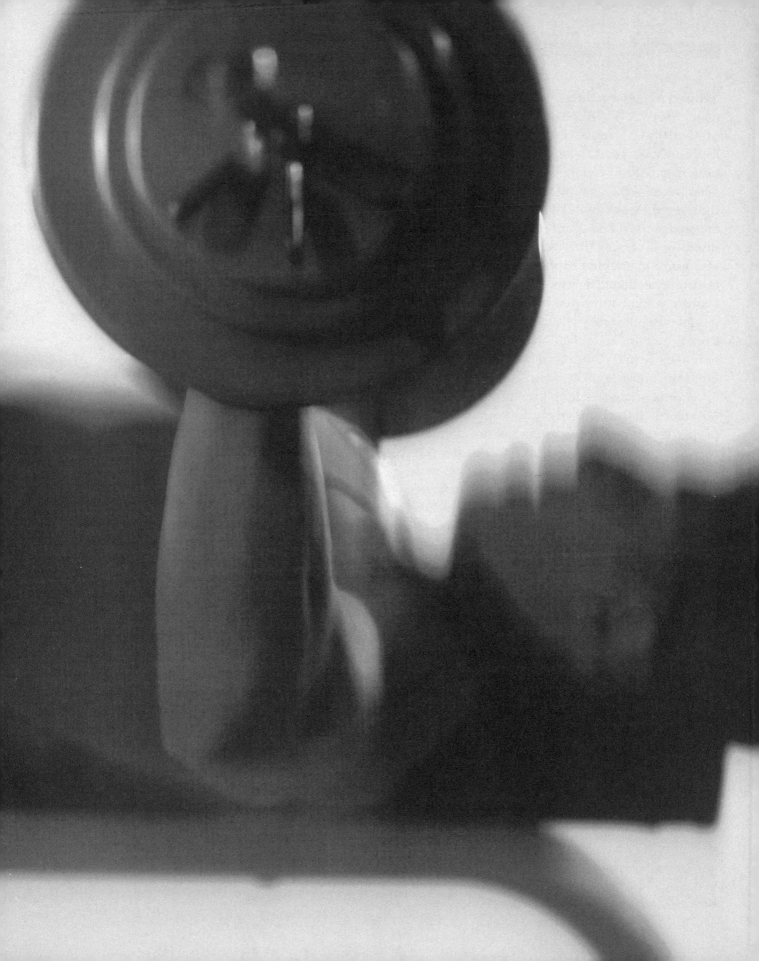

## A BOOK DESIGNED ONLY FOR MEN

Men generally have different goals than women. While most women are more concerned with a slim and toned figure—more specifically one with toned and cellulite-free legs, a defined midsection, and toned arms—most guys want bulging biceps, a powerful chest, ripped thighs and a powerful back in addition to losing the perfect amount of fat necessary to enable people to see a six pack on their midsection. Therefore, by taking this into consideration, we have created a program that will give you just that.

## THE 14-DAY BODY SCULPTING WORKOUT

The 14-Day Body Sculpting Workout is a system that takes a safe and holistic approach to fat loss and muscle toning that enables you to reach your goals in the minimum amount of time. What is so unique about 14 days? Fourteen days is typically the amount of time that it takes us humans to get used to a new habit. Also, 14 days is the amount of time that it takes the body to start getting used to a new training and nutrition scheme. Now, while it is good for us to get used to a new habit (like waking up early in the morning to work out), it is not good for the body to get used to our workout and nutrition program. The reason for that is because once the body adjusts to your workout routine and your current intake of calories, results will cease to come! So in other words, while you will still be working out in earnest and dieting, your body will remain at the same body fat percentage and your muscles will not change any further. This is why after you start a new exercise and nutrition program, you stop getting results after a few weeks.

Why does this happen? The reason for this is because the body likes to remain in a state of homeostasis (balance). In other words, our bodies like to remain the same way that they currently are. So when you start reducing calories in order to lose fat, your body goes ahead and starts losing fat. That is until it reduces its metabolism so that fat loss comes to a standstill. You see, our pre-historic ancestors sometimes would go through periods of famine and only the fat that their bodies had

> **FAQ:**
>
> *Is your 14-Day Body Sculpting Program just a marketing gimmick?*
>
> **ANSWER:**
>
> We are proud to say that the Body Sculpting Bibles are one of the very first books to bring the very powerful principles of periodization training to the commercial market. Back in 2000, periodization training was known only to Olympic and elite athletes. Since 2000, with the release of the first Body Sculpting Bibles, periodization training has become widely known and regarded as the #1 type of training for eliciting remarkable and consistent results.

would keep them alive. Because of this, the body adapted to conserve energy (in the form of fat) in order to always be prepared for periods of low food consumption.

Now, what about muscle? Same thing here. When you start a weight training program, muscle mass comes quickly. However after a period of time of using the same routine the body learns to stay at the same fitness level. It does this in order to conserve energy as the more muscle you have, the more calories you burn. Not a good thing for our pre-historic ancestors to burn a lot of calories when no food was available. Therefore, the body is always attempting to get by with as little muscle as possible.

How can the 14-Day Body Sculpting Workout help solve these problems? This exercise system:

- Changes the parameters (sets, reps, rest in between sets) of weight training routines every 14 days in a logical manner to ensure maximum workout efficiency (more on this later).
- Adjusts the duration of cardiovascular activities every 14 days.
- Varies caloric intake every 14 days.

In addition to the above, we also include mind and visualization techniques that enable you to get the most out of your workouts. Add to that the Zone-Tone, a technique that dramatically increases the mind-to-muscle connection, plus award winning exercise descriptions and you can see why the 14 Day Body Sculpting Workout is designed to help you succeed and reach your goals!

## MORE ON THE 14-DAY BODY SCULPTING WORKOUT

You may have been wondering how a 14-Day Body Sculpting Workout can exist, right? Let's get one thing straight right now. Fourteen days isn't enough time to digest a pasta dinner! Well, maybe we're exaggerating just a bit. However, all programs and/or supplements that promise you a get fit quick fix are just too good to be true and potentially dangerous to your health. We at Custom Physiques, Inc. have created the most dynamic and simple system for creating lean muscle tissue and eliminating unwanted body-fat, for good! We do not believe in starvation diets or long, exhaus-

tive workouts in order to achieve results. We believe in a healthy, systematic and scientific approach to fitness, offering a complete fat loss/muscle-building program providing fast and consistent results. Fast Results? Yes, you heard it right! Did you think we were just going to leave the "14 day" part out? No way! Although it is physically impossible for you to completely change your body shape within 14 days (unless you have a referral to a good plastic surgeon!), you can still make some very respectable changes—to your physical body and your whole self—within that time frame. This book contains the finest fat loss and muscle building information available. How can we be so confident? We realized that we would have to take a different approach to fitness in order to make this program work best. Our strategy was to combine our own breakthrough knowledge with some of the traditional methods of fitness and health, to create the most thorough and complete fitness program ever produced. What you get is a complete and balanced approach to losing fat, building muscle and sculpting the body of your dreams.

We are about to introduce you to a new fitness training philosophy widely accepted by athletes ranging from the Olympic elite to weekend warriors and college athletes. It is called periodization training, which is defined as "a training regimen done a specific way for a specific period of time and then modified and done a different way for a specific period of time." What would be the significance of changing a fitness routine from time to time? Have you ever started a weight training routine, hoping to lose some fat while simultaneously putting on some muscle and found that it was much easier to do so in the very beginning? Do you remember how motivated you were at first and how easy it was to make immediate progress? What happened next? All of a sudden you stopped gaining muscle, you still had those last five pounds of fat attached to your body and because of that, you probably lost your motivation and desire to train. You hit a plateau and no matter how hard you trained or how much you dieted, you just couldn't make any more progress, right? What happened? Your body simply adapted! That's right, your body in an attempt to neutralize and protect your system from further breakdown (tearing down muscle and losing fat), suddenly stopped responding to the catalyst (resistance training and diet).

Periodization training prevents this adaptation. It helps to avoid plateaus, thus increasing and continually creating results. This version of the 14-Day Body Sculpting Workout was completely designed for the man whose goal is to create a more muscular and lean physique. Up until now, you have probably tried every fitness routine, gadget and/or supplement under the sun and still not reached your goals. Well don't lose hope! You will discover shortly just how powerful this program truly is.

We want to help the average guy attain his goal of sculpting a lean and muscular physique. We quickly realized that this would require certain criteria within the traditional periodization program to be customized. We knew that key components of the traditional periodization model such as sports specific training would not be necessary since the program would not be used for sports conditioning. At the same time, we realized that there had to be many specialized additions to help customize the program according to our male

readers' objectives. Our main objective is to provide a direct plan of action for expediting the development of the ideal male physique (a lean and muscular body). We balanced this unique and complete revolutionary training program with the nutrition plan and a healthy mind-set method. The 14-Day Body Sculpting Workout's mind/muscle approach will help you to realize your potential!

We cannot, and will not, promise unachievable results. Unrealistic promises can both sabotage your motivation to get in shape and, even worse, jeopardize your health. Companies that make such far-fetched claims are not concerned with your well being. They only care about what they can get from you—your money. We, on the other hand, are concerned about your health. We are here to help you receive amazing results, and to explain exactly what you should do to become and stay fit and healthy forever.

Both of us have been in situations where our health and self-esteems were in jeopardy. I (James) can remember when I was 14 years old. I was very heavy and very depressed. One day while watching television, I was drawn to a commercial advertisement for a new type of diet pill called the grapefruit diet. The ad guaranteed tremendous results within a very short time period. I was young and vulnerable to such claims. I also felt desperate and immediately decided, without conducting any type of research on the company or product, to rob my piggy bank. That very same day, I sent them my money through the mail. Do you see where this is leading? I received those pills, no questions asked! They had no concern for my health, my age, or my overall well being. I took those pills and luckily, I didn't die. I see kids and adults all the time who make very similar mistakes. They have been struggling for some time, listening to claims that promise instant and miraculous changes to their physical appearance. Do these companies ever stop to think that some people are so frustrated they are blinded by the wonderful claims and left playing Russian roulette with their lives? Do these companies realize that a good portion of these frustrated people happen to be young kids, who from being abused and ridiculed about their physical appearance, become even more frustrated and are even more willing to take any product promising to change their appearance? These kids most likely will not stop to think about the major health implications involved with taking some of these potentially life threatening products. Although there are some great companies out there, who pride themselves on creating safety for their customers, many have very little or no concern for their customers. They fulfill any order they receive, without screening or qualifying one person. We would never and could never hurt or deceive anyone. We have both come from painful childhoods and can both empathize completely with anyone who has a weight problem or any problem that relates to the body and can affect one's self-esteem. Either too heavy or too thin, we have both been through each scenario and because of that, our primary goal is to help anyone who needs or could benefit from our guidance and support. From now on, your new motto must be, "If the product or business has even a trace of uncertainty, move on!" If you don't learn to follow this motto, you will either get taken for your money and/or jeopardize your own health.

Our 14-Day Body Sculpting Workout contains only the safest, top-notch health and fit-

ness information and techniques you need to become fit and healthy. Our program takes into account the importance of physical and mental health, and how they must be combined, in order to reach the pinnacle of good health and fitness. Our program was derived from our over 20-year combined knowledge base of health, fitness and nutrition. What we can do for you in 14 days is to totally supply you with everything you need to reach and surpass your weight loss goals. In two weeks not only will you know exactly what to do, you will actually begin to see remarkable results in a very short time. Even more exciting is the fact that the results you make during that very short time period will be permanent (provided you stick to the program) and only the beginning of your body sculpting success. Our one-of-a-kind program integrates the body and mind, offering you a completely fit body. A body that looks and feels great! Finally, we are most excited to let you know that this will be the last weight reduction and fitness book or program that you will ever need to buy. If your goal is to lose weight and get in amazing shape, welcome to results country: This is the place where you'll find both and then some! So now it's time to get excited, as you begin the 14-Day Body Sculpting Workout, for the body of your dreams. Enjoy!

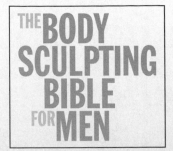
THE **BODY SCULPTING BIBLE FOR MEN**

# Part 1

# The Foundations of Physical Perfection

# Chapter 1
# Common Myths & Misconceptions

For immediate Body Sculpting Bible support & coaching directly from James & Hugo, please visit www.BodySculptingBible.com

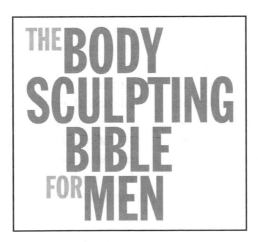

**Myth #14: You need to give all of your attention to your family, which leaves no time for working out.** If you don't start taking care of yourself, you won't be able to care for your family and they may even end up having to take care of you! Giving yourself the time to exercise and stay healthy doesn't mean you're being selfish. In fact, the healthier you are, the better equipped you will be to care for the people you love.

**Myth #15: It's impossible to find the time to work out if you have a baby.** Consider bringing your baby with you -many gyms and health clubs now have child-care services. If your gym doesn't offer this service, find a friend or family member to baby-sit for an hour or so while you work out. You can make it work if you really want to.

**Myth #16: You need to stretch before training with weights.** Not necessarily. You should not do any static stretching (also known as isometric stretching, in which you hold the stretch for a certain amount of time) before weight training. This actually sends a signal to the muscles that they should relax, which is the last thing you want your muscles doing before a set of exercises. You should instead be using dynamic stretches, which warm and ready the muscles for the upcoming workload by performing active stretches with no holding point. You can also prepare the muscles for the lifting activity by performing the actual weight training movement that you are about to perform, using either light weight or no weight.

## UNNECESSARY GADGETS

Let's talk about all of the exercise contraptions we see on TV. Why do we need to pay over $80 to perform an abdominal crunch? The abdomi

nal crunch is perhaps the most simple exercise there is to target the abdominal muscles. Do we need a machine to help us do it? We think not!

Ads for such gadgets promise abs in minutes a day. But did you ever read the fine print on the TV screen? It usually reads that the statements are true as long as you combine the exercise with a sensible diet—which brings us to the next point. You do not need to enslave yourself every day to hours of abdominal work (only 5 to 10 minutes of ab work is sufficient). What really brings out the definition in your midsection is a sensible nutritional program combined with weight training and aerobic exercise. Together, these components burn fat in order for definition to appear. The abdominal work only builds the muscle covered by the fat. Besides, there is no way in which you can reduce the fat in only one section (spot reduction) without reducing it in the rest of your body.

Once again, why would you need to purchase an ab machine? To make the exercise simple? Exercise isn't supposed to be easy! If you expect it to be, you can expect little or no results. Unless you are recovering from a back injury and are not yet strong enough to do a crunch by yourself, save your hard earned dollars for more meaningful things. All you need to perform an abdominal crunch is the right knowledge describing how to execute the exercise correctly and the floor.

If one of your reasons for purchasing an ab machine is to avoid neck strain, this is also not a good reason. If you don't know what you are doing, you can strain your neck with or without the machine.

## FAT BURNING CREAMS

We have all seen commercials that promise to eliminate fat by rubbing the latest cream discovered in some exotic locale. At Custom Physiques Inc. we have talked with many guys who have used such products with no results. Good luck finding any real scientific research on the subject that proves these products work. Again, save your hard earned money.

The only thing that eliminates fat from your body is a systematic approach to eliminating it through the nutritional practices we describe along with a training routine that is designed to tone and eliminate body fat from all angles. That is the only way the battle of the bulge can be won. Don't let anybody mislead you.

---

*FAQ:*

*What if one of these weight loss clinics actually motivates me to lose weight and keep me on track to meet my goals?*

*ANSWER:*

By all means, if you find that you just can't stick to the program and need an outside source to keep you afloat, do what you need to do. We would like to think that anyone can stick to this program and motivate themselves to excel; however life can sometimes get the best of us. If you find yourself needing additional support, do what you need to do to keep on your journey. Your health is worth the extra money, don't you agree?

---

## WEIGHT LOSS CLINICS

Why pay others every month to tell you what to do when you are fully capable of figuring it out yourself after reading this book? We have seen what most weight loss clinics offer, and we are not impressed! Not only do you pay an unbelievable fee (sometimes on a monthly basis) to get a diet that may not be as efficient as it could be (most of these programs are low protein diets); some require you to buy special foods (provided by them, of course, on top of the initial fees they charge.) Others charge you by the pounds you lose. Hey, what a concept! You do the work and you get to pay someone else for your success!

## DRUGS FOR WEIGHT LOSS

If what you want is health and permanent weight loss, don't touch any kind of weight loss drugs. Most are very dangerous (remember Phen-Fen?) and can cause serious side effects such as heart problems and possibly death. Besides, once you stop using them you begin to gain all of the weight back. So what's the use? People criticize bodybuilders for using steroids and everybody preaches how dangerous they are. Well, using weight loss drugs (and this includes those formulas that claim to be natural but contain caffeine and ephedrine) is exactly the same thing! There is nothing different here; it's using dangerous drugs in order to achieve a pleasing cosmetic effect.

When Phen-Fen came out people flocked to their doctors to get a prescription. Unfortunately, many were given the drug despite the fact that research indicated that this drug combination had some serious side effects. The drug was soon pulled from the market.

The only solid and safe solution that takes the weight off permanently is the correct combination of diet, exercise, and rest. Anyone who tries to convince you otherwise is full of it! Therefore, once again, save your money, but more importantly, save your health.

## THE MOST COMMON & FATAL DIETERS' MISTAKE: THINKING THAT EATING LESS IS BETTER

When people think of a diet they think of pain, hunger, and food deprivation. At first, most dieters reduce their food intake dramatically and see that in the first week they lose as much as 10 pounds of weight. They say: "Great! In order to lose more weight I need to eat less." After a few weeks they notice that they are not losing as fast as they had hoped. Frustrated, they start to starve themselves even more. Before we continue, let's stop right here and explain what is going on inside the body.

The first week the person will lose weight as the metabolism gets shocked by the decreased food intake. However, most of the weight lost is derived from water with only 3-4 pounds coming from fat. The second week the body, still not adjusted to the shock, continues to lose weight (though not as fast as the first week). By the third week the body begins to take counter measures in order to adjust to the lowered caloric intake. Think about it; what do you do when your light bill goes up? You probably begin to conserve electricity in order to save money. The body naturally reacts just like you consciously would. When it sees that its metabolic costs are too high (in other words, losing fat because the metabolism is too high) then it decides to save energy and lowers your metabolism in an attempt to keep the fat on. The person experiences a slow down in weight loss or comes to a standstill. The way you save electricity is by turning energy-hungry appliances off, right? The way your body saves energy is by losing muscle, because muscle is the most expensive tissue to maintain.

Let's see what may happen to someone (we'll call him Joe) who is determined to lose weight but does not know how to go about doing so.

As Joe notices that his weight loss comes to a sudden halt, he decides to reduce his caloric intake further. For the first few weeks this in fact works, but afterwards the weight loss comes to a standstill again. After a few cycles of the same thing, Joe continues to spiral downward. At this point most people (99 percent) just forget about the diet and start eating everything in sight. They gain back all of the weight and then some (remember it will be easier for them to gain weight now because they lowered their metabolism by using the wrong dieting practices). However, there is a very determined 1 percent of dieters who will not give up.

These people continue the cycle described above. They begin to look pale, and feel cold. They are hungry all the time but deny it. Sometimes they go without food or water for the whole day. They look at themselves in the mirror and they still see themselves as fat, even though everyone tells them that they are already skinny (very skinny). They are afraid to drink water because they think water will make them gain weight. This terrible condition is called anorexia nervosa, a condition that I (Hugo) suffered from in my early teens. Despite what most people think, this condition is not one that only affects women.

People with this condition are not totally crazy in seeing themselves as fat. Even though they look very skinny in clothes, if you take their fat percentage you will probably see that it is around 20-30 percent. The body has shed plenty of its muscle tissue, but maintained as much fat as possible. Initially, anorexics usually create a goal consisting of a completely different physique, one that is toned, hard and firm. In the hopes of attaining this physique they continue on their downward spiral. However, they never seem to achieve what they originally hoped for, so they decide that the best thing to do is eat fewer calories. See how the cycle is created?

The only cure for conditions such as this is education. We remember that when we were overweight everybody teased us, poked fun at us, and told us to "just stop eating!" People treated us as if we were diseased. Therefore, we decided to take action and started doing what people told us to do: We stopped eating!

However, the only solution for losing weight (fat) and keeping it off while at the same time building a lean and hard physique is eating the correct combinations of food, along with doing weight training and aerobic exercise. So please, never fall into the trap of thinking that eating less will get you good results!

## BULIMIA

Another eating disorder, bulimia (characterized by bingeing and purging) is somewhat of a difficult subject for me (James) to write about because I personally battled with it for a period of time in my life. When I was young, my physique was the last thing on my mind. I did not care about how I looked or what I ate. Being served seconds for lunch and dinner was not enticing for me; it was more like thirds and fourths that got my attention. My mother, who is a registered nurse and an amazing one at that, was not aware of the health implications and effects that too much food would have on my body. Even today, most health practitioners, including medical doctors, are not always aware of some of the implications food can have on a person's body. As I grew older and larger I was forced into realizing I was obese. One day,

**FAQ:**

*Isn't bulimia a problem that only females can get?*

**ANSWER:**

Whenever I tell someone that I was bulimic, they are shocked and say that they never knew that a man could have such a disorder. The truth of the matter is that there are many men who are bulimic. You'd be surprised if you knew how many athletes—and average men—binge and purge. Men are very good at keeping to themselves. We are also not as likely to ask for help as our female counterparts.

Bulimia is not a gender specific disease; it is a problem that exists for us all. Please be advised that bulimia is a deadly eating disorder, and if you are bulimic or have ever considered binging and purging, your life is at serious risk. There is no part-time bulimia; if you think that binging and purging once in a while is ok, you're dead wrong. The effects of disturbing your digestive and nervous systems in such a way will add up and inevitably catch up with you in ways that you'd rather not experience. Please educate yourself on its perils, and please feel free to email me, James Villepigue, for support: info@fitnessbusinesscoach.com. I've been there.

while in Junior High School, a gym teacher pulled me aside and made me step onto the scale. I weighed about 200 pounds at age 12 and 13. He thought that his way of revealing my weight problem to me was productive. He was wrong! The only thing he did was embarrass and anger me.

From that point on, I began to gain more and more weight until finally I was at my all time high of 255 pounds. I was fat and depressed, and had no idea what to do about my problem. I resorted to weight loss pills and liquid diets, which only frustrated me more. My sister, who was also quite heavy, began suddenly to lose weight. I was shocked at how she shed pounds of weight, yet didn't diet or exercise. It was odd, but I started to notice that her

### STEROID MYTH #1: TAKING ANY KIND OF STEROID WILL RESULT IN DEATH

The first thing that we need to understand is that steroids are drugs. Even Tylenol and Aspirin can cause serious problems if you take them in large quantities. All drugs when misused and abused have the potential to kill; it's not only steroids. However, since taking steroids without a prescription is against the law, you may end up facing some jail time (as much as 5 years in Federal Prison) if caught. A good resource that has excellent information on this subject is a website called www.steroid-law.com owned by top expert lawyer on the subject, and fellow lifter, Rick Collins.

### STEROID MYTH #2: STEROIDS ARE EASY TO GET

Another misconception about steroids is that they are easily obtained. As far as accessibility, the truth is that they are illegal substances without a medical prescription, so your accessibility will be through the black market. Needless to say, this raises issues of product purity and authenticity, as well as inaccurate information surrounding their usage since most of the information will be coming from the dealer not the doctor.

### STEROID MYTH #3: ALL STEROIDS ARE PILLS

On the issue of variety, there are many different types of steroid out there. There are injectable steroids and oral steroids. The injectable kind are generally more androgenic (provide male characteristics like hair growth and aggression) in nature and less damaging to organs like the liver. The oral versions are more anabolic in nature and cause more side effects than their injectable brothers as they have to be processed by the liver. Different steroids have different properties so there are some that have more tendencies to build muscle mass while others have a tendency to increase strength. As their properties vary, so do their side effects. Usually the stronger the steroid (especially if oral), the more side effects you can expect.

## THE GOOD SIDE OF STEROIDS

Steroids do increase size and strength. In fact, they do so very significantly. In addition to gains in strength and muscle mass they also seem to provide you with more energy and aggressiveness, things that are conducive to good workouts (but not so in interpersonal relationships). Depending on the steroid used, you may also get cell volumizing effects that promote a bigger pump. Aside from even just the legal risks of steroids, the "good side" comes at a high price.

## THE PSYCHOLOGICAL EFFECTS OF STEROIDS

Based on the fact that steroids give you all of these good effects that bodybuilders constantly look for, it is no surprise that they cause a psychological dependence. Think about it. If you have been taking them for the past eight weeks, assuming good diet and training, chances are that you got pretty good mass and strength gains. You feel unstoppable after the eight weeks of use. Suddenly you taper them off, up until you completely stop their use. A week later after cessation of use you notice that you are not getting good pumps, that your strength is diminishing regardless of your best effort and that your muscle mass is shrinking! Add to that the fact that for the first few weeks after cessation of use you will feel depressed due to low testosterone levels and it is no wonder that there are people out there that never get off from them.

**FAQ:**

*I've had my testosterone levels recently checked and they are much lower than they should be. Am I then a good candidate for steroids?*

**ANSWER:**

This is a common question. If your doctor checked your testosterone levels and found that they are lower than they should be, your doctor should educate you or refer you to someone else well-versed in hormone replacement therapy. You are not a candidate for hormone replacement just because your doctor has diagnosed you with low testosterone levels.

Unfortunately, there are some doctors who give their patients wrong advice—and their patients pay the price. It's sad but true!

## OTHER RISKS OF STEROID USAGE: DEPRESSION AND STEROIDS

Due to the post-cycle low period of testosterone, along with the fact that your estrogen levels will rise, depression at this time will be very real. In order to minimize this, you would need to get with a doctor and jump on many post cycle drugs that will re-establish your natural testosterone production along with suppressing your estrogen levels. If you have an understanding doctor that is willing to help, he may prescribe you with the medications you need. However, chances are that your medical insurance will not cover these drugs due to the fact that the condition was caused due to illegal steroid use. If you do not get these medications, then expect a very bad depression and total loss of gains.

If you do not know what you are doing (i.e. you used steroids with the most side effects, you abused the dosage, etc) then not only will you get bad side effects during the period of use, but you will also get worse side effects after the use. Again, the degree of side effects is directly proportional to the dosage and type

of the steroid and also dependent of the genetic propensity of the subject to get such side effects. Therefore, it would be impossible for me or anyone else to exactly predict what kind of side effects a user might encounter during a period of use. However, one thing is for certain. If you abused the drugs by using super high dosages and for very long periods of time, you may never be able to re-establish natural testosterone production, so you will then need to get with an endocrinologist and possibly stay on low dose testosterone therapy for life.

## POSSIBLE SIDE EFFECTS FROM STEROIDS:

1) Increased liver function

2) Depression of natural testosterone production

3) Increase in cholesterol levels and blood pressure (not conducive to good cardiovascular health)

4) Altered thyroid function

5) Headaches

6) Nose bleeds

7) Cramps

8) Development of breast-like tissue in men (Gynecomastia)

9) Insulin insensitivity (even though Deca Durabolin improves the insulin metabolism)

10) Androgenic side effects such as thinning hair, enlarged prostate, oily skin, water retention, increased body hair, and aggressiveness

11) Stunted growth if you are a teenager

12) Oral steroid specific side effects: In addition to the above, the orals also tend to cause nausea, diarrhea, constipation, and vomiting

13) May accelerate the growth of tumors

Again, keep in mind that different steroids offer different side effects and that everything is dosage dependent, so the list above is a generalized list of side effects.

I am not even going to go into the kind of

side effects that females encounter when they decide to use these drugs, especially the androgenic ones like testosterone. That could be a whole chapter by itself, but I think that most people could imagine what happens when you start introducing abnormal amounts of hormones from the opposite sex into your body.

**Note:** For a better idea of what each particular steroid does, please visit the following link: www.mesomorphosis.com/steroid-profiles/index.htm

## MEDICAL USES OF STEROIDS

I think anabolic steroids have their rightful place in medicine. For instance, I can see their use in patients with extreme muscle wasting conditions like AIDS, for instance. Also, some steroids can be used to eliminate severe anemia. Finally, I have read a lot of European research on the positive effects of low dosages of anabolic steroids like testosterone and Deca-Durabolin on males suffering from clinically low levels. This is called Hormone Replacement Therapy (HRT), and I personally see value in it, as in this case you are just replacing a necessary hormone that the body is no longer producing. This is done all of the time. For instance, if your thyroid is not functioning well, then the doctor prescribes you with thyroid medication.

However, again keep in mind that you are still introducing a foreign substance to the body and HRT does not come without risks. Your doctor can educate you more on that subject.

## MESSAGE TO TEENAGERS

Steroids are not the magical substance that some people make them up to be. Training, diet and rest is what will get you the body that you want. I've seen people that are on steroids and train badly, do not diet and hardly rest,

and as a result, are still small people. Don't expect to take steroids and look like a champion bodybuilder in two weeks because it will not happen.

Teenagers especially should not even think about the use of these drugs because their testosterone levels are already equivalent to what a 300-mg shot of testosterone would increase them to. A lot of complex processes occur on a teen's body that we yet do not even understand so introducing these drugs at this age would interrupt these processes, in addition to killing the best natural production of testosterone that you will ever get. My message to teens is: eat big, train big, and you will get big. These are the best years for good natural growth so do not waste or jeopardize them.

## CONCLUSION

Having said all of the above here is where we will put our two cents worth (here comes the subjective part of this section). We are not going to say: "If you touch these drugs you will die for certain" as by now you should know better. And besides, for your information, there are drugs that are prescribed on a daily basis far more dangerous than steroids, in my opinion. However, keep in mind that unless you are using them under medical supervision for HRT purposes, or for any other medical purpose that your doctor sees fit, then you are breaking the law and you are exposing yourself to whatever you got from the black market and to possible legal issues.

The truth is that most people do not have the expertise to self-administer these powerful agents, and thus, end up risking their health and making those around them miserable. When hormones are introduced into the body, certain chemical reactions begin to occur, and if the subject does not have an extremely thorough understanding of what is happening inside the body, then he is just playing with fire. At best, you get big for a few weeks, assuming that training, diet, and rest are in order, but then it goes away; so what is the use? Besides, is it worth risking jail in order to gain a few pounds of muscle? Also, if you get the drugs from the black market, how can you be assured that the quality is good? How will you know that what you are putting into your body is steroids at all? How can you be sure that if you are using an injectable steroid you will be able to always inject it correctly and without causing either an infection on the site or pinching a nerve perhaps? These are all things that you should think about if there ever comes a time when you are tempted to use the drugs.

Building the body is a lifetime commitment that has to be practiced eagerly day in and day out with the utmost persistence. There are no shortcuts to a championship body; not even steroids I'm afraid. Only hard work combined with a smart training, nutrition, and an effective supplementation system will take you where you want to go.

# Chapter 2
## The Power of the Mind

## Powerful Methods for Achieving Success

For immediate Body Sculpting Bible support & coaching directly from James & Hugo, please visit www.BodySculptingBible.com

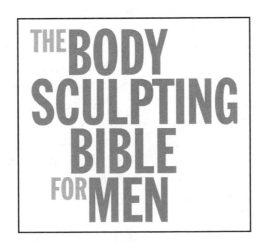

2

## THINGS DON'T ALWAYS HAVE TO BE AS COMPLICATED AS THEY MIGHT SEEM

What you have in your hands right now is a straightforward and logical formula that we have broken down and simplified, making the information easy to comprehend and follow. This manual gives you the most effective sure-fire plan to attain a better looking body, in the shortest amount of time humanly and naturally possible.

The subtitle of this book is "Featuring the 14-Day Body Sculpting Workout" because if you follow the guidelines that we present, you will start to notice amazing changes in your body within a couple of weeks. Please understand that this is not a magic program. We are not claiming that your body will miraculously change overnight. However, by applying the enclosed methods to your lifestyle, along with applying yourself to the program, you will achieve results and then "magic" may just be the word you'll use to describe our program. Often, people who have seen us train ask, "How do you make such noticeable physique changes with such a short workout?" That's just it! That's the underlying formula, the key to your success. Remember, more is not necessarily better, and in the case of this book, definitely not. If you understand how the body works, you will be successful in the shortest time possible. We live in a fast-paced world, where time is a precious asset. We don't have the time to spend long hours in the gym—even a short time in the gym can be a major commitment. Having extra time can greatly enhance your life, allowing you to do some of the things you've otherwise neglected. A basic, yet scientific approach to fitness training is what's needed, and is exactly what you're about to discover with the 14-Day Body Sculpting Workout!

## DIFFERENT ROUTINES: SOME WORK, MOST DON'T!

"What kind of workout routine should I choose?" This is probably one of the most frequently asked questions when it comes to exercise. With so many different routines and so-called "guru philosophies" out there it would surprise us if only a few people were confused about this issue. Deciding what program to choose can be extremely difficult. Even professional trainers and elite athletes frequently have problems choosing a quality program. There are many different programs—some good, some bad, some terrible. The fact of the matter is that some of these programs may in fact work, if you dedicate yourself to them. That is the key word, "dedication." The dedication we mean is the dedication of devoting yourself and your time (remember you are not in the gym to waste time!) to something, to get as much out of it as is humanly possible. To do this, you must define exactly what your training objectives are before and during a fitness session. Without this mindset, you will undeniably fail to achieve optimum results. You must realize that when you're not prepared you cannot expect to receive the maximum response from your actions, and therefore you will not see results. You must know what tools (exercise and technique) to use and what to expect at each workout session in order to receive your desired effect (more muscle tone and less fat). You also must make sure that your response or reactions to the stimulus are as accurate as you expected them to be.

The basic guidelines and training principles of your fitness program must always be based on information that is backed by scientific fact. This particular routine is the exact routine that all of our male clients at Custom Physiques Inc. have followed and they have received phenomenal results. Please understand that the routine alone is not enough to make your dream body appear. You must follow the proper training methods and initial preparation techniques included in this book to help make the program work optimally. Using correct exercise form alone is very important for steady results. If you follow the proper, often neglected, training techniques, form, and principles we describe, this program can be the program that changes your life forever! We do realize that there are currently several schools of thought concerning the best types of weight reduction and body sculpting workouts. We also realize that most of these so-called, state-of-the-art programs lack useful information and will not live up to their claimed benefits.

The 14-Day Body Sculpting Workout is based only on concepts that truly work. We include some traditional principles, which supply the building blocks of all reputable fitness programs, as well as new and exciting principles and techniques that are considered breakthroughs in the field.

## EXPECTATIONS AND DESIRE; EXPECT AND YOU SHALL RECEIVE

Where would we be without our expectations? It happens to be a driving force in our ability to plan effectively. If you want to be a success—in the gym or in the office—you must set goals for yourself. But setting goals is not enough. In order to reach those goals as smoothly and as quickly as possible, you must think about what it is that you expect to receive.

When you begin the 14-Day Body Sculpting Workout, expect optimal results. Expect to receive what you bought this book for. By doing this you are creating a positive mind-set, a vital

component of this program. Once you commit yourself to anything, do not question its power or validity (unless of course it's dangerous). Instead, dedicate yourself to it until you've accomplished your objective. Many of the fitness programs available today would work somewhat if the above mindset were followed. Now imagine what you will accomplish by creating a positive mind-set with this program. You are almost ready to begin your journey to success. Why a journey? Because all of the following techniques can be applied to all aspects of your life! Now let's move on to our first powerful tool for success.

## MIND SCULPTING: VISUALIZATION AND MENTAL IMAGERY (THINK AND BECOME!)

These techniques can help you attain your fitness goals, and improve virtually all aspects of your soon to be (if not already) amazing life!

Before you can sculpt your body into a piece of art, you must first sculpt your mind into a powerful tool. How would you like to guarantee success and accelerate your results exponentially? This next portion of the 14-Day Body Sculpting Workout addresses a very powerful technique that is virtually non-existent in the fitness realm. It happens to be one of the most pragmatic life changing methods used in the history of human potential. The special tool we speak of is known as visualization or mental imagery. In the next few minutes, you are going to learn how to develop and use some fantastic capabilities that lie dormant within each of us. They will allow you to perform remarkable feats that you never believed possible. You can realize your dreams if you focus your thoughts on what you want.

You may wonder how such influences occur. The mind has an all-powerful control over matter: your body is a prime example of this. Do you know that medical doctors consider many illnesses psychosomatic, that is, caused or provoked in part by the patient's own thoughts? Even diseases such as cancer may have psychosomatic origins, since the power of our minds over our bodies is so strong.

Right now you are going to learn how to cultivate a talent for visualization that you already possess within you. This power is more or less developed from one person to the next. But, with the right training anyone can achieve excellent results. Just as exercise develops the muscles, the appropriate physical and mental training will make you a master of visualization. The balance of body and mind exercise is too often neglected, but it is the key to astonishing success!

There are three conditions that you must have in balance for optimum results. The first is **desire**. How can you expect to obtain anything, if you don't want it badly enough? Desire is that fire you feel in your belly when you so badly want something, creating the **drive** and **determination** to achieve. The stronger your desire, and the more sustained it is, the more certainty you add to reaching your goals quickly. In order for your desires to become powerful, you have to feed them with the intense fire of your will and imagination. How? By thinking about them on a daily basis and imagining that your goal has already come true.

By doing this, you will be in the optimal mental state to make your goal a reality. Your mind will attract the events that are capable of producing the results you seek.

The next condition is **discipline**, the essential condition for all personal development and accomplishment. Without this component, you cannot expect to achieve or accomplish

great things. In order to become fulfilled, your mind needs discipline. How can you expect to accomplish or receive anything at all if you're not able to fix your attention on the goal you have set out to achieve? Do you really want to lose weight and get into great shape? The disciplined individual possesses a strong and confident attraction to his goals. The disciplined person succeeds where most fail, and always ends by conquering the obstacles blocking his path. The person who could care less about creating discipline constantly falls prey to failure. No matter how many other great qualities he may possess, success is the exception rather than the rule. Most of the time he ends up where he is by chance; certainly not by choice. So how do you learn and practice discipline? By tirelessly

---

**FAQ:**

*Why do you talk so much about the mind when it's my body I'm concerned with?*

**ANSWER:**

The mind is without question your most powerful asset. Every action you take begins with a thought. Your mind helps control your body and your muscles. When you lift a weight and simply put yourself through the motions, bringing it from point A to point B, you will stimulate your muscles, but not to the degree you could if you put your mind to work. When you really think about and focus on the muscle you intend to stimulate, something much more powerful begins to happen: the mind begins to help further stimulate your muscles, helping your muscles respond at their highest degree possible.

When you visualize yourself in great shape and visualize what it would feel like to be in great shape, your subconscious cannot tell the difference between visualization and reality. In other words, your mind starts to act as if the visualization is reality and begins to adjust to make it a solid truth. This is not science fiction; it is hard science. Training and utilizing the power of the mind can help you achieve more than you ever thought possible.

---

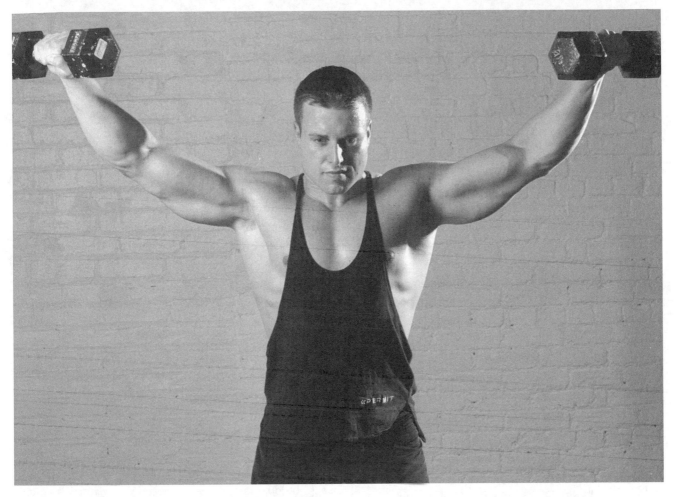

repeating exactly what it is you want to achieve in your life. You must constantly remind yourself of what it is you are out to achieve (more muscle? less fat? better tone? more definition?) from your fitness plan. The same can be done for other aspects of your life. Discipline your mind, apply the principles we've outlined here, and you will realize wonderful results.

The last of the components in the model is **action**! Even if you possess **desire** and **discipline**, without action you will never obtain what you want. Combining action with desire and discipline creates the three musketeers of achievement. Many people have great ideas, foolproof plans, and creative knowledge, yet everything falls apart for them. Why? Because they never act or they never act persistently enough. The difference between a person who knows and one who succeeds resides in the individual's ability to act.

Everything that you read in this book is the fruit of experience born of practice. If you apply the techniques and principles that we have discussed and you put action into the equation, you will meet your goals with astonishing success. Many people wrongly believe that anything that doesn't fit their way of thinking must be false. Unfortunately for them, these people limit themselves by thinking that they are always correct. They never question their own beliefs.

## APPLYING THE VISUALIZATION TECHNIQUE: AN INTRODUCTION TO SELF-HYPNOSIS FOR UNPRECEDENTED RESULTS

Before beginning a visualization session, you must be fully rested. As the body needs adequate rest for exercise and activity, so does the mind for concentration and focus. Have you ever noticed that when you are tired you can't keep your concentration and things don't seem to work? When you feel like this, don't continue trying; take a nap! This allows for optimum concentration, the most important subcomponent of the visualization technique.

Try to set aside a time for practicing the method. It will only take about 15 minutes a day to put the technique into action. But without a set time, procrastination can and will set in, making it impossible to find the time needed. By setting a specified time each day (i.e. right before sleep or upon morning rising) you will condition your mind to be ready and effective every day at the same time. Also, try not to eat prior to the session because it will divert your needed energy (just as you should not eat prior to a workout for circulatory and digestive reasons.) Be enthusiastic about your sessions too. Take pleasure in knowing that you are on your way to your personal best physique.

When practicing visualization, you don't have to force it like exercise. Take it easy and relax! We are not doing bodybuilding exercise, yet the results achieved will blow your mind! The more relaxed you are, the clearer your image will be, thus allowing for more powerful results.

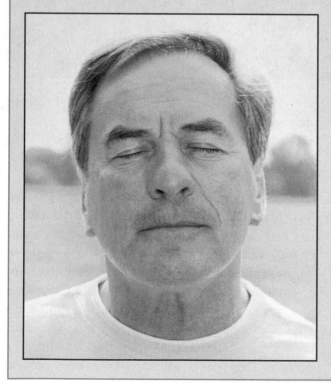

The first step in practicing visualization is to become entirely relaxed and calm. If you have already had some practice with relaxation or self-hypnosis techniques, you should be able to relax very quickly. We will assume that you have no experience with relaxation techniques.

First, direct all of your energies towards obtaining a state of very deep physical and mental relaxation. Your mindset will be that you feel remarkably calm and relaxed. We will now cover in detail a self-hypnosis session to rid your body of tensions and help to relax you completely.

Stretch out comfortably on your favorite recliner or lay in your bed. Next, concentrate on one single point: either directly in front of you or above you (the ceiling, for example). Begin by saying the following sentences either out loud or to yourself, consciously focusing on feeling the physical effects they produce.

"My mind is fully concentrating on my focal point and the harder I concentrate on this point the more my mind and body are relaxed." (Note: Take as much time as necessary to feel the intended effect of total relaxation.)

"My eyes are getting more tired and my eyelids are getting heavier with every passing second." (Focus on your heavy eyelids as you fall deeper into your desired state).

"I want to close my eyes, and I close my eyes."

"I feel totally calm and relaxed. My body is getting heavier and heavier, sinking into my bed (or seat). I can feel myself so, so relaxed. My eyes are now completely closed and I am so, so relaxed, yet focused on my body." (Do not fall asleep; you are relaxed, not sleepy!) "I will now begin to consciously relax my body." (Always begin with your feet, focusing first on your toes and moving body part by body part up towards your head. Proceed as outlined below with the following suggestions.)

"I am concentrating all of my attention onto my feet, which are growing heavier and becoming so, so relaxed." (You may start to feel a tingling sensation as if very slight pins and needles were in your feet and toes.)

"A very comfortable and warm feeling is vibrating throughout my entire body."

"I will now focus on my legs, which are beginning to sink deeply into themselves." (Concentrate on this feeling but do not force it. This should be fun, not work! When you practice regularly, you will automatically fall into the desired state quickly.)

"My stomach is now beginning to feel very heavy, sinking deeper and deeper into itself." (Allow for relaxed and easy breathing to occur. As you progress and move on to each body part, simply allow that part to lazily relax while you concentrate on the amazing feelings of relaxing your body. What you are doing right now may very well change your life forever!)

"My hands and fingers are growing heavier and heavier. They are totally relaxed."

"My chest is now sinking deeper and deeper into itself. With each breath I fall deeper and deeper into relaxation. I feel so, so calm and relaxed; I feel a warm vibration throughout my whole body."

"My neck is growing heavy and feels so relaxed as I allow it to sink deeply into itself. My head is relaxing more and more. I feel no pressure, only the heaviness allowing my head to sink deeply into itself. All of my thoughts are calming and relaxed. I feel as if I am in a dream floating."

"In this mind state, every thought that I wish to focus on is so powerful, so very powerful that nothing can stop it from becoming reality, whatever the obstacles in my way." (Repeat this last sentence mentally three times).

Now form a mental image of exactly what it is that you want to achieve (a totally ripped or defined physique, more muscle, smaller dress size, entering and winning a competition, losing 10 pounds of fat, gaining 10 pounds of muscle), visualizing the object or goal towards which your message will be transmitted. The image must be as vivid and real as possible. Keep it in your mind's eye for about 10 to 15 minutes, without going over 15 minutes.

Think about your message strongly. Do this for 10 to 15 minutes depending on the state of relaxation you have achieved. If you start getting tired or tense, stop, rest, and begin in a few minutes. Think about your message by concentrating all of your attention on it. The more you are absorbed by it, the stronger the effect, thereby creating better success. The more the message is present in your mind during the session, the greater your success. Act with conviction that your message will come true. Don't forget that everything you believe will come true. This is the universal rule. Act with desire, discipline, and faith to achieve. These actions cannot fail to produce the desired results.

What you have just read and experienced is a technique that really does work. We passionately believe in the power of the technique for attaining an abundance of success and achievement in your life. You can apply this powerful visualization technique to any and all aspects of your life. It is universal. Enjoy!

You may find relaxation and visualization foreign; you may not be comfortable with it. However, in order to change your life and make your desires reality, you must be willing to do what may initially be uncomfortable or different. The visualization technique can change your life, but only if you open your mind to change. Don't be afraid of change. You have the power to open up and accept new challenges. Are you capable of letting go and willing to try new things? *If you want to dramatically change your physique and create a more exciting life for yourself, then take some chances, move out of your comfort zone and open your mind and life to new possibilities.* These mind-powering techniques are not commonplace or commercialized. Most teachers, whether it be fitness or academics, are afraid to teach what is not ordinarily taught. They are scared to cross the threshold of beliefs for fear that they will be the first to teach a method and possibly fail. We are not afraid to teach you our methods because we are confident that what we teach works: it has worked for us and thousands of others as well. We are simply revealing what may be the single most powerful life changing tool in existence. Open your mind and begin to make changes where you never thought possible.

Whatever you do, never allow yourself to become this type of person. Always question others and follow your own instincts; but most importantly, act as often as possible!

## THE ZONE-TONE CONCEPT

One of your goals is to get in great shape as quickly as possible, right? If you don't know already, you will soon discover that the mind-to-muscle connection coupled with proper exercise technique and form are crucial if you want to stimulate the necessary muscle fibers needed to create a dynamite physique. While this may seem obvious and common sense, strangely enough, most people neglect the mental aspect behind exercise execution. It is not unusual to go to a gym and see people who are just "going through the motions;" in other words, moving a weight from point A to point B with little stimulation being directed towards the working muscles.

In this section, you will learn another powerful technique that will immediately provide astonishing performance and enhanced results to your physique by teaching you how to develop your mind-to-muscle connection!

We have named this very unique concept the "Zone-Tone" method. It is the art of mentally zoning in and pre-isolating specific muscles just before an exercise is to be executed while at the same time maintaining that zone throughout the execution of the movement. This wonderful technique is very easy to grasp and will deliver enormous benefits to your fitness program. Combining proper form and technique (something that you will learn in the upcoming sections) with the Zone-Tone method will help you reach all of your fitness goals much faster than with conventional practices. You will discover that the level of isolation and stimulation that you feel within your muscles will increase tenfold any time you perform an exercise using this method.

There are several reasons why people fail to create a successful mind-to-muscle connection:

- Lack of human body anatomy knowledge combined with a lack of information available showing how to successfully create a mind-to-muscle connection.
- Misinformation on the part of our teachers or books regarding exercise execution. In other words, people getting the wrong kinds of advice.

- Most people have a difficult time with change—they become accustomed to doing the same thing day-in and day-out. As a result, they refuse to change the way in which they conduct their exercises.
- Lifting gargantuan weights without any concern for proper exercise form and technique, in order to simply satisfy ego.

Of all of these possibilities, perhaps the biggest reason why people are not familiar with the mind-to-muscle connection is the lack of information available on the subject, coupled with a lack of knowledge on basic anatomy. If we asked you where your biceps were, would you be able to point to their exact location on your body? Are you aware that there are actually two biceps muscles, hence the prefix "bi"? Now, the next question is, if we asked you to flex your biceps muscle, could you do it effectively? How about the hamstring muscles located behind your thigh. Could you make that muscle contract really hard? Let's talk triceps; those three relatively small muscles located on the back of the upper arms. If we asked you to squeeze those muscles hard so that they tensed up intensely, could you do so immediately? The answers to these simple questions will soon lead to perhaps the most profound, beneficial and eye opening mental exercise technique the fitness industry has ever experienced. (**Note:** Please do not feel bad if you do not know where these muscles are located. Our job is to teach you where they are and how to use them. **Appendix J** is a simple anatomical chart that contains the location of each muscle group.)

When you're getting ready to do an exercise, do you ever stop to think about exactly what muscles you are about to train? Some of you will say yes and mean it. Some of you will say yes and not tell the whole truth. Most of you will say NO! This is the amazing reality that we are dealing with. We must admit to you that we truly love this fact. We love it, of course, because we are the ones who will teach people how to correctly and effectively transform their physiques 10 times quicker than they previously could have, by simply mastering this method. We love it even more due to the fact that because most of you have never learned how to activate the mind-to-muscle connection while performing an exercise means that you all have a tremendous window of opportunity to make major improvements to your physique!

The key to improving the mind-to-muscle connection is to become attuned to our bodies and enhance this connection to the fullest potential, before and throughout the exercise movement. This means knowing precisely what muscles you are targeting before you start the exercise and moving the muscle from its fully extended position to its fully contracted position (full range of motion), while consciously focusing on feeling the muscles (and only the intended muscles) contract and extend throughout the entire movement. Carelessly going through the motions of exercise is a complete waste of time and a great way to get nowhere very quickly.

## SO HOW DO WE USE THE ZONE-TONE METHOD?

While the Zone-Tone concept might seem like a difficult technique to learn, it is not! You might think that you won't be able to do it effectively or learn to use it quickly, but we will show you

## THE 10 COMMANDMENTS OF BODY SCULPTING PERFECTION

**Commandment #1: Believe in yourself!** If not, you won't be able to achieve your desired results!

**Commandment #2: Write down your goals.** How can you get somewhere if you don't know where you are heading?

**Commandment #3: Set new goals every six weeks.** After six weeks, compare your results against your original goals.

**Commandment #4: Place a calendar on your fridge.** Mark a back slash on the days that you followed your diet without cheating. Make a forward slash on the days that you trained. If you trained and followed a good diet on a given day, you should have an X marked on that day.

**Commandment #5: Place a picture of how you currently look somewhere that you will be able to see on a daily basis.** This picture should provide you with additional motivation to follow this program.

**Commandment #6: Take pictures of yourself every four weeks and place them on the refrigerator next to your "before" picture.** That way, whenever you have a craving and go to the refrigerator you will remember the reason that you are doing this and also get motivated by seeing your progress.

**Commandment #7: Write down the reasons why you are following this program and put them on your refrigerator.** Same benefit as item 6.

**Commandment #8: Keep your house free from any foods that are not good for your program.** Only on Sundays can you bring these foods in the house.

**Commandment #9: Remember to prepare all your meals the day before.** If you bring your food with you to work, you are less likely to give in to your temptations.

**Commandment #10: Remember that only you control what goes in your mouth.** Food does not control you!

that in fact you can! We have taught it successfully to many others and now we will do the same for you.

There are only two simple steps to the Zone-Tone method:

**Step#1: Focus and zone in on the individual muscle/s you intend to train before you begin the exercise.** Before each and every set of an exercise, focus and zone in on the individual muscle(s) you intend to train (for this, knowledge of where each muscle is located is crucial; look at the anatomical chart in Appendix J.) Tense and flex the muscle to be trained as hard as comfortably possible before you even start to execute the exercise. This way you will be sending a message to that muscle, preparing it by completely isolating it even before the exercise begins. By doing so, you have successfully created a mind-to-muscle connection.

**Step#2: Maintain your mind-to-muscle connection during the execution of the exercise.** Throughout the execution of the exercise, deliberately feel the muscle elongate (stretch) and contract, as you move from point A to point B (the full range of movement for a particular exercise). What we really want you to do while you are performing the exercise is to (flex) the muscle as hard as you can in the same way you did on step 1, but with the exception that now you have a weight in your hand. This is crucial as it is of no benefit to activate the muscles before the exercise begins if the mind-to-muscle connection is lost as the movement starts. Most people waste their time by exercising without thinking about what they're doing. They exercise on a physical plane rather than on both the mental and physical planes. This is fine if you are content with average results, but who really wants to be average? On the other hand, if you want to compound your efforts exponentially and undeniably create the body you've always dreamed about having, then you must effectively develop the mind-to-muscle connection.

When you effectively call out to a muscle and prepare it for the oncoming set you create a mind-to-muscle connection. By keeping this connection throughout the execution of the exercise, that one set will produce the results of five sets! Do you realize what this can mean for you? If you implement these principles into your training regimen, you can create unbelievably toned and incredibly defined muscles in half the time! Imagine the type of results that you will get by combining the Zone-Tone method with the 14-Day Body Sculpting Workout and the exercise execution techniques that are later presented in this book! We guarantee that by combining all of these concepts, you will achieve the most astounding and unbelievable physical transformation in the minimum amount of time.

## FURTHER ENHANCING ZONE-TONE'S EFFECT

How would you like to multiply the effects of the Zone-Tone method? Here is a way to compound your efforts with little or no additional time expenditure.

Remember what you did during your meditation and visualization sessions as you focused on relaxing each and every muscle in your body starting with the feet? Well, at this time you have an invaluable opportunity to implement the Zone-Tone method.

## IMPLEMENTATION

Starting with the feet, as you begin to relax and focus upon your toes, slightly wiggle your toes and concentrate on feeling even the slightest movement in each individual toe.

You might actually feel a little strange tingling sensation as you may have never stopped to pay attention to the feeling of these individual parts of your body. You might wonder why we would waste time focusing on the feet first, right? We want to do this so that you become completely familiar and in sync with each and every part of your body. This will eventually give you the ability to isolate any muscle you desire at will. It is very important to remember and focus upon each and every part of your body without neglecting any specific part! As you move on from the feet towards your knees and up, zone in on every body part along the way. Now here's where it can get tricky so pay attention. Simply focusing on the individual muscles of the body is not enough. When you simply think about them you cannot truly get a feel for how they feel when they are in action. To help you hone in and experience the feel for each of these muscles you should do the following:

- As you get to each individual body part, stop and contract the muscle as best as you know how. Do this three to five times and then relax.

- Remember the exact area where you felt that muscle contract and now focus all of your attention and energy on relaxing that same area. You are giving yourself an amazing ability to become in complete control of your entire superficial muscular system and will have the opportunity to call upon their action for maximum muscular efficiency.

Here is yet another technique you should use to further enhance the effects of the Zone-Tone method:

- After you complete each set of an exercise, stand in the mirror and contract the muscles that you were exercising as hard as you can and hold for a count of 3-5 seconds. What will this do for you? It will help you create a stronger mind-to-muscle connection and to accurately identify and call upon those individual muscles during exercise.

We can't tell you enough how important it is to practice the Zone-Tone method both when you're working out and at rest. As with anything, the more you practice the Zone-Tone method, the quicker and more powerful the method will become. Soon you will realize first-hand the astonishing results gained from this powerful concept. Good luck!

## LIFE'S DILEMMAS, SIMPLE SOLUTIONS; SOME PEOPLE MAKE EXCUSES, OTHERS FIND SOLUTIONS

In life we are bound to face adversity or dilemmas at one time or another. When this happens, the key is to not freeze up. This is the problem many people have. Instead of doing something to help solve their problems, they dwell upon them, feel sorry for themselves, and let the problems overtake them. In order to become successful at anything in life, instead of accepting adversity, **combat it!** Instead of feeling sorry for yourself or just dealing with the problem, **find solutions to the problem**! By finding solutions, you never give in to failure. You never admit defeat, and therefore are never defeated. It is only when you admit and give in to failure that you become a failure. The most successful people in the world have learned this philosophy and adapt it to their lives on a daily basis. Finding a solution to a problem is not as hard as it seems. You must use your imagination in order to achieve solutions. You must be willing to do what most people are not willing to do. Namely, you must create solutions by using your talents. Brainstorming is one such talent, in which you write down any and all ideas to help solve your problem. This might be a quick fix, such as changing an exercise or the sequence of exercises you perform during an exercise session. It might be a long-term solution, such as the one you discovered by applying these new principles into your life. The goal here is to be creative and "think outside the box!" Whatever solution or strategy you choose to apply, just make sure it is realistic and based on sound knowledge.

In the next section, you will learn why it is important for you to understand that your subconscious mind cannot tell the difference between a real experience and one that you imagine. Can you imagine the benefits associated with that!

## THE BLUEPRINT FOR A PERFECT BODY

The method below is an extremely powerful tool that can help you accomplish any of your goals (both in and outside the gym). If you're as skeptical as we once were, try to let go of your inhibitions and open your mind to endless possibilities. People don't realize how incredibly happy and successful they can be with just this one technique. So we hope that you make good use of it.

The conscious mind has the ability to conjure up fantastic dreamlike images of the things you most desire. However, it is the subconscious mind (that feeds from the information you program into it with your conscious mind) that can turn your imagined visions into realities. Your subconscious mind reacts not only to what is actually true, but also to what you imagine. Your subconscious mind will store

emotional fantasies or dreams as reality. For instance, if you see yourself with a perfectly lean and muscular body, and truly believe this is possible, you are programming your subconscious mind with your imagination to bring this dream into reality.

Creating a mental blueprint of your dream body with your conscious mind is the first step. But when you program these mental blueprints into your subconscious mind believing that you can have them, or better yet, believing that you already have them, your subconscious mind will go to work for you to devise the methods that will make your fantasy come true. Creating a desired mental picture or blueprint in your mind provides the intellect with a profound principle. The value in creating mental pictures is enormous in that it gives the mind a constructive course of action to follow. It can and will help guide and motivate the practitioner into doing what is necessary in order to succeed. How would you like to see yourself in the next two months? Would you like to lose five inches around your waist? Would you like to gain five pounds of lean muscle for an unbelievably attractive body? Would you like to make a complete metamorphosis of your body shape? If you said yes to any one of these, or perhaps have other desires that you'd like to attain, it is to your utmost advantage to incorporate the "mental blueprints" method into your life. This same technique can be applied to any other aspect of your life as well.

In order to receive the best results from your visualizations, you must learn to create the proper mindset. Creation of the proper mindset method is not a "think positive and everything will be great" type of method. This powerful weapon is fantastic for wiping out any negative thoughts, helping to keep you on the right track to success! Combining the right attitude with the proper training (visualization and blueprint imaging) is the surest way to quickly reach your goals.

The attitudes you project during your daily life can play a significant role in determining future occurrences. In other words, consciously paying attention to your thoughts and changing them, if necessary, into positive thoughts is important for an optimal life and the creation of wonderful things.

Too many people have no faith in themselves. They have no belief that they can actually create better things or a better life for themselves. If you believe in yourself, have strong desires and act upon them with faith, possess desire and diligence, then that dream body, that beautiful house, that nice car, that wonderful life can all be yours. Your subconscious mind will react automatically to give you whatever you program into it, either real or imagined. (Haven't you noticed that when we have a bad dream, the body reacts as if it were a reality; heart rate, adrenaline, and blood pressure go up. The mind cannot distinguish the difference!) Your subconscious mind will not take the trouble to work for you unless you truly believe what you program into it. You must visualize or see yourself the way you want to look. It is also highly important that while transmitting your intended message to your subconscious mind you do so in the spirit that you already possess your dream body (or possess whatever it might be that you wish for). Have confidence in yourself and your goals, making sure that nothing or no one gets in the way of reaching them. You must realize, unfortunately, that many people will not want you to reach your objectives, not always intentionally, but sometimes because of insecurities of their own. You must learn to stay clear of these people and, even more, to stay strong in your convictions. If someone says that you cannot do or achieve certain things, use that negative energy as a way to fuel your determination to get you exactly where you want to be! By doing this, you will conquer any and all obstacles in your way and reach your goals.

Realize that you must use these mental images in order to fuel your determination to help commit yourself and do what you have to do in order to achieve success (e.g.: train, eat right, and rest). Just believing that it is possible to reach your goals is just not enough; we need to take **action** in order to get there.

In conclusion, the secret to achieving success is to program what you want into your subconscious mind by believing in yourself and seeing yourself as you would ultimately like to look or live. Such mental programming will then motivate you to set a plan (in this case a sound workout and nutrition program), follow through with the plan, and persevere. By programming yourself for success, everything you desire can and will be yours.

## THE MANY BENEFITS OF EXERCISE AND CORRECT EATING: YOU WILL GET MUCH MORE THAN YOU HOPED FOR!

Exercise provides many benefits:

**Benefit #1: Increased energy levels.** When you exercise and eat right your energy levels go through the roof as the body is working at peak efficiency. This is due to the fact that the correct combination of diet and exercise produces a hormonal environment that leads to increased energy, fat loss and increased muscle tone.

**Benefit #2: Increased mental focus.** Did you know that exercise actually boosts brainpower? That's right; in fact, the latest research indicates that exercise can help keep the brain sharp well into old age, and might prevent many diseases, such as Alzheimer's disease, along with other mental disorders that accompany aging. If the brain is able to operate in peak condition, imagine the improvements that could be attained with business, decision-making, brainstorming, and every aspect of your life. Think of your brain as you do a muscle. If you train it, it will become conditioned. You train your brain by introducing new challenges like reading new information or learning a new skill such as the many you are now learning while reading this book.

**Benefit #3: Increased self-esteem.** When you begin feeling good about the way you look, your self-esteem automatically goes up. This leads to self-confidence, empowering you with feelings of control, stability and a wonderful ability to make critical decisions under pressure.

**Benefit #4: Increased sense of control over your life.** Once you are able to change the way you look and feel with exercise, you'll notice that you can change anything else that you want in life by using the same basic principles that allowed you to make such a transformation possible (Desire, Discipline, & Action). No longer will you be afraid of setting a goal and not meeting it. If you are able to change yourself, you can change anything else that surrounds you (within reason of course).

**Benefit #5: Reduced chances of heart attack.** By exercising and dieting, you lower your cholesterol, blood pressure and stress levels, greatly reducing your risk of having a heart attack.

**Benefit #6: Reduced chances of osteoporosis.** Correct exercise and diet practices increase bone density, reducing your risk of osteoporosis.

**Benefit #7: Increased strength and stamina.** Naturally, exercise provides you with more strength and stamina that inevitably become extremely useful in your daily activities.

**Benefit #8: Less depression.** Exercise increases your production of endorphins (hormones that make us feel good and happy). Due to increased endorphin production, your chances of getting depressed are greatly reduced. Did you know that it was recently documented in medical journals that the benefits of exercise are equal to that of the benefits associated with taking anti-depressant medication? That's correct, you can receive some of the same calming and balancing effects that prescription medication provides, just by engaging in daily exercise and all without the potential side effects! (The information presented here does not suggest that you stop taking your prescribed anti-depressant medication or any medication prescribed by your medical doctor. It is simply a positive addition to the many benefits associated with exercise).

**Benefit #9: Exercise helps control stress level.** Note that with exercise, worries dissolve while mood rises. Say you had a bad day—the traffic was horrendous, the boss was in a foul mood, the phones wouldn't stop ringing, and you were late for an important meeting. Could you imagine going to bed with all of that accumulated stress? Most people must deal with the stresses surrounding them, but think back to how we discussed finding solutions rather than letting dilemmas get the best of us. Exercising right after work (for those of you who like late afternoon training sessions) is a great natural therapy that helps to release your stress, while secreting those powerful endorphin hormones that make us feel amazing.

## TURN OFF THE STRESS LIGHT!

If you feel like you are stressed and it's time to go to sleep, try this technique to help you "turn off the stress light." When you lay down in bed, first relax your entire body by quickly going through the steps of the relaxation technique you learned in **"Applying the Visualization Technique,"** beginning on page 30.

Once you feel physically relaxed, mentally picture a light bulb in your head that is turned on. You can clearly see in your mind's eye how bright that light is. You can also see in your mind's eye the on/off switch for the light, located on the wall right next to the light. Now imagine that this light represents your mind which is currently turned on and so very bright. The bright light indicates that there is a lot of activity going on, and, the more stress

---

**FAQ:**

*I've read your techniques concerning Zone-Tone and Turn off the Stress Light, and I'm having difficulty actually making them work for me.*

**ANSWER:**

Harnessing the power of your mind can sometimes be challenging. Just like exercising the body, you must practice your mental form and technique in order to truly harness the power of your mind. When you have perfected form and technique for both mind and body, the exercise begins to feel effortless and fluid. Then, you can trust that every movement you make is doing exactly what it should, and you are getting the most out of your training. It may take some time to get the hang of this, but with practice and dedication, your mind can quickly become you biggest and most valuable asset.

---

you are dealing with, the brighter the light will be.

Now, think strongly about how that light switch located on the wall can either be left in the "turned on" position or simply "turned off." If you leave the light turned on, the activity will continue. Maybe you need to think and put some things into perspective.

If you wish to rest, putting all of your thoughts and stresses to sleep, then you need to turn that light off! That's right, in your mind's eye, put your finger on that light switch and get ready to turn off that light, which represents all of the thoughts in your mind.

You must focus strongly on making the connection between that light and your mind's activity. When you turn that switch to the off position, the bright light you see in your mind's eye will automatically go black, and with it will cease all activity in your mind.

Let yourself fall deep into relaxation once you see the darkness. At first, you might need to repeat the turning off the light switch process a few times before you feel the strong connection take place, but don't force it! The whole process will eventually become quite natural, and you will soon find the technique nothing short of remarkable. In fact we've been using the technique for several years now, and it never fails to work wonders for helping us fall asleep quickly. The next day you'll be refreshed and ready to tackle anything the day throws at you. One of the most important things to avoid while training is sleep deprivation. You can read about the side effects associated with this problem on page 111.

## THE FORMULA FOR SUCCESS

Since we are engineers it is hard for us to write a book containing no formulas. Consider the following formula for success in changing your appearance; it is based on determination.

$$S = D \times (T+N+R)$$

S is the success that you achieve in your program, D is your determination to succeed, T is your training, N is your nutritional program, and R stands for rest.

After examining the formula above, it is easy to see why just purchasing a sophisticated gadget or a couple of magic pills at the health food store is not going to cut it. In order to achieve permanent weight loss all of the factors described above have to be present and in perfect harmony. Follow one but not the other, and your success will be negatively affected.

Each component in the formula above can only have two values. A value of 1 is given to a component if it is followed completely. A value of 0 is given to any component that is not followed or just followed halfway. Therefore, if every single component is followed, you get a maximum value of 3. In this case, you would get the fastest results possible from your program. If you stop following one of the components inside of the parenthesis, then you get a lesser value and sub-optimal results. However, if you don't have any determination, you get a value of 0, your whole program fails, and you don't get any results. The reason? *Determination is by far the most important factor in determining the amount of success you will achieve in your Body Sculpting Workout*.

## THE FIRST COMPONENT: DETERMINATION

Determination is the first component of the formula for good reason. Of the four components that make up the formula, this is the only one that is more important than the others. If you are not determined enough to make the sacrifices necessary to get in shape, nothing is going to happen. You can have all the knowledge that we have on how to get in superb shape, but if you don't apply it, all you have is wasted knowledge. You need to want to change your appearance as badly as you would want to breathe if you were drowning. You also have to believe in yourself and know that you can do it. You must not doubt your ability to change. **If you have doubts, you will fail!** You will also need tunnel vision; in other words, focus on your goal and no matter how much adversity you encounter, stick to your plan, follow through, and get there. It is not an easy path. In a day and age where skepticism and negativity rule, roadblocks will appear (such as people telling you that you will not succeed or putting your program down). Every time you encounter a negative situation, use it to your own advantage. Use it to fuel your desire to achieve your goal. Don't let anybody put you down! This is important stuff. This not only applies to changing your appearance; this applies to every aspect of your life! If you set your mind to something and want that something badly enough, you can attain it, no matter what the circumstances may be. Set a goal, develop an action plan and follow through with it—no matter what happens—until you reach that goal. In this book we give you a proven plan to change the way you look. Whether you want to lose a few pounds of fat and put on 15 pounds of lean muscle or lose 100 pounds of fat and put on 5 pounds of lean muscle, we provide you with a road map on how to get there. Use your desire and put the plan to work for you.

## THE OTHER COMPONENTS OF THE FORMULA FOR SUCCESS

In the next few chapters we will cover the topics of training, nutrition, and recuperation. Due to the enormous amount of information necessary to thoroughly cover these topics, we have decided to dedicate a full chapter to each one of them. **Chapter 3** covers your training plan, **Chapter 4** discusses your nutrition plan and delves into the importance of supplements and **Chapter 5** is dedicated to the often neglected components of rest and recovery.

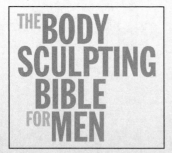
THE BODY SCULPTING BIBLE FOR MEN

# Part 2

# The Building Blocks of Body Sculpting

## FIRST THINGS FIRST

Before you move any further in this book, you should first ask yourself what has brought you here. This may seem like a silly question, but it's not. In order for this program to help you achieve your body sculpting goals, you first need to identify your exact reasons for wanting to create a perfect

A seemingly crazier question may be: are you *really* ready to get your body in amazing shape? We have always believed that there is a time and a place for everything. Have you ever wondered what makes the difference when someone finally quits smoking after so many failed attempts? Or how a person can finally lose 200 pounds after trying for years without success? The answer is surprisingly simple: **Those people were ready!**

Being ready is just as important as being able. Once you are truly ready to begin, you'll find that your fitness goals will finally become a reality. Sound familiar? We've watched people shovel in a five-course meal on Tuesday night and then wake up on Wednesday morning and eat healthy for the rest of the year, dropping dozens of pounds in the process and enjoying a life they never thought possible before. How? Simple: they'd had enough; they were finally ready. I've watched people slouch past the gym every day for years before they finally came inside; but once they did, they all had one thing in common: they were ready for action!

Creating your ultimate body is not as simple as just wanting to create your ultimate body. It requires a time commitment, sacrificing some of your favorite foods, rearranging your schedule, embracing a new philosophy and, let's face it, a lot of blood, sweat, and tears. We are not going to lie to you. To make such a commitment, to draw that proverbial line in the sand between your old life and your new, you simply

have to be ready. Otherwise, it's all just pomp and circumstance.

Call it intuition, but we can always tell which of our clients will succeed and which won't. This judgment doesn't have anything to do with how they look, how much money they have, how old they are, how close they live to the gym, what kind of sneakers they wear, or what they do for a living. It all boils down to whether or not they're ready.

Don't just take our word for it, though; let's turn to science for evidence. According to a study done by Sarah Whitehead, and reported in the February 2005 *Journal of Sport Sciences*, research has shown that the enjoyment of exercise and the willingness to go it alone (e.g. without a friend) are both related to our level of physical activity and participation in sports. The research revealed that the more a person finds pleasure in exercise and the more his desire to exercise comes from within, the more likely he is going to engage in physical activity.

Another study, done by Amanda Daley and Gaynor Parfitt, and reported in the June 1996 *Journal of Occupational and Organizational Psychology*, found that exercise improves both mood and job performance.

Both studies support our theory that when you embrace health, fitness, and nutrition you don't just look better; you feel better! You don't just lose weight; you gain confidence. These are scientific studies delving into the matters of sports and fitness and yet they have both revealed that your physical and mental realities are interdependent.

Mind and body are not mutually exclusive; where one benefits, the other benefits. The better you feel, the better you perform; the better you perform, the better you feel. Like a snowball rolling downhill, the benefits just keep increasing until one day you look up to find the best looking you that you can be staring back in the mirror. If you haven't yet felt this, stick with us and we guarantee that you soon will!

## READY, SET, GO! DISCOVERING YOUR READINESS!

We all think that strong muscles and proper nutrition are the backbone upon which your perfect body is built. Yes, they're absolutely important, but your intentions and attitude toward your fitness lifestyle are two of the most important factors when it comes to your decisions about finally being ready to get in great shape.

In order to achieve success you must first decide exactly what you want to attain from it, verbalizing your goal and visualizing it, picturing what you want in your mind, and keeping that image firmly before you, every moment, until your goals are brought to fruition.

Naturally, in order to receive you must give something, so it's necessary to decide what you are going to give. Fair enough? First and foremost, be willing to invest a feasible amount of time, as there are no shortcuts in achieving a beautiful physique. When you are an all-natural athlete, one of the most rewarding gifts is the empowerment in knowing that you and you alone are fully responsible for all of your wonderful body sculpting results! Therefore, results cannot be expected to appear in five minutes.

However, by investing your time equally between the most important elements of your fitness lifestyle—weight training, cardiovascular, nutrition, rest and recuperation, supplementation, and mindset—nothing short of miraculous results are quite achievable.

Your intention guides all of these pieces to help them work together. Clearly, intent is critical to success. So, what exactly is intention? According to Princeton University, it is "an anticipated outcome that is intended or that guides your planned actions". Your intention for this book is likely to look better than you ever have, right? Yes, that's certainly a broad way of looking at it, but we want you to have a more specific and direct intention. Perhaps your intention is to lose 20 pounds of fat and to add 2-5 pounds of muscle to your frame in 1½ months. That's a specific intention; a very direct and realistic goal, combined with an exact time frame.

In order to define your intention, we have discovered an exercise that is most effective and should always be used when focusing your intention. While many of us confuse intention with purpose, it is important to note that intention and purpose are not the same. So first we need to make the distinction between intention and purpose.

The difference between the two is that purpose is achieved through reflexes, and intention is achieved through planning.

It might be helpful to look at it this way: If I were to tap you on the knee with a hammer, your leg would automatically move; this is the same as purpose. Purpose revolves around seeing a stimulus and reacting to the stimulus. Intention would be similar to asking why the hammer is hitting the knee and discovering why your leg moves when hit. Intention is a much deeper conflict and will, in fact, help you in your quest for a fulfilling fitness regimen.

Exercise involves concentration on the goal at hand. For instance, if you are beginning an exercise such as a bench press, you should look at the weights and grow intent on using them to build your muscles. Think to yourself, "If I do this bench press I will work my upper body and will further develop it by breaking down and rebuilding the muscle tissue." Do not use purpose, which would be saying, "If I do this bench press my chest muscles will start burning and I'll be sore when I am done."

The distinction in this case may be accurate,

but recognizing the short-term nature of purpose will help you focus on the bigger picture. Use intention exercises to understand the underlying goal of the exercise, not just the reaction to the exercise.

So, how does one go about creating this point of finally being "ready"?

You must begin by recognizing that right now is the most important point of your life!

Get up off the couch, get your kids up off the couch, get your brothers, sisters, cousins, friends, and foes off that couch! Our country depends on this, folks!

Now, let's hit the fast forward button...

## FAILING FORWARD

Most of you reading this book may have already attempted to follow a workout and diet regimen. It's easy to look back on past failures and dwell on the reasons why you or those programs failed to get you in shape.

Here's the deal: In order for any program to work, the negative must be banished from your mind. The only way to do this is to forget the past. Do not accept the past, forget the past! Accepting the past will make you think that it is just fine that you have failed in your physical fitness pursuits. It is not fine that you have failed because you are more important than to have failure run your thoughts.

At first it is hard to do this. A good way to practice this is to forget about recent problematic situations that you cannot control by dwelling on them and move on. If you are late for work one day, then set a goal and do not let it happen again. If you go out to dinner with friends and feel totally overwhelmed with temptation to resist those fried mozzarella sticks, remember that you are in control and that you and only you can sabotage your commitment. Do not sit and ponder on what has happened in the past. In doing this, you will say to yourself, "maybe my diet and exercise

program has failed, but this new program will not fail because my failure is in the past."

By not getting caught up in the past, one can see failure as a necessary step in achieving any goal. One cannot know success without also becoming acquainted with failure. Just be prepared for the next time and build up your willpower.

This technique can be used throughout your exercising career. If you fail to meet your ideal performance goals, then just forget about your failure that day and try it at the next workout session. If you fail at the next workout session, then forget about your failure and then try it at the third workout session. It's all about getting back in the saddle and not giving up!

Approach anything that you have failed at before as though you are trying it for the very first time. By exercising daily and following various nutrition guidelines, you will begin to notice that any type of setback has little or no effect on your motivation to succeed.

If you want your reality to be filled with success, then only think about the successes. If, however, you focus on failures, your physical fitness reality will be filled with failure and self-doubt.

Fail forward and you will realize your greatest fitness potential!

**Here is a list of ways that you can avoid fitness failure and make your Body Sculpting goals a reality:**

1. Create a scare tactic for yourself.
2. Find an accountability partner.
3. Make sure that your regimen includes the "Five Muscular Tiers," which are: Resistance Training, Cardiovascular Training, Nutrition, Supplementation, and Rest & Recuperation. By following the Body Sculpting Bible Program, you will fulfill this requirement.
4. Don't start your fitness regimen on New Years Day. It's a trend and trends end. Start it either before or after the holiday. Even a week apart is better than starting on this infamous day of destined fitness failures!
5. Be realistic with your goals. If you shoot too high, you could easily become frustrated and quit. Shoot for a doable goal, e.g. "I will lose three pounds by the end of this week" or "I will take my treadmill training to another level this week by increasing the speed by ½ MPH and adding a one-grade incline."
6. Make a pact with your family members. If you don't, self sabotage is imminent. If you all make fitness a part of your lives, all of your lives will surely be enriched.

Sticking to a fitness regimen (a.k.a. commitment) has been proven to be the absolute most challenging thing for people who constantly seek to shape up. It's the reason why fitness is a multi-billion dollar industry and it's not about to decrease anytime soon.

So, why do so many people, possibly including you, fail with health and fitness goals? There are a few reasons why, but one of the biggest reasons is the "Buy In". In other words, unless you really have a powerful reason to get in shape and you're willing to put in the blood, sweat, and tears necessary to make it a reality, you are guaranteed to fail at it, case closed!

So, how do you create a "Buy In"? It may sound harsh, but one way is with scare tactics. You tie your reason for getting in shape to a fact such as, if you don't shape up, you'll likely end up getting sick and will die young. You do it by admitting to yourself that if you don't take care of yourself your family will likely lose you. You do it by being honest with yourself about the fact that the only way that anyone will be attracted to you is if you are attractive! You do it by not BS-ing yourself into thinking that people who are in good shape aren't treated better than those who are not! Listen, we hate these facts as much as many of you will (especially considering that we both were once obese) and we are sure we'll hear some of your rants about how wrong we are, but sadly enough, these are facts and it is what it is.

Another way to combat fitness failure is by having an accountability partner. Choosing a training partner who has similar goals as you is a great way to stay in the game and to make your goals a reality

# Chapter 3
## Training

For immediate Body Sculpting Bible support & coaching directly from James & Hugo, please visit www.BodySculptingBible.com

**3**

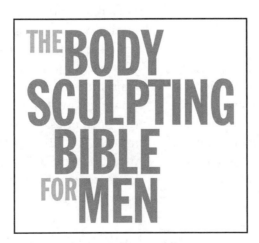

Training is the first component inside the parenthesis of the formula for success. The way you train will ultimately determine the way you look. This is how you will be able to sculpt your body into a work of art.

There are two types of training: Anaerobic exercise (e.g. weight training), which uses glycogen as its main source of fuel, and aerobic exercise (e.g. walking, bike riding, etc), which uses oxygen as its main source of fuel. We will discuss each separately and then go into detail about each type.

## WEIGHT TRAINING

The anaerobic training that we will be using is weight training. Weight training is the number one way to resculpt your body. It is far superior to any other form of exercise because it is the only one that can give shape to your body and increase your metabolism permanently. This is vital since a slow metabolism is at the root of obesity. We find it ridiculous that some fitness authorities don't adhere to this simple yet very true concept. It is ludicrous how some "fitness experts" believe that aerobic exercise is the key to the perfect physique. **These "authorities" are wrong** and should educate themselves by learning the facts.

### GOALS

Without goals we are dead in the water. We have nowhere to aim and nowhere to go. Therefore we need to set goals in order to achieve success.

Our body sculpting goals are going to be the following:

**Gain:** 10-25 pounds of muscle (or more depending on how muscular you want to look) in order to tone up and increase the metabolism.

**Lose:** Enough fat to get down to 10-12% body fat (or less than 10% but no less than 6% depending on how defined you would like to look).

Depending on where your physical fitness level is at this moment, it may take you longer than six weeks to achieve these goals. However, don't feel bad about that, as the important thing is that you will be moving forward and you will achieve these goals very quickly by being persistent and consistent with your fitness program. Besides, remember that by doing nothing, in a year from now your body will look the same as it looks now—or worse.

Now that you know where you're headed, let's see what the characteristics of a good weight-training program are.

## CHARACTERISTICS OF A GOOD WEIGHT-TRAINING PROGRAM

In order for weight training to be effective, the following rules should be followed:

**Sessions should be short: 60 minutes maximum.** The maximum amount of time a weight training session should last is 60 minutes. After 60 minutes, the levels of muscle building and fat burning hormones (like growth hormone and testosterone) begin to drop. In addition, the glycogen (stored carbohydrates) in your system, which is the fuel that your muscles use to contract, is depleted. If you weight train more than 60 minutes, you will actually be wasting your time since you will no longer have the hormones or the fuel necessary to produce muscle growth. Continue to train past 60 minutes and you will get impaired recovery, which leads to overtraining, a condition where your body does not recover from its weight training sessions. This leads to loss of strength and muscle mass.

**The rest between sets should be kept to a minimum; 90 seconds or less.** Keeping your rest time in between sets and exercises to a minimum not only allows you to perform a prodigious amount of work within the 60-minute weight training window, but also helps improve your cardiovascular system and most importantly maximizes the output of growth hormone, a powerful fat-burning/muscle-building hormone. Also, this rest interval promotes a muscle voluminizing effect in which water goes inside the muscle cells (not outside) and makes the muscles look more firm and toned. Do not confuse this with water retention outside of the muscle cells, which is what makes us look puffy and fat.

**Sets of each exercise should consist of 8-15 repetitions.** There are many reasons for this. First and foremost, it has been shown that it is within this range that growth hormone output is maximized. As we already know, this is a good thing since this hormone does exactly what we are looking for (it increases muscle and decreases body fat). In addition, since you are performing so many repetitions, you get a great pump (blood rushing into the muscle) that provides nutrients to nourish muscle cells and helps them recover and rebuild faster. Finally, performing 8-15 repetitions reduces the possibility of injury dramatically since you will need to use a weight that you can control in order to perform the prescribed amount of reps. (Note: This rule does not apply to the calves and abdominals as these muscles usually respond better to higher repetition ranges, in the order of 15-25 reps.)

**Training must be progressive.** Progression means one more repetition than the last time the exercise was performed or a little bit more weight

---

**FAQ:**

*Can I ever go below or exceed the 8 to 15 repetition range?*

**ANSWER:**

Absolutely! For all intents and purposes, the rep ranges that we recommend are for the workouts in the book. There may be times that you would benefit greatly by either doing more or fewer repetitions. It all depends on your goals and routine.

---

if you are able to do more than 15 repetitions for a particular exercise. It is important to understand that you will not be able to increase weight or the number of repetitions every session. However, progression comes in many forms; like performing more work within the 60-minute period. The overall goal of a training routine is to ensure progression over a period of time to bring about continuous improvements in muscle tone and definition.

**Training must be varied.** This principle is vital to ensure continuous gains in strength and muscle tone as well as to prevent boredom. Variation does not necessarily mean changing all of the exercises in your program. Variation can occur in the form of using different techniques to stimulate the muscle, changing repetition and set parameters, and even changing the rest in between sets. It can also be something as simple as changing the width of your grip placement on the bar to help isolate specific muscles. As you will soon see, the 14-Day Body Sculpting Workout makes full use of this principle, since every two weeks your routine changes, providing you the variation that your body needs to keep moving forward.

**Training must consist primarily of free-weight basic exercises.** Only free weight basic exercises provide the fast results you are looking

*FAQ:*

*I see all the regulars at the gym using machines. Are machines better than free weights?*

*ANSWER:*

Free weights allow the muscles to be stimulated on many different levels. In order to prevent the free weights from wobbling around while you lift them, there are additional stabilizing and balancing muscles assisting during the exercise, and you are fully working the entire muscle.

When you're exercising using a machine, you are restrained to a predefined range of motion. There are no stabilizing muscles involved, and you are strictly concerned with getting the weight from point A to point B. The bad side of this is you aren't getting the bonus of having additional muscles stimulated. The good side is that machines are great if you have an injury and need to isolate a muscle to avoid stressing it. You also may simply feel that you are being stimulated more with a machine than with free weights.

The best thing to do is use both free weights and machines. You can get the best of both worlds. As for the gym regulars: if you pay close attention, you'll find that they are lifting their fair share of free weights.

*FAQ:*

*You write about how important it is to make your workouts short. Why is this better than longer workouts, where I can really work my body harder with the extra time?*

*ANSWER:*

Your body is not meant to endure long periods of stress. The more stress you put your body through, the more it will break down and won't have the ability to recuperate. The best strategy for the best workout and results is to train as hard as you can as quickly as you can. Think of it this way: you have a certain amount of energy that you will use during your weight training session, and it's not going to last forever. You begin to use this energy the moment you start to exercise. Thus, your objective should be to direct your energy towards lifting as intensely as possible.

Ability to exercise intensely will vary from person to person, but most people have a specific amount of time that allows them to get the best workout. Powerful muscle building and fat burning hormones are released, and your body is ready for results. When you go beyond this time block, you get diminishing returns, or your energy levels deplete and your focus wanders. When this happens, your muscle glycogen has been spent and toxins begin to release into your bloodstream. Have you ever seen a boxing match, where both opponents are fresh and ready to do battle at the very beginning of the fight? They come out and they are strong, powerful, and fierce! The second round comes around and they still have that fuel to sustain their attack, but when the third round arrives, their drive is restrained and conserved. What has happened?

They have blown their power energy. At the beginning of the round, their muscle glycogen is at peak levels, adrenaline is spilling over, and focus is sharp. It's these beginning rounds that are the most valuable. The same principles apply to weight training. Come out fierce, give it all you've got, and get it done before you run out of steam.

for because they recruit the most muscle while you are performing them. Besides, the body is designed to be in a three dimensional universe. Whenever you use a machine you limit your body to a two-dimensional universe and consequently you limit the amount of muscle fibers that are going to do work. Not all machines are bad, however. Some definitely have a place in our weight-training program because they allow us to isolate the muscle in a way that no free weights would allow us to do. However, our program should be mostly based on barbells, dumbbells and exercises where the body moves through space (such as the dip, the pull-up and the squat). The best exercises for each body part are the following:

## BACK

### BASIC EXERCISES

Wide-grip pull-ups (or pull-downs if unable to perform pull-ups) to front, close-grip chin-ups (or close-grip pull-downs if unable to perform chin-ups) with palms facing your body, chin-ups with a neutral grip with palms facing each other (or close-grip pull-downs with a V-Bar if unable to perform neutral grip chins), one-arm rows, two-arm rows, pullovers, bent over barbell rows.

### ISOLATION EXERCISES

Stiff-arm pull-downs, low-pulley rows

## CHEST

### BASIC EXERCISES

Incline bench press (and its dumbbell version), flat bench press (and its dumbbell version), chest dips, push-ups

### ISOLATION EXERCISES

Chest flys (incline and flat versions), incline cable crossovers

## THIGHS AND BUTTOCKS

### BASIC EXERCISES

Barbell squats (and dumbbell version), ballet squats (and dumbbell version), lunges, leg press.

### ISOLATION EXERCISES

Leg extensions

## HAMSTRINGS

### BASIC EXERCISES

Stiff-legged deadlifts (and its dumbbell version), leg press (feet high on the platform), lunges (how far you extend your leg when you do this exercise determines which leg muscle is activated the most. The farther away from the torso that you extend your leg, the more you hit the hamstrings).

### ISOLATION EXERCISES

Lying leg curls, standing leg curls, seated leg curls

## SHOULDERS

### BASIC EXERCISES

Military press (and dumbbell version), upright rows (and dumbbell version)

### ISOLATION EXERCISES

Lateral raises, bent-over lateral raises, rear-delt machine

## BICEPS

### BASIC EXERCISES

Dumbbell curls, barbell and dumbbell preacher curls, incline dumbbell curls, hammer curls, reverse curls, E-Z bar curls

### ISOLATION EXERCISES

Concentration curls

## TRICEPS

### BASIC EXERCISES
Barbell and dumbbell lying triceps extensions, barbell and dumbbell overhead triceps extensions, triceps dips, close-grip bench press (and dumbbell version)

### ISOLATION EXERCISES
Triceps pushdown, triceps kickbacks

## CALVES

(Note: For calves and abdominals there is really no distinction between basic and isolation exercises)
Standing, seated, and donkey calf raises, calf raises on leg press machine, one-legged or two-legged calf raises with dumbbells

## ABDOMINALS

Crunches, leg raises, and knee-ins, trunk curl and crunch, V-ups

## AEROBIC TRAINING

Aerobic training such as walking or running on a treadmill is a good way to accelerate the fat burning process (as long as it is not overdone and is used only in addition to a good weight training program). It should never be used as a substitute for weight training since it does not permanently increase your metabolism and does not have the ability to reshape your body.

*FAQ:*

*Should I only weight train and leave the cardio to runners and endurance athletes?*

**ANSWER:**

Absolutely not. Some fitness professionals will say that it is ok to only weight train, especially if your routine is made up of supersets. However, it's best that your fitness routine have a balanced approach and heart-healthy aerobics/cardio training is crucial.

In order for aerobic exercise to be effective, it needs to be performed within the fat burning zone. The fat burning zone is the zone at which you are doing just the right amount of work to burn fat. Your pulse (how fast your heart is beating per minute) determines this zone. It is important to remain in this zone for a certain period of time. Work harder or longer than what the formula recommends, will quickly lead to exhaustion which will prevent you from continuing to perform the activity for a prolonged period of time. On the other hand, too low of an effort will not prompt your body to start its fat burning mechanisms.

To determine your fat-burning zone, use the following formula:

Fat burning zone = (220-Your Age) x (.75)

For example, a 20-year-old man would need to reach a pulse in the neighborhood of 150 beats per minute in order to be in the fat burning zone. It is important to remember that this is not an absolute figure, but an approximation. As long as you stay within 10 beats of the number that the formula provides, you can rest assured that you will be burning fat.

Another important point is that in order for aerobic exercise to be an optimal fat burner, it needs to be performed at the appropriate times.

There are two ideal times where aerobic exercise is most effective in burning fat. The first ideal time is first thing in the morning on an empty stomach after drinking 16 to 24 ounces of water in order to prevent dehydration. Exercise performed at this time burns 300 percent more body fat than at any other time in the day because your body does not have any glycogen (stored carbohydrates) in the system to burn. Therefore, it has to go directly into the fat stores in order to get the energy necessary to complete the activity. The other time that aerobic exercise is effective is immediately after a weight training session as your glycogen stores have already been depleted. Because of this, once you start doing your cardio, you will start burning fat as soon as you elevate your heart rate since it is the only fuel available.

When aerobic exercise is not performed first thing in the morning or right after the weight training workout it takes your body approximately 20 to 30 minutes to start burning fat because that is how long it takes the body to deplete its glycogen stores and switch to a fat-burning environment. Therefore, it is not as efficient to perform aerobic exercise alone at other times of the day because you would need to work out for 20-30 minutes just to get to the fat burning stage and then continue to work out for an additional 20 minutes to burn fat. This would mean a grand total of 50 minutes a day. In our opinion, aerobic exercise shouldn't be performed more than 6 times a week for 40 minutes maximum each session, in order to avoid losing muscle mass. Remember that more is not always better, and this is especially true when it comes to aerobic exercise. As you will see, for this program (unless you are interested in bodybuilding competition), the most you will be doing is three sessions lasting between 20 to 40 minutes each.

Good forms of aerobic exercise include riding a stationary bike, fast walking (this can be done on a treadmill), climbing on a stair stepper, swimming, using a fitness rider or rowing machine, using any good cardio tapes like Tae-Bo, or any other form of cardiovascular activity that raises your heartbeat to the fat burning zone.

## PUTTING IT ALL TOGETHER

Now we will learn how to put all this knowledge together in a workout program that will yield the results. We present three different workouts. The one you should choose will depend on your previous training experience and your fitness goals.

The first workout (*the Break-In Routine*) is to be used by men who have never done weight training before. This program is a break-in program that will not only allow you to get in shape quickly, but will also condition you to get in the shape necessary to be able to use the 14-Day Body Sculpting Workout.

The second workout (*the 14-Day Body Sculpting Workout*) is for men who have been weight training for at least 10 weeks and want to get into awesome shape (gain 10-25 pounds of muscle and reduce body fat to 10%).

---

**FAQ:**

*There is a lot to remember as far as reps, sets, rest times, as well as proper form. Can't I just stick to an easy routine?*

**ANSWER:**

If you want to make radical and long-lasting changes to your body, you need to stick to the entire program and all of its details. No one said this was going to be easy. Once you get the hang of it, I promise that it will become second nature to you! All of the little details help to make this program the most effective and powerful routine available.

---

The third workout (*the Advanced 14-Day Body Sculpting Workout*) is the most advanced workout to be used only by men who either have an interest in bodybuilding competition or just want to look like a bodybuilder (gain 25 pounds of muscle or more and reduce body fat to 6%). This last workout requires at least one year of weight training experience in the gym and is the most time consuming of all workouts. It will emphasize all angles of the muscle in order to produce the most stunning Body Sculpting effect. Therefore, this workout is reserved for the most serious fitness guys out there.

Before we present the 14-Day Body Sculpting Workout, let's discuss a few terms that you need to understand in order to execute the routine.

**Repetitions or reps:** The amount of times that you perform an exercise. For instance, imagine you are performing a bench press. You pick up the bar, lower it, pause and lift it up. That action of executing the movement for one time counts as one repetition. If you perform that same movement a second time, then that is your second repetition and so on and so forth.

**Sets:** A set is a collection of repetitions that culminates in the muscle reaching muscular failure. Muscular failure is the point at which, due to a buildup of lactic acid in the muscle, it becomes impossible to perform another repetition with good form.

**Rest Interval:** The amount of time you rest between sets. For instance, a rest interval of 60 seconds means that after you finish your first set, you will remain idle for 60 seconds before going on to the next set.

Now that we have discussed these important terms, let's discuss the main techniques that make the 14-Day Body Sculpting Workout so effective.

**Modified Compound Supersets:** In a modified compound set, you pair exercises, usually for opposing muscle groups or for opposing muscle movements (e.g. push vs. pull). First you perform one exercise, rest the recommended amount of seconds, and then perform the second exercise (for instance, first do biceps, then do triceps). Then rest the prescribed amount of time again and go back to the first exercise. A modified superset for Dumbbell Curls and Triceps Pushdowns in which you perform 4 sets of each exercise will look like the following:

You will be resting a total of 2 minutes plus the amount of time that it takes you to perform the other exercise, so you actually are resting a given muscle between 2.5 and 3 minutes. Using this technique of pairing exercises in a **modified** superset fashion not only saves time and keeps the body warm, it also allows for faster recovery of the nervous system between sets. This allows you to lift heavier weights than if you just stay idle for 2-3 minutes waiting to recover. An additional benefit of this technique is that it saves time and limits rest to a maximum of 90-seconds in between sets.

## SAMPLE MODIFIED COMPOUND SUPERSET

| EXERCISE | PAGE NO. | REPS | SETS | REST |
|---|---|---|---|---|
| MODIFIED COMPOUND SUPERSET # 1 | | | | |
| Back—Dumbbell One-Arm Rows | 168 | 15-20 | 2 | 90 seconds |
| Chest—Push-Up (against the wall if unable to perform on the floor) | 208 | 15-20 | 2 | 90 seconds |

**Supersets:** A superset is a combination of exercises performed right after each other with no rest in between. There are two ways to implement a superset. The first way is to do two exercises for the same muscle group at once (like dumbbell curls immediately followed by concentration curls). The drawback to this technique is that you will not be as strong as you usually are on the second exercise. The second and best way to superset is by pairing exercises of opposing muscle groups (antagonists) or different muscle movements such as back and chest, thighs and hamstrings, biceps and triceps, shoulders and calves, upper abs and lower abs.

When pairing antagonistic exercises, there is no drop of strength whatsoever. As a matter of fact, sometimes your strength increases because the blood in the opposite muscle group helps you perform an exercise. For instance, if you superset dumbbell curls with triceps extensions, the blood in the biceps helps you do more weight during the triceps extensions. Because of this, we will only perform supersets where opposing muscle group or opposing muscle movement exercises are paired. Supersetting not only allows you to do more work in a shorter period of time, but it also increases endurance, creates an incredible pump (especially when you pair antagonistic exercises), and helps burn fat by elevating the heart rate to the fat burning zone (which also gives you cardiovascular effects). Also, because of the stress created by this technique, growth hormone levels go through the

| SAMPLE SUPERSET | | | | |
| --- | --- | --- | --- | --- |
| EXERCISE | PAGE NO. | REPS | SETS | REST |
| SUPERSET # 1 | | | | |
| Back—Dumbbell One-Arm Row | 166 | 10-12 | 3 | No Rest |
| Chest—Push-Up | 206 | 10-12 | 3 | 60 seconds |
| (against the wall if unable to perform on the floor) | | | | |

roof. Remember that this hormone is responsible for fat loss and enhanced muscle tone.

**Giant Sets:** Giant Sets are four exercises done one after the other with no rest in between sets. Again, there are two ways to implement this. You can either use four exercises for the same muscle group or perform two pairs of opposing muscle group exercises. For the purposes of this book whenever we do Giant Sets, we will perform two pairs of opposing or different muscle group exercises with no rest (the exception is in abdominal work in which we will alternate between lower abs and upper abs).

A Giant Set for biceps and triceps in which you perform 4 sets of each exercise is shown on the top of page 60.

Giant Sets provide you with more of the same benefits that supersets have to offer. This is the most intense and powerful technique that we will use in our 14-Day Body Sculpting Workout. We need to be cautious when using Giant Sets since they are considered an extremely intense exercise protocol. Although the human body is capable of handling great intensity and stress, you should never push it to the edge. The Giant Sets protocol is very powerful and results-oriented training method, but should be used sparingly. In our program the

| SAMPLE GIANT SET | | | | |
|---|---|---|---|---|
| EXERCISE | PAGE NO. | REPS | SETS | REST |
| **GIANT SET #1** | | | | |
| Back—Dumbbell One-Arm Row | 168 | 8-10 | 4 | No rest |
| Chest—Push-Up | 208 | 8-10 | 4 | No rest |
| (against the wall if unable to perform on the floor) | | | | |
| Back—Two-Arm Row | 170 | 8-10 | 4 | No rest |
| Chest—Flat Dumbbell Fly (performed on the | 198 | 8-10 | 4 | 60 seconds |
| floor if no access to an exercise bench) | | | | |

Giant Sets protocol will only be used for about two weeks. Have you ever heard the saying that "too much of a good medicine is bad?" This certainly applies to Giant Sets. This is really strong medicine in the fight against fat. Use it for more than two weeks and your body will no longer be able to recover; the nervous system will get burned out and will reach a state of overtraining, where your body can no longer recover from the workouts.

Now that we have discussed the three techniques that are the basis of the 14-Day Body Sculpting Workout, let's see what the routines look like.

## HOW DOES THE 14-DAY BODY SCULPTING WORKOUT WORK?

The 14-Day Body Sculpting Workout is based on your body's physiology. It usually takes your

**FAQ:**

*Why 14 days?*

**ANSWER:**

We found that our 14-day periodization program worked because its duration wasn't too long (so you would get bored) and it wasn't too short (so you wouldn't be constantly changing programs). It was "just right." The program has helped literally hundreds of thousands of people throughout the world make and keep amazing changes to their bodies.

body 14 days to get used to a new practice, whether that practice is a diet, a new exercise program, or just getting up earlier in the morning. Getting used to a new practice, such as waking up early to exercise, is a great thing. However, getting used to an exercise program is not as great. Why? Once your body gets used to it, it will stop responding and your results (i.e. fat loss and increased muscle tone) will come to a screeching halt. That is the reason why most people who go to the gym experience great results initially, but later see and feel themselves going nowhere. The key to experiencing continued results is variation. However, it cannot be haphazard variation. You must have a planned scheme that will guarantee continual results; a scheme such as the one offered by the 14-Day Body Sculpting Workout.

For the first two weeks you will use modified compound supersets. During this period, the body gets stronger as rest periods are abundant and repetitions are at a higher range (12-15). Working out this way allows the nervous system to recover and the body to increase its strength. In addition, the high repetitions allow the body to start building more capillaries (necessary for the delivery of nutrients to the muscle cell) and to prepare the joints for the heavier weights to come.

On weeks three and four you will start using

supersets, a more intense technique that creates higher demands on the central nervous system, along with heavier weights and fewer reps (10-12) with a slightly higher number of sets. The increased volume and the shock to the body created by the increased stress of the weight training routine causes an increased output of growth hormone (a hormone that greatly enhances fat loss and muscle tone), and an increase in metabolism.

When your body starts adapting to this routine, you further increase the intensity by increasing the number of sets again, using heavier weights (8-10 reps) and by using Giant Sets. Once again the body is shocked, growth hormone output goes through the roof and the metabolism is jolted.

The routine is so intense that if you were to maintain it for more than two weeks you would enter a state of overtraining (where your body cannot recover from the demands imposed by the intense routine). When your body has reached a level that gets fairly close to overtraining, you will give it a chance to recover for the next couple of weeks by going back to week one where you use fewer sets, higher reps, and have ample amounts of time to recover in between sets by using the modified compound superset technique. Are you going backwards? Not at all! With this program you are always moving forward. Even though you are going back to a less stressful type of training with less volume, you will notice that you will now be stronger on the same exercises. You will be able to use greater weight for the 12-15 repetition range for the following reason: in order for the body to prevent itself from going into overtraining during the two weeks of high volume and giant sets, it naturally built up its nervous system energies to the highest level possible as an emergency measure. Now that you have backed off on the

stress, you'll have all of this extra energy that the body will utilize to get even stronger and more muscular. That is how your strength will increase. After two weeks of modified compound supersets, once again you'll begin to increase the stress on the body by continuing this results-producing cycle.

Why is it necessary to get strong and why should you lift heavier weights? Because building up your strength through progressive resistance training is the key to increased muscle tone and accelerated fat loss. Remember, if your strength stays the same, your body will look the same and you may as well consider yourself moving backwards.

## CHOOSING THE BEST TIME TO WORK OUT

We recommend you work out in the morning as soon as you wake up. Drink 16 ounces of cold water before you start the workout and an additional 30 to 60 ounces during the activity. This is essential to prevent dehydration. We recommend working out first thing in the morning on an empty stomach because you will burn 300% more body fat this way. In the morning your body doesn't have any carbohydrates to burn. In the absence of carbohydrates, your body goes straight to the fat stores (triglycerides) in order to get the energy necessary to do the work. Another good reason to work out in the morning is that growth hormone levels are at their highest levels (remember that growth hormone is one of the hormones responsible for muscle growth and the one that influences fat loss the most). Working out in the morning will allow you to expedite the fat loss process for dramatic results. However, we do understand that certain obstacles such as work constraints and other situations might not permit everybody to train in the morning. In this case, do your cardio or weight training three hours after any meal (if your last meal was at 3:00 pm, then your exercise session should be at 6:00 pm).

If you follow the **Advanced 14-Day Body Sculpting Workout** you will be doing cardio and abs first thing in the morning and weight training at some other time during the day. However, if this is impossible due to your schedule, then perform abs before the weight training workout and cardio right after the weight-training workout. (**Note: If you do decide to workout in the morning, please make sure that you properly warm up and stretch. This will not only ensure that you are wide awake but will also prevent injuries and potential accidents.**)

## WORKOUT CLOTHING

When you go to the gym, you should wear comfortable clothes that allow your body to move freely. Rigid clothes, such as jeans, are definitely out of the question. You also need to choose clothes based on the climate you live in and environmental conditions. You should wear extra layers of clothing if your environment is cold to help keep your body temperature on the warm side and prevent possible injuries. Wear nice comfortable cross training shoes along with a thick absorbent pair of socks. Never train in your bare feet or with sandals; you could seriously injure your feet if you ever dropped a plate on them.

## HOW FAST SHOULD YOU LIFT THE WEIGHT?

Many people in the fitness industry have had difficulty in deciding: "Should I lift the weight fast? Should I lift the weight slow? Should I move the weight fast or slow on the positive (concentric) portion of the rep? Should I move fast or

slow on the negative (eccentric) portion of the rep?" We have done the research on these questions and will now explain each one in detail.

We have found that slow lifting is usually only good for beginners who have never lifted a weight. It helps them to learn and master the movement and prevents them from using bad exercise form. However, as you become more advanced, science and our own experience indicate that you should lift the weight as quickly as possible without sacrificing form and without involving momentum (jerking and bouncing of the weights.) You create more force by lifting fast, and therefore, more muscle fibers need to be activated. By ensuring that you are not using momentum to help you move the weight, you can be sure that the force generated during the movement will be created solely by your muscles and not inertia. This is what helps stimulate your muscles to grow, creating the tone and shape that you desire. While some might believe that super slow lifting is beneficial because it is difficult to perform and painful, it is not the best way to stimulate muscle growth. Super slow lifting accumulates too much lactic acid within your muscles and fatigues them before they reach real momentary muscular failure.

Science tells us that Force = Mass (in this case, the weight you are lifting) multiplied by Acceleration (the increasing speed at which you lift the weight). Therefore, the best way to lift weights is to lift them fast, with total control of the weight and without relying on momentum. Since you won't be jerking the weights or using ballistic movements during exercise, the risk of getting injured is not any greater than the risk of getting injured lifting slowly.

If you are lifting a weight that only allows you to do 8 repetitions, if you're looking in the mirror, it will look like you are lifting the weight

**FAQ:**

*I've read that varying your lifting speed can actually be beneficial.*

**ANSWER:**

It definitely is. Just like the 14-Day Body Sculpting Program changes every 14 days, which makes sure your muscles are never expecting what's coming, you can change your lifting speed to increase results. The speed you lift the weight from point A to point B can have huge effects on your muscles, as it can increase the amount of concurrent time your muscles are under tension during each set. The key here is to switch things up from time to time.

slowly even though you are lifting it as fast as possible. The heavier the weight the slower you will be able to move it, even though you are trying to accelerate it as fast as you can. This is amazing! We are sure you've heard people's concerns about how lifting heavier weights is dangerous, right? It is actually the opposite. When you lift lighter weights, you have the ability to move the weights very quickly and sloppily because little stress is put upon the muscles, tissues and joints. This creates a greater risk for injuries to occur. When you lift heavier weights, you are forced to go slower with the weights and to use controlled form during movement. Lifting heavier weights will stimulate more muscle fibers while limiting the chance for injuries (assuming that the maximum amount of weight lifted is one that allows for a minimum of 8 repetitions; heavier weights may indeed cause connective tissue injury).

## MUSCLE SORENESS

Muscle soreness is caused by micro-trauma to the muscles and is a good indicator that the workout you performed was effective. If you have never exercised before, you will experience higher levels of soreness than usual at the beginning of your program. That is okay. As your body gets used to the exercise program the muscle soreness will subside to tolerable levels. You just need to persevere through those first few weeks. Do not confuse this type of soreness with overtraining.

There are several degrees of soreness that you should be aware of:

- Delayed Onset Muscle Soreness (DOMS)
- Typical Mild Muscle Soreness
- Injury-Type Muscle Soreness

The first type of soreness is delayed onset muscle soreness (DOMS). The term DOMS refers to the deep muscular soreness usually experienced two days after (not the day after) the exercise has been done. DOMS prevents the total muscular contraction from occurring within a muscle. This type of severe soreness is caused when you either embark on an exercise program for the first time or when you train a body part harder than usual. It can last for a couple of days for an advanced well-conditioned athlete or for as long as a week for a beginner. If this type of soreness is affecting you and it is time to work out again, the best thing to do is not to rest but to exercise the affected body part in an active recovery routine.

In active recovery routines all of the loads are reduced by 50 percent, and the sets are not taken to muscular failure. For example, if you are to perform an exercise for 10 repetitions, divide the weight that you usually use for that exercise by two and that is the weight that you will use for your active recovery routine. Also, stop performing the exercise even though you may not reach muscular failure at the tenth rep. The reason for this type of workout is to restore full movement in the muscle, helping to remove the lactic acid and other waste products building up within the muscles. It also forces high concentrations of blood into the damaged area of the muscles and nourishes the muscles for repair and growth. We find that doing this is always beneficial; by the next day you will not be as sore or stiff as you ordinarily would have been if you had skipped a workout in order to wait for the pain to subside.

The second type of soreness is the typical mild muscle soreness experienced the day after a good workout. While scientists are still unable to pinpoint the true cause of such soreness, the explanation generally accepted is that it is caused by micro-trauma at the muscle-fiber level and by an excess of lactic acid. At any rate, what's important is that this is good soreness considering it is of a mild nature and muscle function is not impaired as it is with DOMS. The pain generally lasts a day for advanced athletes and up to three days for a beginner. This soreness, on average, indicates that you had a good workout the day before because you created the trauma necessary to trigger adaptation (e.g. muscle growth). When you are no longer experiencing this type of soreness, it is a good indication that your body has successfully adapted to the training program. This is not one of the goals you will be striving for, as it leads to no gains. This is the reason why our program changes on a consistent basis.

The third type of soreness is the one caused by injury. This soreness is entirely different in nature from the ones described above, as it is usually immobilizing and triggers very sharp pain within the muscles and/or joints. Depending on the nature of the injury, the pain might either be experienced constantly or only when the joints are moved or the muscles con-

> **FAQ:**
>
> *What should I do to warm up my muscles before weight training?*
>
> **ANSWER:**
>
> First, remember that there is a huge difference between warming up and stretching. Warming happens before you begin your weight training, and stretching should occur either after you've done a full body warm-up, or at the end of your weight training session.
>
> Warming up is something that we seldom see discussed in fitness books. We've spoken to hundreds of people who just don't realize the benefits and safety reasons for warming up. Have you ever had a day where your body felt achey? It could be something as simple as stress that makes your low back and neck feel tight. When you're tense, you may have trouble squatting down to the ground without any weight at all!
>
> We might feel like we can lift our max weight right at the beginning, but this is the wrong approach and a very hazardous one. You must warm up your muscles and the surrounding joints and connective tissue that you intend to stimulate to ensure safety and prepare your body for high intensity training.

tract. These injuries often become apparent as soon as they happen. Other times they appear either the day after and even sometimes days after the activity. If you suddenly become injured, the first thing that you should do is apply the RICE principle (Rest, Ice, Compression, and Elevation).

After consulting a doctor, he or she might allow you to continue training, carefully working around the injury (in other words, utilizing exercises that work around the injured muscle(s), without over stepping the range of motion that triggers the pain). More serious injuries, such as a muscle tear, may involve complete rest of the injured and surrounding areas and, depending on the severity, possibly surgery. The best way to prevent this type of injury, pain, and soreness, is by cycling your exercise parameters and by constantly practicing good form.

## BREATHING WHILE PERFORMING AN EXERCISE

The correct way to breathe while performing an exercise is to exhale while you are forcing the weight up (the concentric phase or muscle contraction) and to inhale while you are lowering or releasing the weight (the eccentric phase or the negative portion of the exercise). For example, if you are doing a bench press, you exhale while you push the weight up away from your body and inhale while you lower the weight down towards your chest.

> **FAQ:**
> *I am concerned that I am not breathing correctly during exercise.*
>
> **ANSWER:**
> The most important thing to do is just make sure you're breathing! Don't hold your breath. Lots of people (especially beginners) can quickly become overwhelmed with all of this new information to retain. Stop worrying so much about what you're not doing right and just do the best you can. When it comes to breathing, your body has a wonderful ability to make sure you're breathing so you don't pass out.
>
> When you are weight training, the rule is to exhale during the exertion and inhale during the descent. If you mess up here and there, just practice!

## WARMING UP BEFORE TRAINING AND STRETCHING

People always ask us, "What is the best time for stretching?" Our answer is, the best time for stretching is after your body temperature has increased and the blood has begun circulating within the muscle. This is achieved by performing exercise that raises your heart rate and circulates the blood at an increased rate. If you fail to adequately do this, you run the risk of tearing a muscle or causing bodily injury. Are you up for an experiment? Wet a rubber band with water and put it in the freezer. After two hours, take it out and try to stretch it to its limit. Pay attention and you will discover that the rubber band easily breaks. The same process can easily happen to your muscles if you stretch them without sufficiently warming them up. Having said that, before you begin the weight training

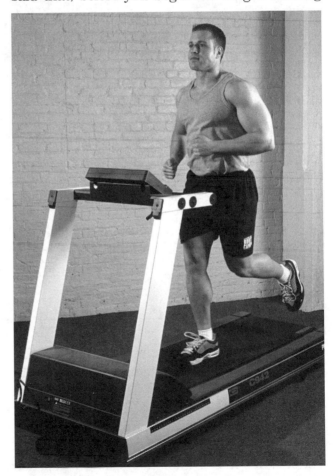

*Perform approximately fifteen minutes worth of aerobic activity to get the blood flowing and to increase your body temperature.*

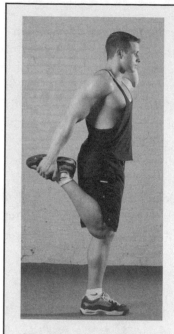

*Stretch your **thighs** by grasping a pole with one arm and bending the opposite leg, bringing your foot toward your buttocks (you grasp the pole with the left hand, then bend the right leg). Grasp your ankle with the free hand and slowly lift your foot as comfortably as possible. Hold this position for a count of five and repeat with the other leg.*

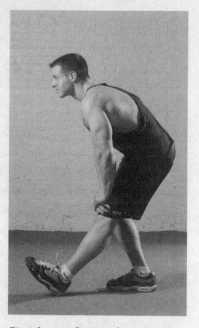

*Stretch your **hamstrings** by stepping forward with your left heel while bending your right knee. Keep your left leg straight and toe pointed up. Placing your hands on your left thigh, bend forward at the waist and feel the stretch in your hamstring. Hold this position for a count of five and repeat with the opposite leg.*

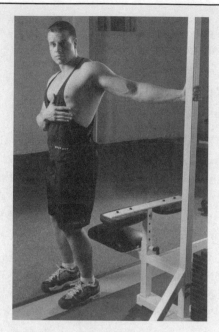

*Stretch your **chest** by grasping a stationary pole with one of your arms, ensuring that this arm is parallel to the ground. Slowly turn away from the pole and allow your arm to be as far behind the body as possible. Ensure that you do not overextend your chest by just going as far away as is comfortably possible. Hold this position for a count of five and repeat with the other arm.*

workout, spend 15 minutes warming up followed by light stretching. Just go through the next few steps.

## SELECTING THE WEIGHT FOR EACH EXERCISE

The weight you select for each exercise depends on the amount of repetitions that you need to do for a particular set. If you need to do between 10-12 repetitions for one set, then you need to pick a weight where you fail (the point at which completing another repetition becomes impossible) between 10-12 reps. This takes a bit of practice, but after a while you will become extremely accurate when it comes to choosing the correct weight for a particular repetition range. If you pick a weight that allows you to do more than 12 repetitions, you'll need to increase the amount of weight being lifted. If you reach failure before hitting the tenth rep, you'll need

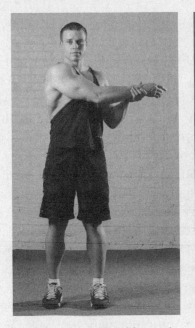

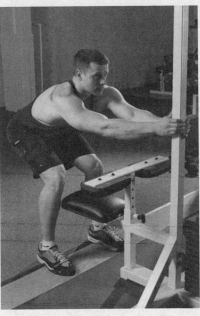

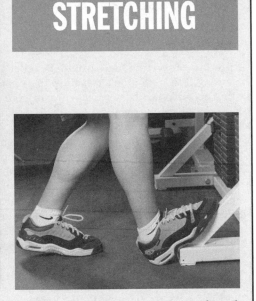

## STRETCHING

*Stretch your* **shoulders** *by grasping one of your wrists with the opposite hand. Without moving your torso, begin to pull your arm as far as possible. Hold this position for a count of five and repeat with the other arm.*

*Stretch your* **back** *by grasping a pole with both arms, bending your knees, and sitting back in order to fully extend your arms and achieve a stretch in your lats and lower back. Hold this position for a count of five.*

*Stretch your* **calves** *by grasping a pole with both arms, standing on a raised surface, and placing one foot on the edge of the surface in order to allow your heel to go down as far as comfortably possible. Hold this position for a count of five and repeat with the other leg.*

to decrease the amount of weight being lifted. For example, if you were doing four sets of an exercise, as you continue to work through the sets, fatigue will set in and you may not be able to continue using the weight that you chose to lift during the first set. When you get to the point where you can no longer lift a particular weight for a pre-determined repetition range, simply decrease the weight and prepare yourself for the next set.

### FAQ:

*I am getting a lot of mixed messages about stretching: do it, don't do it. What's the definitive answer?*

### ANSWER:

Stretching is great! There is just a time and place to do it. Stretching is essential to make sure your body is flexible and mobile. If you sit for long periods of time, then you know how quickly you can become stiff and achey. Stretching allows the muscles, joints, and connective tissues to remain limber and mobile. Don't forget that weight training is itself a form of stretching. It's false that bodybuilders aren't flexible. I have seen lots of huge guys and girls do full Chinese splits!

It takes work to become and maintain your flexibility. Just make sure that you are fully warmed up before stretching. You can stretch between sets or at the end of your workout.

# OVERTRAINING

Overtraining is caused when the body is taxed beyond its ability to recover. The main causes may include long workouts, an overload of training volume (too many sets and reps), a bad diet lacking nutrients, lack of sleep, etc. People experiencing this condition might notice such symptoms as a loss of muscle mass, weakness, trouble sleeping, loss of appetite, a lethargic and constant tired feeling, and feelings of depression.

It is impossible to overtrain with our weight training program (assuming you follow the nutrition and rest practices prescribed) because after you stress the body's recuperative capabilities to the maximum (by doing supersets for two weeks and then moving on to Giant Sets for two more), you back off into the less stressful modified compound supersets. In addition, you get a rest day after every day of lifting (unless you are using the advanced version) and you also get the weekends off. During rest days, you concentrate on fat burning aerobic exercise (which aids in the recuperation process by removing the lactic acid created by weight training) instead. We use Sunday as our total inactivity day; you can choose any day of the week as your rest day. This day serves to rest the body and the mind. Finally, the ample nutrients provided by the diet, along with the recommended supplements, eliminate the possibility of getting overtrained.

Provided that you follow the training program as laid out, in conjunction with the nutrition and rest components, overtraining is a state of mind and does not exist.

# SKIPPING WORKOUTS

**Skipping workouts is unacceptable.** You hear it all the time, people constantly making excuses about how they have no time to exercise. Unless you are in a situation where you are on call 24 hours a day and are being utilized at least 23 hours out of the 24, then we are more than sure that you can find the time to train. The fact of the matter is that some people don't want to spend the time exercising, so instead, they make excuses about how busy they are. We don't care if you only have 15

> **FAQ:**
>
> *How much time should I wait between warm-up sets?*
>
> **ANSWER:**
>
> You shouldn't rest a lot. The time it takes you to change the weight or take a drink of water will be approximately 30 to 60 seconds, which is fine. Don't let too much time pass, as your muscles will get cold and you could quickly stiffen up and risk injury.

minutes to allocate towards exercise, it's still 15 minutes of exercise! If you are interested in completely changing the way you look and feel, all the excuses in the world can not hold you back from doing what it takes to fit a workout into your schedule. All you need is the vision, the motivation and the determination to do so.

Skipping workouts will severely jeopardize your toning and fat burning efforts, in addition to destroying your bodysculpter's mindset. However, if for some reason you are not able to train (let's say because all the gyms in the world are closed on that day, and you have no gym at home and don't know anyone with one), then remember back to what your grandparents used to say, about how they had to walk over 5 miles just to get to work, in the snow, with no shoes or socks! In all seriousness, if you skip a workout one day, simply make up the skipped session the next day. This might mean training twice in one day (doing your cardio session in the morning and weights in the afternoon) or sacrificing your Sunday rest day. If you skip a workout for whatever reason, don't beat yourself up about it. Just realize that tomorrow is a new day and you will be able to make up the skipped session. However, don't make a habit of skipping training sessions, as skipping sessions will ultimately limit the results you expect to receive.

# Chapter 4
## Nutrition

For immediate Body Sculpting Bible support & coaching directly from James & Hugo, please visit www.BodySculptingBible.com

4

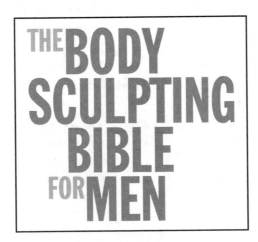

The second component of the formula for success is nutrition. Nutrition is what gives us the raw materials for recuperation, energy, and growth. Without a good diet, your dreams of achieving your ideal body will never be reached. Please pay close attention to the following sections.

If you truly wish to succeed and reach all of your body sculpting goals quickly with no delays, then you must make sure to follow the nutritional guidelines. Too many people neglect to follow these guidelines and because of that, never reach their goals of creating a beautiful physique. You could train like a madman but if you fail to pay attention to your nutrition, you will fail.

Let's discuss the characteristics of a good nutrition program, beginning with the nutritional basics.

## NUTRITION BASICS

There are three macronutrients that the human body needs in order to function properly:

## CARBOHYDRATES

Carbohydrates are your body's main source of energy. When you ingest carbohydrates your pancreas releases a hormone called insulin. In addition to regulating our blood sugar, insulin is very important because:

- It grabs on to the carbohydrates and either stores them in the muscle and liver for future use (this is called glycogen which is stored carbohydrates) or stores them as fat.
- It grabs on to the amino acids (protein) and shelters them inside the muscle

cell for recovery and repair. This is called increasing protein synthesis.
- While the above is an oversimplification of the many actions of insulin, for our purposes of discussion those are its main functions.

Most people who are overweight and are on low-fat/high-carbohydrate diets are in that condition because they eat an overabundance of carbohydrates. Too many carbohydrates cause your body to release huge amounts of insulin. When there is too much insulin in the body, your body naturally turns these excess carbohydrate calories into fat, thus creating a human fat storing machine. Therefore, it is important that we eat the right amount and types of carbs.

## COMPLEX AND SIMPLE CARBOHYDRATES

Carbohydrates are divided into two categories: complex carbs and simple carbs.

The **complex carbohydrates** are hundreds of sugar units linked together in single molecules (reason they are called complex) and typically give you more sustained energy (provided they have a medium to low Glycemic Index (GI) as they take more time to be broken down by the body. **Note:** Complex carbohydrates with a high GI behave more like a simple sugar, which is digested quickly.

There are two types of complex carbs, which you will be eating in small portions frequently throughout the day:
- **Starchy carbs** provide you with raw energy that your body can use. Good sources are oatmeal, grits, brown rice, lentils, sweet potatoes, and cream of wheat.

## GLYCEMIC INDEX

In order to understand the proper carbs to consume, you must understand the details of the Glycemic Index. The Glycemic Index (or GI for short) is a measurement of how quickly your blood sugar rises after ingesting a carbohydrate. Basically, once you consume a carbohydrate and it gets digested, it gets turned to glucose (blood sugar). Blood sugar is used by the body to manufacture ATP (Adenosine Tri-Phosphate), which is the molecule that the body uses to power up all of its functions. You can think of ATP as your body's fuel, as without ATP, your organism would not be able to function.

The way that GI works is that each food is assigned a value, typically from 0-100, based on how fast blood sugar increases in the next two hours after consuming a carbohydrate. A value of 100 would represent a food that increases blood sugar very rapidly, such as a straight glucose drink. A value of 59, like the one from brown rice, means that the blood sugar response is moderate. Therefore, for the purposes of blood sugar control and fat loss, brown rice is a much better choice than a glucose drink.

That is because how quickly a carbohydrate is turned into glucose and released in the bloodstream affects the amount of insulin that the pancreas will release to control blood sugar levels. Too quick of a conversion and your insulin levels skyrocket, a bad situation if you are trying to lose body fat since fat loss cannot occur in the presence of high insulin levels. Such a hormonal environment triggers fat storage. Therefore, it stands to reason that if a carbohydrate is released slowly into the blood stream, then less insulin is released and fat loss is maximized.

So is controlling GI the main key to losing body fat? Yes and no. Understanding the effect of foods on your blood sugar is important as several studies have shown that eating low GI carbohydrates throughout the day suppresses appetite and provides more stable energy levels as blood sugar is better controlled (**Note:** sudden drops in blood sugar make you feel hungry and lethargic). In addition, eating low GI foods allows for more consumption of food without body fat storage and for a leaner you due to body fat loss.

### What's a Low-GI Food?

While there are many opinions out there on what a low GI food is, typically a food under 55 is considered low, a food under 70 is medium, and anything over 70 is high. However, we must understand that what you eat in conjunction with your carbohydrates will affect your GI. Every time you eat a protein with a carbohydrate the total GI of the meal will go down since protein is a very complex molecule and thus slows down the digestion of the carb. Fats also have this effect. Since you will not be eating just a carbohydrate in the Body Sculpting Bible nutrition plan, then the raw GI number should only be used as a guideline. Besides, GI does not provide us with the whole answer as to which carbohydrate is best for us in order to lose fat.

### What GI Does Not Take Into Account

An important reason why we cannot take GI as the only measure of whether a carbohydrate that we choose will help us lose fat or not is because GI does not take into account the different ways in which the body handles complex carbohydrates from starches like brown rice (or grains like oatmeal) vs. a simple carbohydrate like an apple.

- **Fibrous carbs** cannot be absorbed, but are rich in vitamins and minerals. In addition, fiber cleans up your intestines, which allows for better absorption of the nutrients that you get from digestible foods. Mixing fibrous sources with starchy sources lowers the rate of digestion of the starchy carbs, thus lowering their GI. Good sources are: asparagus, squash, broccoli, green beans, cabbage, cauliflower, celery, cucumber, mushrooms, lettuce, red or green peppers, tomato, spinach, and zucchini.

**Simple carbohydrates** are made up of one, two, or three units of sugar (at the most) linked together in single molecules, and thus, give you immediate energy as they are released more readily in the body. Good sources are: apples, pears, cantaloupes, oranges, cherries, strawberries, grapefruit, lemon, nectarines, and peaches. Higher sugar fruits like grapes or bananas are best for after a workout if desired.

Though the glycemic index categorizes most fruits as low GI, as you will see, the simple sugar found in fruits called fructose is metabolized differently than the sugars from starches. To understand how the process differs, first let's see how the body uses glucose.

If blood glucose levels are low, the body uses the glucose it gets from foods and burns it immediately for energy. This is one of the reasons why after a workout, the body utilizes carbohydrates so efficiently. Now, assuming that there is no immediate need for energy, glucose is then converted into glycogen and stored in the liver or the muscles. The liver can hold roughly 100 grams of glycogen but the muscles, depending on how muscular you are, may store

between 200-400 grams. The key point to remember: the glycogen from muscles can only supply energy to the muscles when they are contracting (so muscle glycogen gets depleted badly during a weight training workout). Liver glycogen, however, can supply energy to the entire body. It is key to remember this in order to understand how fructose does not help with fat loss.

The way that the body gets fat when there is an excess of carbohydrates is that if all of the glycogen stores in the body are full, then the extra glucose is converted to fat by the liver and stored as adipose tissue (bodyfat), probably around your waist.

Now that you understand how glucose is used and how fat can be stored in situations where all glycogen levels are full, let's go back to the fruits. What happens with fructose is that the muscles do not have the enzyme required to turn fructose into glycogen. The liver does, so fructose replenishes the liver. It does not take much to replenish a liver of glycogen as it can hold around 100 grams only. Therefore, if you overdo the fruits, you will fill up your liver glycogen and this causes the body to release an enzyme signaling the body that glycogen stores are full. Since the liver has to supply energy for the whole body, the body uses its glycogen stores as the fuel gauge. When the tank is full, so to speak, that is when any extra fuel gets stored away. Because of this, we suggest that fruits are limited and even eliminated if on an aggressive fat loss diet. By the way, if you are wondering why most fruits can be so low GI and still cause so much damage is because fructose leaves the liver as fat and fat does not raise insulin levels.

## CARBOHYDRATE CONSUMPTION RECOMMENDATIONS

It is recommended that you eat mainly medium (less than 65 GI) to low (less than 55 GI) glycemic complex carbs throughout the day, as they are responsible for creating consistent energy levels for peak performance and daily functions.

If you must eat fruits, minimize your consumption to two servings per day at times where some of your liver glycogen has been depleted. The best times are the morning with breakfast and right after a workout. This will help to speed up the recuperation time and aid in the production of lean muscle tissue. Ingesting simple carbs throughout the day is not recommended as if your liver glycogen is full, then you will risk storing body fat.

Now that we have covered all that there is to know regarding carbohydrates, let's talk about the major building blocks in the body, which are proteins.

## PROTEIN

Every tissue in your body is made up of protein (i.e. muscle, hair, skin, and nails etc.).

Proteins are the building blocks of lean muscle tissue. Without it, building muscle and burning fat efficiently would be impossible. Protein helps to increase your metabolism every time you eat it by 20 percent, and it time-releases carbohydrates (glucose) by lowering their glycemic index, so you get sustained energy throughout the day.

During the 14-Day Body Sculpting Program you should consume between 1-1.5 grams of protein per pound of lean body mass (In other words, if you are 200 lbs and have 10% body fat, you should consume at least 180 grams of protein, since your lean body mass = 180 lbs).

Most people should not consume more than 1.5 grams per pound of lean body mass as this is unnecessary and the extra protein will be turned into glucose and used for energy, excreted out of the body, or provide excess calories that may get turned into fat. (Note: While protein itself is very unlikely to be stored as fat, a consistent caloric intake much higher than that required for your body to function will lead to an increase in body fat over time).

Good examples of protein include: salmon, lean ground turkey, flounder, grouper, halibut, cod, round steak, chicken breast, tuna fish (spring water), turkey breast, whey protein, and egg substitutes.

All proteins are low in glycemic index and by combining a carbohydrate with a protein, the combined glycemic index of the whole meal goes down as a result. The proteins included here were selected due to their low fat content and their digestibility.

**NOTE:** Avoid deli meats as they are high in sodium. If you are eating salmon, eliminate two servings of good fats.

## FATS

All the cells in the body have some fat. Fats are responsible for lubricating your joints. In addition, hormones are manufactured from fats. If you eliminate the fats from your diet, your hormonal production will drop and a whole array of chemical reactions will be interrupted. Your body will start accumulating more body fat than usual to keep functioning. Because your testosterone production is halted, so will the production of lean muscle mass. Therefore, in order to have an efficient metabolism, we need to consume a small amount of certain fats.

There are three types of fats: saturated, polyunsaturated, and monounsaturated.

**Saturated Fats** are associated with heart disease and high cholesterol levels. They are found to a large extent in products of animal origin. However, some vegetable fats are altered in a way that increases the amount of saturated fats in them by a chemical process known as hydrogenation. Hydrogenated vegetable oils are generally found in packaged foods as they extend the shelf life of the food item. However, in return, these fats, when consumed, cause your body to be resistant to insulin (which in turn causes issues in controlling your blood sugar) and also increase your cholesterol dramatically.

Coconut oil, palm oil, and palm kernel oil, which are also frequently used in packaged foods, and non-dairy creamers are highly saturated. These oils are also many times hydrogenated. If you read the ingredient label of an item and see that it says "partially hydrogenated (name of oil)", then immediately put that item back in the shelf. Consider partially hydrogenated oils poison to your body.

**Polyunsaturated Fats** make up most of the fats in vegetable oils, such as corn, cottonseed, safflower, soybean, and sunflower oil. Also, flaxseed oil and fish oils are polyunsaturated. These last two fats are usually high in the Omega 3 Essential Fatty Acids (EFAs). What are Omega 3 EFAs? Omega 3 EFAs are one of the two essential fats that the body needs. "Essential" means that the body cannot produce it on its own and therefore must be obtained from diet. The other kind of EFAs the body needs are the Omega-6 oils. Flax and fish oils are high on the Omega 3 EFAs, which help improve immune system, energy production, insulin sensitivity, and hormonal production. In addition, they have been shown to have anti-lipogenic properties (help prevent fat storage) as

well as help to burn body fat, and assist in improving recovery by having anti-inflammatory properties and by protecting muscle from being broken down. Omega-6 oils are also beneficial to the body by reducing post training inflammation. These oils, however, are more easily found in most vegetable oils, margarine, poultry and eggs so we don't see a need to supplement them further.

**Monounsaturated Fats** have a positive effect on the good cholesterol levels. Sources of these fats are virgin olive oil, canola oil, and peanut oil.

20% of your calories should come from good fats. Any less than 20% and your hormonal production goes down. Any more than 20% and you start accumulating plenty of fat.

Good sources of fat are non-processed vegetable oils such as canola oil, safflower oil, natural peanut butter, olive oil, flaxseed oil, and fish oils.

## WATER

Water is by far the most abundant substance in our body. Without water, an organism would not survive very long. Most people that come to us for advice on how to get in shape, almost always underestimate the great value of water.

Water is good for the following reasons:
- Over 65% of your body is composed of water (most of your muscle cells are composed of water).
- Water cleanses your body of toxins and pollutants that can make you sick.
- Water is needed for all of the complex chemical reactions that your body performs on a daily basis. Processes such as energy production, muscle building, and fat burning all require water. A

lack of water would interrupt all of these processes.

- Water helps lubricate the joints for increased mobility and decreased joint pain.
- When the outside temperature increases, water serves as a coolant to lower body temperature to where it is supposed to be.
- Water helps control your appetite. Have you ever felt like you were still hungry after eating a huge meal? This might very well be an indication that your body is beginning to dehydrate. You will notice that by drinking water at that time, your cravings will miraculously stop.
- Cold water increases your metabolism and aids in the breakdown of body fat.

In order to determine how much water your body needs each day, multiply your lean body weight by .66. This indicates how many ounces of water your body needs in a day for optimum function.

## CHARACTERISTICS OF A GOOD NUTRITION PROGRAM

Now that we have discussed the main nutrients that your body needs day in and day out to function, let's discuss what makes up a good nutrition program:

**Your nutrition plan should be based on eating small and frequent meals throughout the day.** Why? Because when you feed your body several times a day, your metabolism greatly increases. In addition, whenever three hours go by without any food consumption, your

# Nutrition Chart and Glycemic Index

| STARCHY CARBOHYDRATES | | | |
|---|---|---|---|
| Eat with all 5-6 meals throughout the day. Around 50-54 grams of carbohydrates per serving. 1 serving per meal. | | | |
| **FOOD ITEM** | **SERVING SIZE (MEASURE DRY)** | **GLYCEMIC INDEX** | **DESIRABLE** |
| Old Fashioned Oats | 1 cup dry | Low | Highly |
| Cream of Rice | 1/2 cup dry | High | Good After Workout Only |
| Cream of Wheat | 8 tablespoons dry | Medium | Good |
| Baked Potatoes | 8 ounce cooked | Medium | Good |
| Sweet Potatoes | 8 ounce cooked | Medium | Good |
| Rice (Brown Whole Grain) | 1 cup cooked | Medium | Good |
| White Rice | 1 cup cooked | High | Good After Workout Only |
| Spaghetti | 8 oz cooked | Low | Good in GI but too many carbs for a small serving. |
| Whole wheat flour bread | 4 slices | High | Not a great choice but ok in moderation. |
| Corn | 1-1/2 cup | Medium | Good |
| Peas | 2 cups | Medium | Good |
| Low GI=1-55 Medium GI=56-69 High GI=70-100 | | | |

## SIMPLE CARBOHYDRATES

If you must, eat 1 serving with Breakfast and 1 after workout as even though they are low to medium in GI, too many simple sugars from fruits in the diet throughout the day can prevent fat loss. If your post workout meal is breakfast, then just consume 1 serving per day of fruits.

Around 20 grams of carbohydrates per serving. If breakfast is the post workout meal: 1 serving per day with post workout meal. If post workout meal is not breakfast: 1 serving with breakfast and 1 serving with post workout meal.

| FOOD ITEM | SERVING SIZE | GLYCEMIC INDEX | DESIRABLE |
|---|---|---|---|
| Apples | 1 | Low | Good |
| Oranges | 1 | Low | Good |
| Grapefruit | 1 | Low | Good |
| Cherries | 14 | Low | Good |
| Pears | 2/3 | Low | Good |
| Bananas | 2/3 | Medium | After Workout Only |
| Lemons | 2 | Low | Good |
| Cantaloupe | 1/2melon | High | After Workout Only |
| Strawberries | 2 cups | 1 cup | Good |
| Apricots | 6 | Medium | After Workout Only |
| Grapes | 1 cup | Low | Good |
| Mango | 2/3 cup | Medium | After Workout Only |
| Papaya | 1 cup | Medium | After Workout Only |

Low GI=1-55 Medium GI=56-69 High GI=70-100Low GI=1-55 Medium GI=56-69 High GI=70-100

## FIBROUS CARBOHYDRATES

Eat at least 1 serving with lunch and 1 serving with dinner though more can be consumed if desired; consider these free foods as they do not get absorbed.

Around 10 grams of carbohydrates per serving. At least 1 serving at lunch and 1 serving at dinner.

| FOOD ITEM | SERVING SIZE (MEASURE COOKED) | GLYCEMIC INDEX | DESIRABLE |
|---|---|---|---|
| Broccoli | 1 cup | Low | Good |
| Green Beans | 1 cup | Low | Good |
| Asparagus | 12 spears or 1 cup | Low | Good |
| Lettuce | 1 head raw | Low | Good |
| Tomatoes | 2 cups chopped | Low | Good |
| Green Peppers (chopped) | 1-1/2 cup raw | Low | Good |
| Onions | 1/2cup | Low | Good |
| Mushrooms | 1 cup | Low | Good |
| Cucumber sliced | 3 cups | Low | Good |
| Cauliflower | 2 cups | Low | Good |
| Spinach | 4 cups | Low | Good |
| Cabbage | 2 cups | Low | Good |
| Carrots | 1/2 cup sliced | High | After Workout |

Low GI=1-55 Medium GI=56-69 High GI=70-100

## PROTEINS

Eat with all 5-6 meals throughout the day. Around 40-46 grams of protein per serving. 1 serving per meal.

| FOOD ITEM | SERVING SIZE (MEASURE COOKED) | GLYCEMIC INDEX | DESIRABLE |
|---|---|---|---|
| Chicken breast (skinless) | 6 ounces | Low | Good |
| Turkey | 6 ounces | Low | Good |
| Veal | 6 ounces | Low | Good |
| Top Sirloin | 6 ounces | Low | Good |
| Tuna | 6 ounces | Low | Good |
| Wild Alaskan Salmon | 6 ounces | Low | Good |
| Egg Whites (in carton) | 2 cups | Low | Good |
| Whey Protein | 2 scoops | Low | Good |
| Orange Roughy | 6 ounces | Low | Good |

## GOOD FATS

Around 10 grams of fats per serving. 1 serving at lunch, dinner, and any other meal except post workout meal.

| FOOD ITEM | SERVING SIZE | GLYCEMIC INDEX | DESIRABLE |
|---|---|---|---|
| Fish Oils | 2 teaspoons | Low | Good |
| Flax Oils | 2 teaspoons | Low | Good |
| Extra Virgin Olive Oil | 2 teaspoons | Low | Good |
| Natural Peanut Butter | 4 teaspoons | Low | Good |

All fats are low in glycemic index and by combining a carbohydrate with a protein the combined glycemic index of the whole meal goes down. The fats included here were selected due to their high essential fatty acids content and their health properties.

NOTES: Avoid cooking with flax oil as the heat degrades the oil. Bake and broil instead of frying. Also, if eating salmon, eliminate 2 servings of good fats as salmon is high on EFAs.

The complete list of the glycemic index and glycemic load for 750 foods can be found in the article "International tables of glycemic index and glycemic load values: 2002," by Kaye Foster-Powell, Susanna H.A. Holt, and Janette C. Brand-Miller in the July 2002 American Journal of Clinical Nutrition, Vol. 62, pages 5–56. <http://www.ajcn.org/cgi/content/full/76/1/5>

body switches to a catabolic state (a state in which your body starts burning muscle for energy!). The body actually believes that it is starving and in an attempt to protect itself from starvation, begins to feed itself by cannibalizing on your lean muscle tissue! It also lowers its metabolic rate (rate at which the body burns calories) and begins to store ingested calories as fat for future use. Bad scenario to be catabolic! The diet industry has made us think that the key to losing fat requires an extreme restriction of calories. You can see how much this theory has worked as America continues to gain weight!

Another reason to eat frequent meals is to manage blood sugar, insulin, and energy levels. Larger infrequent feedings result in larger releases of insulin with blood sugar crashes resulting in low energy levels 30 minutes to an hour after the meal is eaten. In addition, whatever extra calories the body cannot use at that time are stored for future use as body fat. Also, when you fall into the state of low blood sugar, you get lethargic and may crave sweets.

Smaller, more frequent feedings spike the metabolism and maintain a more stable blood sugar pattern that results in better utilization of nutrients, more stable energy and reduced cravings (or even no cravings) throughout the day.

During the 14-Day Body Sculpting Program you will be eating between five to six meals a day (or six to seven if you are following The Advanced 14-Day Body Sculpting Program) at 2-½ to 3- hour intervals.

**Your meals should contain carbohydrates, protein and fats in the correct ratios.** When you eat a meal that does not make up the proper balance of nutrients (for example an all carbohydrate meal; such as a pasta meal), you will not yield the desired results. Every macronutrient has to be present in order for the body to absorb them and use them properly and efficiently. Without boring you with the effect of food on the body's biochemistry, let's just say that if you solely eat carbohydrates as a meal, your energy levels will crash in about 30 minutes and your body will store any carbs that were not used as body fat (this is a large oversimplification of what really happens inside the body but as previously stated this is not a biochemistry book). Conversely, if you only eat protein all the time, you will lack energy. Therefore, by eating a meal with one serving of starchy carbohydrates, a serving of fibrous carbohydrates and a serving of protein, you will have most of the macronutrients that your body needs. Once you add a tablespoon of either extra virgin olive oil or flaxseed oil to one of your vegetable servings of the day, then you have covered all of your macronutrient requirements.

**No smoking and limited alcohol consumption.** Both offer health problems which are not in line with what you are trying to accomplish. Alcohol in particular adds 7 empty calories per gram to your diet, which is not a good situation when you are trying to control your caloric intake.

**Increase your intake of protein.** Proteins are the building blocks of all living organisms. If you are trying to build a structure such as the Empire State Building any construction contractor will tell you that they will need way more raw material to build such a large structure than to build a regular house. The same thing happens with body sculpting. Several researchers have discovered that the protein needs of people engaged in weight training activity exceed those of sedentary people. While most researchers are still debating on the amount, most of us in the field agree that 1-1.5 grams of protein per pound of lean body mass is just about right for any hard training person. "Now what about kidney damage?" some may ask. Well, according to research conducted in the year 2000 called "Do Regular High Protein Diets Have Potential Health Risks on Kidney Function in Athletes?" published in the International Journal of Sports Nutrition (Jacques R. Poortmans and Oliver Dellalieux. International Journal of Sports Nutrition, 2000, 10) higher protein intakes do not pose a threat to healthy kidney function. Having said that, the same is not true if you already suffer from a kidney condition.

**Reduce your intake of bad fats and bring on the good fats.** Bad fats are things like butter, cooking oils, and saturated fats such as the ones found in meats. However, ensure adequate intake of good fats such as flaxseed oil, extra virgin olive oil and natural peanut butter. One tablespoon of flaxseed oil a day covers all of the essential fatty acid requirements of most people.

**Reduce your intake of sugars.** Foods laden with sugar cause a sharp rise in insulin levels. Insulin is a good hormone when it is not present in excess as it carries the amino acids from the protein into the muscle cell so that they can be used for growth and repair. It also carries the carbohydrates into the liver and muscle cells for storage as glycogen (stored carbohydrates) that can be used for future occasions. However, in excess, once the body's reserves of carbohydrate storage are full, insulin turns these carbs into fat!

In addition, the excess insulin production will also take the carbs away from the blood stream too quickly creating a situation of low blood sugar. In this case you feel tired, groggy, and usually crave sweets. It is a vicious cycle that guarantees fat gain and possibly insulin resistance and diabetes later on. So this means that you need to eliminate all sorts of junk food from your diet. That alone will cause you to eliminate empty calories that are not used by the body and are turned into fat. Also, foods that are high in sugars and fats are the worst as when both of these macronutrients are present it is extremely easy for insulin to carry triglycerides (fats) into the adipose tissue stores (fat cells). Also regular sodas are out as well as fruit juices. Fruit juices you say? Yes. Most fruit juices are really high in sugars typically in the order of 30-40 grams per 8-ounce servings! In addition, do you know that three 8-ounce glasses of orange juice are enough to fill up your glycogen stores? Remember that once liver glycogen is full, any extra blood sugar gets stored in places that won't make you look great in a bathing suit.

**If you are interested in gaining muscle, have the correct post-workout nutrition meal.** The most important meal is the post-workout meal. This meal should consist of a high glycemic complex carb and preferably some sort of fast-released liquid protein such as whey isolate. Surprised? Well, only after a workout it is beneficial to have a large release of insulin as in this manner glycogen levels get replenished quicker, and repair and growth occur. If you cannot do away with fruits, this is the time to have a serving of simple carbs as well. There are many post workout preparations that are effective as long as there is minimum fat and fiber in the meal as both fats and fiber reduce the speed at which the food is released. A good example of a post workout meal is cream of rice with whey protein isolate. Cream of rice has a high glycemic index that it makes it perfect to create the high insulin environment needed for glycogen replenishment after a workout. A trick that we learned from Mr. Central Florida Todd Mendelsohn (from www.musclebuildingdiet.com) is that you can have a serving and a half of cream of rice (1/3 cup uncooked) mixed with whey protein isolate (a very fast released protein) as the ideal meal after a workout. It will replenish all glycogen stores immediately as well as provide the body with the amino acids that it needs. By replenishing glycogen store and providing the body with the amino acids that it needs at this crucial time, you accelerate your body sculpting results tenfold!

## DESIGNING YOUR BODY SCULPTING DIET

Now that we have discussed what foods to eat and in which amount, we can move on and design our diet. However, we realize that not everyone is at the same level. Some of you may already be following a program that is close enough to what we recommend here while others find this information to be completely new to them. Because of that, we have created three levels from which to start.

If you are completely new to this, please choose the Break-In Body Sculpting Diet Plan. By slowly changing your diet in this manner, you will not find the changes so overwhelming. If you already follow a set diet and you just need to fine tune it, then just go straight to the Body Sculpting Diet Plan. If you have been following a great diet for a while, already look great and want to take it to another level, such as the look of a fitness or figure competitor, then follow the Advanced Body Sculpting Diet Plan. Please keep in mind that the Advanced Body Sculpting Diet Plan is more restrictive as it is designed with the goal of achieving an incredible level of fitness and leanness.

## BREAK-IN BODY SCULPTING DIET PLAN

Usually people associate diets with starvation plans or days of agony and pain. However that is not the correct definition of a diet. The word diet refers to the food choices that we make on a daily basis. In this book, we are going to teach you a program that you will be able to use for the rest of your life to help keep you in tip-top shape. The reason our diet works is because of our food choices, the timing of meals and the back and forth switching in caloric intake. We don't expect you to change overnight. As a matter of fact, this is the reason why we feel that 99 percent of dieters fail. Our goal is to have you succeed just as we did. While it is possible for some people to make drastic changes in a small amount of time, we realize that most people do better by making incremental and progressive changes that will eventually get them to reach

their desired goals. That is the way that we are going to teach you to change your "diet." Small incremental steps with huge rewards!

## BABY STEPS, GIANT RESULTS: THE NO-PAIN, ALL-GAIN PLAN TO A PERFECT DIET

In keeping with our 14-day philosophy, we will make incremental changes to your diet every two weeks. Remember that this is how long it takes to create a new pattern as well as how long it takes the body to get used to something new. Every 14 days we are going to set a new goal. Each goal will build upon the success of the previous one. It is imperative that you use your determination and all of the Chapter 3 techniques in order to ensure the success of the program. By achieving each goal every two weeks you will end up with the diet that will yield the consistent fat loss/muscle toning results that you are looking for. In other words, you will end up with the exact same diet that we discussed on the sections above!

### (Weeks 1-2) Cut the fat.

For the first two weeks, we just want you to start looking at the labels of the foods that you consume and try to start cutting out as many fats as possible. Make some instant changes in your current routine, for example:

If you fry things, start steaming and broiling as a healthy alternative.

If you use salad dressing with a high fat content, substitute them for low fat or non-fat choices.

Select lower fat choices for meats. For instance, if you consume corned beef, substitute skinless chicken or turkey. If you consume chicken with the skin, start removing the skin (this has the most fat). If you like red meats, then buy the lean cuts.

Your taste buds will get used to your new low-fat eating habits in the two-week period.

## (Weeks 3-4) Eliminate refined sugars.

Now it's time to eliminate the refined sugars from your diet. Where are the refined sugars? They are everywhere! Therefore, in order to accomplish this goal, do the following:

- Eliminate regular sodas because they contain large amounts of sugars. Instead, drink diet sodas (however, they contain Aspartame and some research indicates that high consumption of Aspartame may cause cancer and many, many other potentially serious side effects in the long term. It may be a good idea to switch to a non-carbonated beverage).
- Eliminate the use of table sugars.
- Eliminate the consumption of sweets (except on the day that you have your cheat meal).

## (Weeks 5-6) Incorporate an abundant amount of water.

Start drinking much more water than you have previously consumed. We have already explained the reasons for consuming water. In order to accomplish this goal, do the following:

Substitute water for all types of drinks (including diet sodas and fruit juices, even if they claim to be natural). Every time you get thirsty, drink water.

Drink at least an 8-ounce glass of water with every meal.

Drink approximately 16 ounces or more of water during your workout.

## (Weeks 7-8) Caloric intake control and macronutrient management.

During these next two weeks we will get closer than ever to the ideal diet. The good news is that after these two weeks, dieting will cease to get more complicated, and you will continue to see some truly unbelievable results.

In order to jump on the fast track for results, without hesitating, do the following:

Start following the Low-Calorie Diet Prescribed in the Body Sculpting Diet Plan section.

Write down everything that you eat, along with the serving sizes.

Use the tables found in the Choosing What To Eat section (or Appendix B) in order to select your foods and know what your serving sizes look like.

For instructions on how to proceed after week 8, read the Caloric Cycling section presented in the Body Sculpting Diet Plan section.

# THE 14-DAY BODY SCULPTING DIET PLAN

## CALORIC CYCLING

Congratulations for making it this far, guys! By now, between the training and the diet you have seen some extremely favorable changes in the way that you look and feel. Great! Now, we will give you the secret for creating even more powerful and consistent results. The secret is called caloric cycling. By incorporating the following cycling principles in your diet, you ensure that you'll never reach the nasty fat loss plateaus that most dieters encounter.

In the training section, we discussed how the body will quickly get used to an exercise program and stop responding to the routine. When this happens your results cease and your efforts are simply wasted. The same principle applies to your diet.

In order to keep your metabolism efficiently burning body fat and building your body, caloric cycling will play an essential role in the program. As a matter of fact, recent research points to the fact that you lose faster (up to twice as fast) by cycling your calories than by not cycling them.

**Here's how to cycle calories:**

If you have been on the Break-In Plan, follow the High-Calorie Diet found below (right) for the next two weeks.

Go back to the Low Calorie Diet found below for the following two weeks.

Alternate every two weeks in this manner for fantastic results.

Continue writing down everything that you eat as well as the serving sizes in order to ensure that you don't go over the allotted macronutrient intake per meal.

Presented below is the 14-Day Body Sculpting Diet Plan. For the first two weeks, you will follow the Low Calorie Diet and for the next two weeks, you will follow the High Calorie Diet.

## WEEKS 1-2: CALORIES:LOW (Approximately 2400 calories)

Around 250 grams of carbohydrates (mostly complex with simple carbs being saved for after the workout)

Around 250 grams of protein

Around 40 grams of fats

### MEAL #1 (7:30 AM) BREAKFAST (POST-WORKOUT)
Choose 1 serving of Proteins
Choose 1 serving of Starchy Carbs
Optionally, you may choose to add 1 serving of Simple Carbs in the form of Fruit, if you can't live without them.

### MEAL #2 (10:30 AM) MORNING BREAK SNACK
Choose 1 serving of Proteins
Choose 1 serving of Starchy Carbs
Choose 1 serving of Good Fats

### MEAL #3 (1:30 PM) LUNCH TIME
Choose 1 serving of Proteins
Choose 1 serving of Starchy Carbs
Choose 1 serving of Fibrous Carbs
Choose 1 serving of Good Fats

### MEAL #4 (3:30 PM) AFTERNOON BREAK SNACK
Choose 1 serving of Proteins
Choose 1 serving of Starchy Carbs

### MEAL #5 (6:30 PM) DINNER
Choose 1-1/2 serving of Proteins
Choose 1/2 serving of Starchy Carbs
Choose 1 serving of Fibrous Carbs
Choose 1 serving of Good Fats

## WEEKS 3-4 CALORIES: HIGH (Approximately 2800 calories)

310 grams of carbohydrates (mostly complex with simple carbs being saved for after the workout)

310 grams of protein

40 grams of fats

### MEAL #1 (7:30 AM) BREAKFAST (POST-WORKOUT)
Choose 1 serving of Proteins
Choose 1 serving of Starchy Carbs
Optionally, you may choose to add 1 serving of Simple Carbs in the form of Fruit, if you can't live without them.

### MEAL #2 (10:30 AM) MORNING BREAK SNACK
Choose 1 serving of Proteins
Choose 1 serving of Starchy Carbs

### MEAL #3 (1:30 PM) LUNCH TIME
Choose 1 serving of Proteins
Choose 1 serving of Starchy Carbs
Choose 1 serving of Fibrous Carbs
Choose 1 serving of Good Fats

### MEAL #4 (3:30 PM) AFTERNOON BREAK SNACK
Choose 1 serving of Proteins
Choose 1 serving of Starchy Carbs

### MEAL #5 (6:30 PM) DINNER
Choose 1-1/2 serving of Proteins
Choose 1 serving of Starchy Carbs
Choose 1 serving of Fibrous Carbs
Choose 1 serving of Good Fats

### MEAL #6 (8:30 PM) LATE SNACK
Choose 1-1/2 serving of Proteins
Choose 1/2 serving of Starchy Carbs
Choose 1 serving of Fibrous Carbs
Choose 1 serving of Good Fats

## DON'T STRIVE FOR ABSOLUTE PERFECTION, STRIVE FOR CONSISTENCY

Many times we see dieters that start out doing great. However, there comes a day that for some reason or another they lose a workout or they blow their diets. After that day, they become so discouraged that they continue missing workouts or destroying their diets with self-sabotage. Many weeks go by before they get back on track (if ever). In the meantime, muscle size fades and the fat pounds pile up. Please remember the following: we are all human and we are entitled to make mistakes. Always strive for perfection, but if for some reason things don't go as well as they should on a given day, pick up and then move on. Forget about it and jump right back into your program. If you blow a meal one day, don't make it any worse by eating incorrectly all day long. If you miss a workout, don't wait until next Monday to start over. Just continue with your program the way it is laid out. Pick up from where you left off! In the end, your determination and consistency will enable you to win the battle of the bulge.

## TROUBLESHOOTING YOUR CALORIC INTAKE

The optimum fat loss per week is 2 pounds. Any more than two pounds a week and you will lose muscle, which will result in the loss of muscle tone, which in turn yields a saggy look and a significantly lower metabolism. Having said that, we need to point out the fact that while most men burn between 2400 to 2800 calories, some have a higher than usual metabolism.

Therefore, some guys may find themselves losing more than 2 pounds a week at the prescribed number of calories and others may find themselves gaining weight. If this is the case, don't panic! If you find you are losing too much, simply add 1 serving of carbs, 1 serving of proteins, and 1 serving of good fats to your diet (both on low and high calorie weeks). In this manner, your diet will fluctuate between 2850 and 3250 calories. After two weeks you should assess how this is working, by measuring your lean body mass. If you are still losing weight after two weeks, again increase your food intake by an additional serving of carbs, proteins and fats. Repeat the process until you reach the caloric intake that allows for a 2-pound fat loss while at the same time adds muscle tone/size.

The reverse applies if you are suddenly gaining weight. If you are gaining, cut your calories by 1/2 serving of just carbs and proteins for both the lower calorie diet and the higher calorie diet. You'll notice that we did not cut the calories by quite as much (since we cut no good fats), as your metabolism might only need a 200 calorie deficit. If you find that you are still gaining, even after the 200 calorie cut, you may than decrease your calories by the additional 200 calories. Don't jump the gun though! Give your body the opportunity to adjust.

## ADVANCED BODY SCULPTING DIET PLAN

Some of you guys want to attain an extreme level of fitness; a level achieved by only a hand-

---

### CAUTION

The diet plans in this book are designed for men with sedentary lifestyles. If you are into marathon running or any sort of high endurance sport, then you may need to double or even triple the amount of carbohydrates that are prescribed in this program.

---

ful of men that choose to take the Body Sculpting Lifestyle to the next level.

If you fall in this category and want to look like a competitive bodybuilder, then this section is for you. Be warned however that in order to achieve such look, an extreme amount of discipline is required. You have to keep in mind that the more extreme you want to look, the more disciplined and restrictive you need to be about your nutrition. You will also have to spend more time in the gym as well, following a routine like the Advanced Body Sculpting Workout where you do weights and cardio for 6 days a week.

If this still appeals you, then the diet strategy provided in this section is just right for you and will provide you with the desired results.

## CARBOHYDRATE CYCLING FOR EXTREME BODY SCULPTING

The key to convincing the body to go extremely low in body fat is to deprive it of carbohydrates temporarily. In this manner, your body has to use more fat than usual in order to meet its energy needs. Now, we are not talking about a zero carbohydrate diet or anything along those lines. We are talking instead of creating a state of moderate carbohydrate depravation followed by a state of moderate carbohydrate loading in order to prevent the metabolism from adjusting downwards (as if you did low carbs all of the time the body would adapt by lowering its metabolism to prevent further fat burning). So if you compared your glycogen stores (stored carbohydrates in the liver and muscles) against the gas tank of a car, you would want to run with the tank in medium at all times. How is this accomplished? By having a low-carbohydrate day followed by a medium-carbohydrate day and then followed by a high-carbohydrate day.

Day 1: Low Day
Day 2: Medium Day
Day 3: High Day
Day 4: Start Over At Day 1.

## HOW TO DETERMINE YOUR LOW, MEDIUM, HIGH CARBOHYDRATE DAYS

In order to determine how many carbohydrates you will need on any given day, you'll need to know what your lean body mass is.

### Lean Body Mass (LBM) = (Total Weight – Fat Weight)

You can calculate your fat weight by using a pair of skin fold calipers on yourself (such as the Accu-Measure) or by having a trainer at your health club (if you are a member at one) check it for you. As an alternative, go to Appendix F: Tracking your Progress, where we present some formulas that you can use.

Once you have your LBM, you can use the formulas below to figure out the carbohydrate grams you need per day.

### Low Carbohydrate Day = LBM x 0.5
### Medium Carbohydrate Day = LBM x 0.88
### High Carbohydrate Day = LBM x 1.5

The carbohydrate sources you will be choosing from will be mostly low to medium glycemic starchy ones (except for the cream of rice after a workout which is high glycemic) as these sources work best for insulin release control, loading muscle glycogen, and energy purposes. For best results, stick to the carbohydrate choices presented in the Approved List.

## STARCHY CARBOHYDRATES APPROVED LIST

Around 25-27 grams of carbohydrates per serving. Amount of servings depends on whether it is a low, medium or high carbohydrate day.

| FOOD ITEM | SERVING SIZE (MEASURE DRY) | GLYCEMIC INDEX | DESIRABLE |
|---|---|---|---|
| Old Fashioned Oats | 1/2 cup dry | Low | Highly |
| Cream of Rice | 1/4 cup dry | High | Good After Workout Only |
| Cream of Wheat | 4 tablespoons dry | Medium | Good |
| Baked Potatoes | 8 ounces cooked | Medium | Good |
| Sweet Potatoes | 8 ounces cooked | Medium | Good |
| Rice (Brown Whole Grain) | 1/2 cup cooked | Medium | Good |

## HOW TO DETERMINE YOUR PROTEIN LEVELS

Because you will be training hard, you will need 1.5 grams of protein per pound of LBM split over 6 meals per day in order to preserve and enhance muscle tone.

Protein Grams = LBM x 1.5

As far as protein choices, all of the ones discussed in the nutrition section are fair. However, due to the fact that you will need more protein, the serving sizes are bigger.

## PROTEINS

Eat with all 6-8 meals throughout the day. Around 28-30 grams of protein per serving. 1 serving per meal.

| FOOD ITEM | SERVING SIZE (MEASURE COOKED) | GLYCEMIC INDEX | DESIRABLE |
|---|---|---|---|
| Chicken breast (skinless) | 4 ounces | Low | Good |
| Turkey | 4 ounces | Low | Good |
| Veal | 4 ounces | Low | Good |
| Top Sirloin | 4 ounces | Low | Good |
| Tuna | 4 ounces | Low | Good |
| Wild Alaskan Salmon | 4 ounces | Low | Good |
| Egg Whites (in carton) | 1-1/4 cup | Low | Good |
| Whey Protein | 1-1/4 scoop | Low | Good |
| Orange Roughy | 4 ounces | Low | Good |

## HOW TO DETERMINE YOUR FAT GRAMS

In the absence of carbohydrates, one's needs for good fats increases. In addition, remember that good fats help to preserve muscle tissue, produce energy and also aid in the burning of body fat. To determine how many grams of good fats your body needs, here is the formula:

Good Fats = LBM x 0.3

As far as good fats choices, all of the ones discussed in the nutrition section are fair.

## GOOD FATS
Around 5 grams of fats per serving. 1 serving in breakfast, lunch and dinner.

| FOOD ITEM | SERVING SIZE | GLYCEMIC INDEX | DESIRABLE |
|---|---|---|---|
| Fish Oils | 1 teaspoon | Low | Good |
| Flax Oils | 1 teaspoon | Low | Good |
| Extra Virgin Olive Oil | 1 teaspoon | Low | Good |
| Natural Peanut Butter | 2 teaspoon | Low | Good |

## BODYWEIGHT CHARTS

If all of the math above is making you dizzy, no need to worry as the table below provides you with all of the macronutrient requirements that you need depending on your LBM and also on whether you are doing a Low, Medium or High Carbohydrate Day.

| | Carbs (g) | | | Protein (g) | Fats (g) |
|---|---|---|---|---|---|
| LBM | LOW DAY | MEDIUM DAY | HIGH DAY | | |
| 90 | 45 | 79 | 135 | 135 | 27 |
| 95 | 48 | 84 | 143 | 143 | 29 |
| 100 | 50 | 88 | 150 | 150 | 30 |
| 105 | 53 | 92 | 158 | 158 | 32 |
| 110 | 55 | 97 | 165 | 165 | 33 |
| 115 | 58 | 101 | 173 | 173 | 35 |
| 120 | 60 | 106 | 180 | 180 | 36 |
| 125 | 63 | 110 | 188 | 188 | 38 |
| 130 | 65 | 114 | 195 | 195 | 39 |
| 135 | 68 | 119 | 203 | 203 | 41 |
| 140 | 70 | 123 | 210 | 210 | 42 |
| 145 | 73 | 128 | 218 | 218 | 44 |
| 150 | 75 | 132 | 225 | 225 | 45 |
| 155 | 78 | 136 | 233 | 233 | 47 |
| 160 | 80 | 141 | 240 | 240 | 48 |
| 165 | 83 | 145 | 248 | 248 | 50 |
| 170 | 85 | 150 | 255 | 255 | 51 |
| 175 | 88 | 154 | 263 | 263 | 53 |
| 180 | 90 | 158 | 270 | 270 | 54 |
| 185 | 93 | 163 | 278 | 278 | 56 |
| 200 | 100 | 176 | 300 | 300 | 60 |
| 205 | 103 | 180 | 308 | 308 | 62 |
| 210 | 105 | 185 | 315 | 315 | 63 |
| 215 | 108 | 189 | 323 | 323 | 65 |
| 220 | 110 | 194 | 330 | 330 | 66 |
| 225 | 113 | 198 | 338 | 338 | 68 |
| 230 | 115 | 202 | 345 | 345 | 69 |
| 235 | 118 | 207 | 353 | 353 | 71 |
| 240 | 120 | 211 | 360 | 360 | 72 |
| 245 | 123 | 216 | 368 | 368 | 74 |
| 250 | 125 | 220 | 375 | 375 | 75 |

## DESIGNING YOUR DIET

Designing your Advanced Body Sculpting Diet Plan is easy.

First, divide your protein requirements by 6. That will give you the grams of protein that you will need per meal. If the resulting number is a decimal, just round to the nearest tenth. So for instance in the case of a guy with 185-lbs of LBM, 278 (185 x 1.5 to get protein requirements) divided by 6 equals 46.3, so in this case, just have 46 grams of protein per meal.

Now divide the amount of carbohydrates by 50. This will give you the approximate amount of carbohydrate servings that you need per day. Follow the same rounding protocol as described above for proteins. If you only are allowed 2 servings, then add them to Meal 1 and your Post-Workout Meal (PWM). If Meal 1 is your Post Workout Meal then you just need to add the second serving to Meal 3. If you have three servings of carbs, then add them to meals 1, 2, and your Post-Workout Meal. Again, if Meal 1 is your PWM, then you would have carbs at meals 1, 2, and 3. Continue this same pattern for the amount of servings that you have.

For fats, divide the grams of fats by 10 and that gives you the number of teaspoons of EFAs that you need in your diet, keeping in mind that if salmon is consumed, two of those teaspoons can be eliminated. As long as you do not add these to your PWM, then you can add them to any of the other meals.

For vegetables, there is no need to count, so just add them at will to at least two meals. On low carb days, feel free to add them to all of your carb free meals.

## DIETING TO ADD MUSCLE MASS

The Body Sculpting Diets in this book are designed to help men add some muscle while stripping body fat at the same time. For those guys who have a faster metabolism and are just interested in gaining muscle, as their body fat is already low, then all of the advice in this section applies to them with the following modifications to the training and nutrition programs.

### EATING TO GAIN MUSCLE WEIGHT

Eating to just gain muscle (as opposed to gaining muscle and losing body fat) follows the same prescriptions above except that the total caloric intake will be higher, for most people in the order of 2600 calories for two weeks and 3100 for the next two. If the person trying to gain is an ectomorph (a naturally skinny person who has trouble gaining weight) then the caloric range may be as high as 3000 for two weeks and 3500 for the next two.

Two sample meal plans guaranteed to pack on the muscle are presented on the next page.

## WEEKS 1-2: CALORIES: MEDIUM (Approximately 2600 calories)

### MEAL #1 (8:30 AM)
**Carbs 54 grams; Protein 45 grams; Fats 17 grams**

| | |
|---|---|
| 1 cup egg substitute | 160 calories |
| 1 cup of dry oats | 300 calories |
| 1 tablespoon flaxseed oil | 130 calories |

### MEAL #2 (10:30 AM)
**Carbs 40 grams; Protein 40 grams; Fats 8 grams**

| | |
|---|---|
| Protein Drink | 390 calories |

### MEAL #3 (12:30 PM)
**Carbs 50 grams; Protein 48 grams; Fats 8 grams**

| | |
|---|---|
| 8 ounces chicken (weighed prior to cooking) | 120 calories |
| 1 cup salad | 80 calories |
| (lettuce, tomato, carrot, cucumber, green peppers, etc.) | |
| 10 oz baked potato | 200 calories |

### MEAL #4 (2:30 PM)
**Carbs 40 grams; Protein 40 grams; Fats 8 grams**

| | |
|---|---|
| Protein Drink | 390 calories |

### MEAL #5 (4:30 PM)
**Carbs 45 grams; Protein 48 grams; Fats 5 grams**
(Pre-Workout Meal; to be eaten at least two hours before the workout)

| | |
|---|---|
| 8 oz chicken, turkey breast or tuna | 240 calories |
| (weighed prior to cooking) | |
| 1 cup brown rice | 180 calories |

### 6:30-7:30 PM WEIGHT TRAINING WORKOUT

### MEAL #6 (7:30 PM)
**Carbs 42 grams; Protein 50 grams; Fats 0 grams**
**(Bring this meal to gym)**

| | |
|---|---|
| 50 grams of protein from whey isolate product | 200 calories |
| 7 tablespoons of cream of rice | 175 calories |

### DAILY TOTALS
**Calories:** 2565; **Carbohydrates:** 271 grams;
**Protein:** 271 grams; **Fats:** 46 grams

## WEEKS 3-4 CALORIES: HIGH (Approximately 3100 calories)

### MEAL #1 (8:30 AM)
**Carbs 81 grams; Protein 50 grams; Fats 20 grams**

| | |
|---|---|
| 1 cup egg substitute | 160 calories |
| 1.5 cup of dry oats | 450 calories |
| 1 tablespoon flaxseed oil | 130 calories |

### MEAL #2 (10:30 AM)
**Carbs 40 grams; Protein 40 grams; Fats 8 grams**

| | |
|---|---|
| Protein Drink | 390 calories |

### MEAL #3 (12:30 PM)
**Carbs 50 grams; Protein 48 grams; Fats 8 grams**

| | |
|---|---|
| 8 ounces chicken (weighed prior to cooking) | 120 calories |
| 1 cup salad | 80 calories |
| (lettuce, tomato, carrot, cucumber, green peppers, etc.) | |
| 10 oz baked potato | 200 calories |

### MEAL #4 (2:30 PM)
**Carbs 40 grams; Protein 40 grams; Fats 8 grams**

| | |
|---|---|
| Protein Drink | 390 calories |

### MEAL #5 (4:30 PM)
**Carbs 48 grams; Protein 48 grams; Fats 5 grams**
(Pre-Workout Meal; to be eaten at least two hours before the workout)

| | |
|---|---|
| 8 oz chicken, turkey breast or tuna | 240 calories |
| (weighed prior to cooking) | |
| 8 oz sweet potatoes | 200 calories |

### 6:30-7:30 PM WEIGHT TRAINING WORKOUT

### MEAL #6 (7:30 PM)
**Carbs 42 grams; Protein 50 grams; Fats 0 grams**
**(Bring this meal to gym)**

| | |
|---|---|
| 50 grams of protein from whey isolate product | 200 calories |
| 7 Tablespoons of cream of rice - 175 | |

### MEAL #7 (9:30 PM)
**Carbs 18 grams; Protein 40 grams; Fats 5 grams**

| | |
|---|---|
| Protein Drink | 390 calories |

### DAILY TOTALS
**Calories:** 3125; **Carbohydrates:** 341 grams;
**Protein:** 316 grams; **Fats:** 57 grams

## Do I Need to Measure my Food Intake and Log it in a Diary Forever?

Not at all. Typically you will notice that after the first six-week cycle you pretty much know how much food you need to take in everyday. The reason for measuring and keeping track of the foods that you eat during the first six weeks is to give you an idea of how much food you need in order to get in shape. Without tracking at the beginning of the program, it would be impossible to determine the correct quantity of nutrients your body needs in order to lose weight and tone up. However, since after six weeks you already know how much food you need, you can start building your meals based on a visual inspection alone. However, just be cautious not to progressively put more food on the plate. If you start to see that your weight is beginning to climb, track your food intake for the next three days and see how much you are deviating from what you should be having.

## The Sunday Reward

If you are not following the Advanced Body Sculpting Diet, you may cheat on your diet for one meal on Sunday (e.g. FORGET CALORIE COUNTING and eat whatever you want—within reason of course—for that one meal). You can only reward yourself in this way if you have stayed on track the rest of the week. One cheat meal a week may actually be beneficial since it confuses your body and increases metabolism. By cheating, you prevent your body from adjusting to the diet, which would lower your metabolism. It also removes the psychological fear that you will never be able to eat bad foods again. However, having said that, we must caution that some people (us included) find it hard to go back to good dieting if they incorporate cheat foods in their diets once a week. They fall

into a non-stop bingeing rage with these foods that may last for weeks. Do not feel bad if you fall into this category. It is natural to crave foods that are bad, considering that they taste so darn good. If you fall into this category and feel tempted or need to still build your will power of resistance, then stick to a healthy diet and stay away from cheat meals until you have reached a confident level of empowerment. We have actually learned to do just fine without cheat foods at all.

## The Importance of Preparing Food Beforehand

Preparation is crucial to the success of your dietary program. If you are not prepared, you will fail! Life is too hectic nowadays to be eating five or six times a day without a little bit of preparation.

One thing you can do is to prepare your food the night before and store it in individual containers that have a section for complex or simple carbs, a place for fibrous carbs and a place for protein. You also can prepare protein shakes the night before and store them individually in containers that you can purchase at the grocery store. When the following day comes, all you have to do is take out the container that has breakfast, heat it up and eat. Then grab the container for lunch and two protein shakes, put them in the cooler and go to work. Take a water bottle everywhere you go. No need to dehydrate while at work. When you come home, take out the container for dinner, re-heat it, eat it and prepare the food for the following day.

If you think you will be able to stick to the plan without being prepared, you place yourself at risk. You will either end up eating the wrong kinds of food, or missing meals. You will defi-

## TIPS FOR CHOOSING FOODS

1)   Always try to use natural foods.  Avoid using canned or pre-prepared types of foods as they usually contain too much fats, sodium and carbs.

2)   Always choose low-fat protein sources.  If you eat really low fat meals, don't worry about incurring a fat deficiency since the supplements program takes care of the need for essential fatty acids.  Besides, there are trace amounts of fats even in the low fat protein sources that we choose.

3)   If you choose to include skim milk in your diet, remember that it not only has protein (8 to 9 grams for every 8 ounces of milk) but also simple carbs (12 to 13 grams for every 8 ounces of milk).  Therefore, count milk as both.  Note that since the carbs in milk are simple carbs, this food item should only be used in the post workout meal.  Guys interested in competing or following the Advanced Body Sculpting Diet should, however, eliminate any dairy products from the diet as these products tend to make you retain water and the lactose in them makes it harder to get to the desired low body-fat percentage required for contest condition.  In addition, whole-wheat products should also be minimized during this phase as they may contain pytho-estrogens that makes it harder to lose fat.

4)   Try to include fibrous carbs in at least two meals.

5)   Post-Workout Meal should contain high glycemic complex carbs combined with fast released proteins such as whey protein isolate.  Fats and fibers should be eliminated from this meal ideally to facilitate maximum insulin release and thus improve recovery and muscle growth.

nitely spend more money, because eating out is not cheap. Therefore, remember to be prepared!

### MEAL FREQUENCY AND WORK

Choose from among these alternatives to make sure you get your five or six meals in each day:

- Have lunch and dinner as real meals and keep the rest of the meals as either meal replacement protein shakes or protein bars; preferably meal replacement shakes as most protein bars have too much fats and sugars.

- Have real food for your breakfast, lunch and dinner and meal replacement protein shakes for the other two meals.
- Have all of your meals as real meals by convincing your boss to allow you to have three 20-minute breaks instead of a full hour lunch, so you can eat all of your meals.

### EMOTIONAL EATING

In our fast-paced, high-stress society many people resort to emotional eating for comfort. This is a dangerous activity; if this happens very often, the weight will begin to pile on. Also dan-

## BEVERAGE TIPS

Many dieters, due to their lack of nutrition knowledge, can literally just blow their diets without realizing that they're doing it. The culprit? Drinking the wrong types of beverages.

- Drink plenty of water daily. Your recommended fluid intake should be 0.66 x body weight in ounces per day.
- Absolutely no regular sodas or fruit juices, even the ones that claim to be all natural, as there are way too many simple carbs in these beverages. For example, the average soda contains 40 grams of sugar while an 8-ounce serving of the average fruit juice contains between 25-35 grams of simple carbs! Therefore three 8 ounce glasses of orange juice would fill up your liver glycogen immediately!
- Crystal Light beverages, and decaffeinated tea/coffee are OK as long as they are used in moderation; your main beverage should be water.
- Try to avoid all alcohol. An occasional glass of red wine is OK provided that you are of legal drinking age.

gerous is the fact that emotional eating usually occurs at night after work.

If you feel like you engage in emotional eating, remember that you need to write down everything you eat during the first eight weeks of this program. During the first eight weeks, it should be easier to resist the temptation to eat emotionally because you will need to document it in your log. If you are past the original eight weeks, then ask yourself, "Am I eating this because my body needs it or is it because I need it emotionally?" In cases like this, stop to think about what is most important for you. Is it the food or your goals? You know what the right choice is. If it's late at night, just go to bed and rest assured that the craving will go away by the time the morning comes.

### PROTEIN SHAKES

It's better to eat as much real food as possible, but if you are too busy to fix five to six real meals, you can substitute meals with a shake.

You can have either a meal replacement packet mixed with water or a scoop of protein mixed in skim milk with a teaspoon of flaxseed oil. However, make sure that you eat at least two real meals a day, and keep in mind that the more real food you eat, the better results you get, as real food increases your metabolism more than shakes.

### QUICK AND EASY RECIPES

Here are some healthy recipes, many created using protein powder, which you can incorporate into your meal plans. The following recipes are healthy recipes that you can add to your diet program. However, if you include them in your diet, be sure t measure your portions and count how many carbohydrates and proteins you are taking in. In this manner, you make sure that you are taking your portion of protein and your portion of carbs. Remember that for

---

## COOKING TIPS

If you want to achieve your Body Sculpting goals, proper food preparation is essential! Follow the guidelines below to ensure proper food preparation:

- Eat vegetables raw or slightly steamed. If boiling, be careful not to overcook or you will lose the nutritional value of the vegetables.
- Do not fry. Always broil, grill, steam or bake (broiling, grilling and steaming are better as they allow fat to drain while cooking).
- Trim all fat from meat and remove skin from poultry prior to cooking.
- Do not use salts, butter, oils, or sugar while cooking. Experiment with herbs, non-salt seasonings, lemon juice, vinegar, garlic and pepper, even a touch (1 Tbsp; not a bottle) of some white or red wine. Occasional use of salsa, low sodium soy sauce, catsup, and mustard to enhance meats and vegetables is OK if used sparingly (1 Tbsp). Minced white or green onions are also excellent for seasoning.

---

men a portion of carbs is roughly 40 grams and a portion of protein is about 40 grams.

## N-LARGE 2 LEMON SMOOTHIE

Blend 3 scoops of Prolab's vanilla N-Large 2 powder in 16 ounces of skim milk. Add 7 lemons and some ice cubes to the mix and blend for 30 seconds on high speed to a minute.

Calories: Approximately 758
Carbohydrates: 119 grams
Protein: 57 grams
Fats: 6 grams

## N-LARGE 2 STRAWBERRY/CHERRIES SMOOTHIE

Blend 3 scoops of Prolab's strawberry N-Large 2 powder in 16 ounces of skim milk. Add 1 cup of cherries and some ice cubes to the mix and blend for 30 seconds on high speed to a minute.

Calories: Approximately 750
Carbohydrates: 114 grams
Protein: 57 grams
Fats: 6 grams

## N-LARGE 2 ORANGE SMOOTHIE

Blend 3 scoops of Prolab's vanilla N-Large 2 powder in 16 ounces of skim milk. Add 2 oranges and some ice cubes to the mix and blend for 30 seconds on high speed to a minute.

Calories: Approximately 770
Carbohydrates: 122 grams
Protein: 57 grams
Fats: 6 grams

## SWEET POTATO CAKES

### INGREDIENTS

| | |
|---|---|
| 4 oz | of sweet potatoes |
| 1 | scoop of protein powder (vanilla is preferred) |
| 5 | egg whites |
| | Splenda (optional) |
| | cinnamon (optional) |

### DIRECTIONS

1. Fully cook the sweet potatoes
2. Mix all the ingredients together
3. Cook the mixture on a skillet just like you would cook pancakes

## SWEET POTATO MUFFINS

### INGREDIENTS

| | |
|---|---|
| 8 oz | plain mashed sweet potatoes |
| 2 cups | dry oatmeal |
| 1 cup | egg whites |
| 1 | whole egg |
| 1 tbsp | of vanilla |
| 1/4 cup | splenda |
| | cinnamon |
| | muffin pan |

### DIRECTIONS

1. Mix all ingredients in a mixing bowl
2. Spray muffin pan with non-stick spray such as Pam
3. Pour mixture into muffin pan
4. Bake at 350 degrees Fahrenheit for approximately 30 minutes

## PORTABLE PANCAKES

### INGREDIENTS

| | |
|---|---|
| 1/2 cup | dry old fashioned oats |
| 5 | egg whites |
| | Splenda (optional) |
| | cinnamon (optional) |

### DIRECTIONS

1. Mix all the ingredients together
2. Let mixture soak for 5 minutes
3. Cook the mixture on a skillet just like you would cook pancakes

Notes: You can top these with all-natural peanut butter, sugar-free jelly, or fruit of your choice

## HOMEMADE PROTEIN BARS

### INGREDIENTS

| | |
|---|---|
| 2 cups | dry old fashioned oats |
| 4 | scoops of whey protein powder |
| 1/2 cup | all-natural peanut butter |
| Approx. 6 T | water |

### DIRECTIONS

1. Mix all ingredients in a large mixing bowl (easiest to do by hand)
2. Dough should be fairly stiff and formed into bars on wax paper
3. Either freeze for 30 minutes or chill in refrigerator until ready to eat

## HOMEMADE GRANOLA

### INGREDIENTS

| | |
|---|---|
| 1/2 cup | dry old fashioned oats |
| 1/4 cup | water |
| 1 t | vanilla extract |
| 3 | packets of Splenda |
| | cinnamon (optional) |

### DIRECTIONS

1. Mix the oats with splenda and cinnamon
2. Add in the water and then the vanilla
3. Spray a piece of aluminum foil with non-stick cooking spray such as Pam
4. Spread oat mixture onto foil and enclose
5. Bake at approximately 250 degrees for 10 minutes
6. Open the aluminum foil and mix/stir the oats to break up the pieces
7. Bake for an additional 5-10 minutes or until desired crunchiness

## EATING ON THE RUN: FAST FOODS

In today's times, the fast paced living of our society can really tax our abilities to plan and prepare. This preparation certainly includes the scheduling of food consumption. If for one reason or another, our time constraints don't allow us to take the time to prepare all of the food we need for the day, or if we simply run out of food, there is a solution. You can go to fast food restaurants. Now, aren't fast foods bad if you are trying to get in shape? Well, the answer is "no" as long as you choose wisely.

The rules for eating in fast food restaurants (or any other type of restaurant) are:

- If it is not your cheat day (see The Sunday Reward section), refrain from fatty choices such as french fries.
- Drink between 8-16 ounces of water before you get to the restaurant and then drink an additional 8-16 ounces while you eat. This will prevent you from feeling hungry and falling to temptation. If you find that temptation is strong remember two things:
  a) There is nothing better than being in shape.
  b) You control everything that goes into your mouth. Food does not and should not control you!
- Always combine a serving of low fat protein (in the case of fast food restaurants, this is either skinless chicken or turkey) with a small serving of carbs. Remember that if you are eating a chicken or turkey sandwich, the bread will count as the carbs.
- Salads in addition to a serving of protein and a serving of starchy carbs are always good since they provide fiber and fill you up. However, avoid using high-fat/high-sugar dressings.
- Refrain from using high carbohydrate sauces or mayonnaise.

Now that we know the rules of fast food eating, let's look at some healthy meals you can choose at some of the major fast food chains:

In Arby's you can have either a Light Chicken Deluxe Sandwich with extra lettuce and tomato (no mayo) or a Light Turkey Deluxe Sandwich. They also have an excellent roast chicken salad that will not harm you unless you fill it up with high fat dressing.

In Bennigan's try the chicken platter, which includes a serving of spicy rice along with vegetables and two chicken breasts.

In Boston Market for protein you can have a serving of turkey breast or chicken breast. For carbs you can have a small serving of steamed vegetables along with potatoes, or corn, or rice pilaf or fruit salad. If you'd rather have something quicker, then go for the chicken or turkey sandwich.

In the Golden Corral try their chicken (remove the skin) with their steamed rice and green beans.

In Hardee's order either a chicken fillet sandwich or grilled chicken salad.

In Kentucky Fried Chicken have a quarter chicken (no skin) for protein and a small serving of mashed potatoes, or garden rice, or red beans for carbs.

In Long John Silver's you may have a flavor-baked chicken or fish for protein and a small serving of plain baked potato or green beans.

In McDonald's you can have either a McGrilled Chicken Classic or a Chunky Chicken Salad.

In Subway order a Roast Turkey Breast Sub, a Veggie Sub or a Roast Beef Sub. Remember the rules that we already discussed: NO EXTRA OILS OR MAYO etc. Also, there is no need to order a sub larger than 6 inches.

In Taco Bell order any of the following: a Light Chicken Burrito, or a Light Chicken Taco, or a Light Bean Burrito, or a Light Soft Taco Supreme, or a Light Taco Supreme, or a Light Taco, or a Light Soft Taco.

Finally, in Wendy's have either a grilled chicken sandwich or a grilled chicken salad.

Well, there you have it. If you find yourself in another restaurant that we haven't discussed don't panic! Just ask for whatever chicken plate they have and if it comes with skin just take it off. Basically, if you stick to the five rules discussed above, no matter where you find yourself, you won't have a problem finding something to eat. Bon Appetite!

## TUNA-CAKES

### INGREDIENTS

| | |
|---|---|
| 1 | egg white |
| 1/4 cup cottage cheese | |
| 1 can | flaked light tuna |
| | herbs of your choice |
| | onion |
| | green pepper |

### DIRECTIONS

1. Mix all of the ingredients in a mixing bowl
2. Heat skillet so that it is hot when you pour mixture onto it
3. Pour into skillet and cook like pancakes

## EGG WHITE SALSA

### INGREDIENTS

egg whites measured to your needs
onions
green peppers
Mrs. Dash seasonings (any flavor)
salsa

### DIRECTIONS

1. Heat skillet so that it is hot when you pour mixture onto it
2. Pour chopped up onions and green peppers onto skillet
3. Sprinkle seasonings onto veggies
4. After heating veggies, pour whites over them
5. After fully cooking the mixture remove from the pan
6. Spoon salsa (2 T) on top of veggies and enjoy!

## HEALTH-CONSCIOUS ICE CREAM

### INGREDIENTS

| | |
|---|---|
| 1 cup | cottage cheese |
| 1/4 | packet Crystal Light® |
| | Small bowl or cups |

### DIRECTIONS

1. Mix cottage cheese and crystal light flavoring in a small bowl or individual dishes
2. Place mixture into the freezer
3. Let sit in freezer for approximately 1-2 hours
4. Enjoy your frozen treat

## PHYSIQUE-FRIENDLY POPSICLES

### INGREDIENTS

Crystal Light
water
popsicle molds

### DIRECTIONS

1. Follow instructions on Crystal Light mixture
2. Pour Crystal Light drink into popsicle molds
3. Place popsicles into the freezer
4. Enjoy your cold treat without ruining all of your gym efforts

## ADDITIONAL IDEAS FOR A SWEET TOOTH:

Sugar-free jello, flavored tea with Splenda or stevia, frozen bananas, and any protein powder treats mentioned above

## SUPPLEMENTATION

Many people incorrectly believe supplements are the most important part in helping you to gain muscle. However, supplements are simply additions to a good nutrition and training program. Supplements do not make up for improper training, or lack thereof, and a crappy diet. Supplements only work when your diet and your training program are optimized.

Nutritional supplements protect us from nutritional deficiencies. Your new exercise programs' increased activity levels make your body require greater amounts of vitamins and minerals, and increase the chances of your suffering a nutritional deficiency without supplementation. Remember, even a slight nutrient deficiency can sabotage your muscle growth.

Unfortunately, we cannot rely solely on food to provide us with all the vitamins and minerals that our body requires. This is largely because the processing food goes through even before it arrives at the supermarket: cooking, air, and light have already robbed your foods of the vitamins that they normally offer. If you are deficient in one or more essential nutrients, your body may not be able to build muscle and burn fat properly.

However, not all supplements are equal. The use of supplements depends on both your goals and your budget. Below we have described the different categories of supplements and have discussed which ones you will need to use at all times.

## MULTIPLE VITAMIN AND MINERAL FORMULA

This type of supplement is essential to ensure that our bodies operate at maximum efficiency. On a very simplistic level, without these vitamins and minerals, it is impossible to covert the food we eat into hormones, tissues and energy.

Vitamins are organic compounds (produced by both animals and vegetables), and enhance the actions of proteins, causing reactions such as muscle building, fat burning, and energy production. There are two types of vitamins:

- **Fat-soluble vitamins** are stored in fat and if taken in excessive amounts will become toxic. (Such as A, D, E, and K.)
- **Water-soluble vitamins** are not stored in the body. (Such as B-Complex and Vitamin C.)

Minerals, inorganic compounds not produced by animals or vegetables, assure that your brain receives the correct signals from the body, for the balances of fluids, muscular contractions and energy production as well as for the building of muscle and bones. There are two types of minerals:

- **Bulk minerals** are called such because the body requires them in great quantities and often in the measure of grams. (Such as calcium, magnesium, potassium, sodium and phosphorus.)
- **Trace minerals** are required by the body in tiny amounts, usually in the order of micrograms. (Such as chromium, copper, cobalt, silicon, selenium, iron and zinc.)

### SOURCES:

You must be very careful with the vitamin and mineral formula you choose. Some don't always contain what the labels claim, and some come from poor sources and are not absorbed very well by the body. Keeping that in mind, try to stick to this tried and true recommended formula list below. Other reputable companies on the market include QNT Sports, Twinlabs, EAS, Weider, Labrada, Shiff, Optimum Nutrition, Advanced Nutrition, and Champion Nutrition.

- the Super Spectrum Vitamin/Mineral formula (available at Dave Draper's site: www.davedraper.com)
- Vitamin Shoppes' Health & Fitness Nutrients For Active People (Vitamin Paks)
- GNC's Ultra Mega
- Country Life's Multi-100
- Ultra Two by Nature's Plus

### QUANTITY:

Take as directed.

## PROTEIN SUPPLEMENTS

**Weight Gainers** are protein shakes consisting mainly of whey proteins. Some also include milk or egg proteins. Characterized by their extremely high carbohydrate content, weight gainers were very popular back in the 90s but their popularity has died mainly because many people do not have the metabolism of a hardgainer, and a high carbohydrate diet leads quickly to fat gains rather than muscle mass gains.

### SOURCES:

Any health food store or drug store.

### QUANTITY:

The carbohydrate content is designed for a fast release, and is best in the mid-morning, mid-afternoon, and post workout meals. Weight gainers can be mixed with fruit juice or skim milk, and if you are trying to increase the calorie content, this use of flaxseed oil and fruits is useful. However, if you do not have the metabolism to support this, it's probably best to avoid these.

**Meal Replacement Powders (MRPs)** are lower in calories and have far less carbohydrates than weight gainers. Most powders are composed of whey proteins, but there are many new formulas now on the market that consist of a protein blend of whey and milk proteins. The carbohydrate component used to be maltodextrin, with 25-27 grams of carbohydrate per serving, but the new generation of formulas use slow-release carbohydrates like brown rice and oats to make the product lower in glycemic value. Essential fatty acids and a vitamin and mineral profile have also been added.

## SUPPLEMENT RECOMMENDATIONS SUMMARY

**Essential to Take**
- MultiVitamin (taken with breakfast)
- Essential Oils and Monounsaturated Oils (as per nutrition guidelines)
- 1 gram Vitamin C (taken with breakfast, lunch, and dinner)
- Whey Gain, Whey Protein Powder, or Meal Replacement Powder (to mix with skim milk or water for protein shakes)
- 200 mcg of Chromium Picolinate (post-workout with protein shake)

**Highly Recommended**
- 2.5 grams of Creatine (before and after workout)
- 3 grams of glutamine (post-workout or before bed on non-workout days)

**Note:** Nitrobolic Extreme contains these two ingredients along with nitric oxide boosters and pre-workout energizers.

**25 Years of Age and Older: To Increase Testosterone Levels**
- 1 serving of ZMA (with evening meal)
- 4 capsules QNT USA Testek in the morning and later in the day
- 4 capsules Labrada Nutrition Humano Growth at bedtime

**NOTE**: There is no need to take all of these supplements at the same time. You can get great benefits from doing six weeks of one, six weeks of another, and so on. But if you have the finances to use them all, there are no adverse effects from doing so.

**Other Useful Supplements**
- Fat burning stack: 4 caps of Riptek first thing in the morning and again 6-7 hours later on an empty stomach. (**Note:** Riptek increases your metabolism naturally via the use of a pepper extract called Capsimax.)
- Pre-Workout stack: 1-2 scoops of Labrada's Super Charge one month alternated with 1-2 scoops of QNT USA Hydravol on the following month.

For any questions on supplements, please feel free to visit our Fan Page at www.facebook.com/bodysculpting-bibles or our site at www.bodysculptingbible.com.

## ALL ABOUT PROTEIN AND BIOLOGICAL VALUES (BV)

It is nearly impossible in today's world to eat six perfectly balanced meals required to get in shape daily. Thus, these supplements can be used as "fast food." They are easy to prepare and the formulas that are available on the market today are as good as a milkshake from any fast food chain. There are many categories of protein supplements, so let's first talk about the different sources of protein.

Each source of protein is measured by its quality, by Biological Value (BV). BV measures how well the body absorbs and uses the protein. The higher the BV, the more nitrogen your body can absorb, use, and retain. As a result, proteins with the highest BV promote the most lean muscle gains. Whey protein ranks with the highest BV value, a104. Egg protein is second with 100, and milk proteins come in third at 91. Beef protein rates an 80 and soy proteins at 74. Because bean proteins are a plant-based protein, they rank a 49.

**Whey Proteins (Whey Concentrate/Whey Isolate)** are a great protein source. They have been recorded to improve sports performance by reducing stress and lowering cortisol levels, improving immunity by increasing glutathione (GSH) which also helps reduce overtraining, and improving liver functions in some forms of hepatitis. It also helps to reduce your blood pressure and it can help fight HIV.

**Whey Proteins** are also highly digestible and have an even better amino acid profile than egg whites. However, not all whey is created equal. The whey that gives you the benefits described above has to be micro-filtered at very low temperatures to allow production of high protein contents with no undenatured protein, and a minimum of fat, cholesterol, and lactose.

There are whey isolates and whey concentrates. Whey isolates are sub-fractions of whey absorbed rapidly into the system. While excellent for post-workout nutrition, whey isolate is a poor choice for supplementation during the day because if the body does not need all the amino acids released into the bloodstream, it will use them for energy production, not muscle building. Whey isolate also does not have many of the health-enhancing properties, as the process required to produce whey isolate destroys many of the health/immune system-enhancing sub-fractions. In conclusion, for during the day use, a product consisting mainly of whey concentrate is your best bet while for after the workout, a whey isolate product will be a better choice.

**Egg Protein** is a super bio-available protein second only to whey. It is a slower released protein than whey, which makes it perfect for daytime use. I often mix egg and whey protein for one of the most bio-available protein shakes available.

**Milk Proteins (Calcium Casseinate/Micellar Casein)**. Similar to egg proteins, this highly bio-available protein source has slightly less BV, and is designed to slowly release into the blood stream. The natural, undenatured protein in milk is micellar casein, which provides a steady release of amino acids, making this an excellent choice for a long-lasting muscle protecting protein.

**Beef Proteins** are slow released proteins that rate an 80 on the BV scale. While I am unaware of any protein supplement in powder form on the market that is derived from beef proteins, there are beef liver tablets. Beef proteins are abundant in blood-building iron and also B-vitamins, both factors that contribute to better nutrient use and energy production.

**Soy Proteins** have positive health benefits for both men and women. Studies show they may reduce the risk of hormone-dependent cancers (breast, prostate, etc), and possibly protect from other cancers as well. Soy has been well known to reduce high cholesterol and ease the symptoms of menopause. Soy also helps prevent osteoporosis by building up bone mass. Because of this, we recommend 1 serving of soy protein per day for women, but only for its health benefits. In the muscle-building department, soy is not useful; its BV value is 74, and because it has estrogen-like substances, it might reduce testosterone use, and for men, could be anti-constructive.

## SOURCES:

Any health food store or drug store.

## QUANTITY:

1 packet mixed with water per serving.

**Protein Powders** are powders that consist mainly of protein (typically whey protein, but you can also find blends). They typically contain no more than 5 grams of carbohydrates and 20-25 grams of protein per scoop. Calorie-wise, they could be anywhere from 100-125 calories.

## SOURCES:

Any health food store or drug store. For specific brand recommendations, please visit our Fan Page at www.facebook.com/bodysculptingbibles or our site at www.bodysculptingbible.com.

## QUANTITY:

2 scoops mixed with 8 ounces of skim milk per serving.

**Protein Bars** are bars made out of any of the protein sources mentioned above. The carbohydrate mix usually is a combination of glycerin (sugar alcohol, and not really a carbohydrate) and sugars. Bars generally contain fats which are less than desirable. Use these bars only in cases of extreme emergency when there is nothing better available to eat.

## SOURCES:

Any health food store or drug store.

## QUANTITY:

A serving is just one bar. For specific brand recommendations, please visit our Fan Page at www.facebook.com/bodysculptingbibles or our site at www.bodysculptingbible.com.

## GOOD OILS: FISH OILS, FLAX OIL, EXTRA-VIRGIN OLIVE OIL, AND PEANUT BUTTER

If you follow a very strict low-fat diet you'll find that you begin to start having trouble keeping your strength up and losing fat. It is really easy to incur a fat deficiency when your diet is really clean. To fix this you should also be taking in good oil, or fat supplements.

**Fish oils** are best obtained through a consumption of salmon a minimum of three times a week. Fish oil caps are good, but you need at least 10 per day in order to get even 10 grams of fish oil.

**Flax Oil** is best obtained from buying the whole ground flaxseed meal, which needs to be refrigerated at all times. Do not cook with this oil if you choose to use it instead of the meal, as it is light and heat sensitive. It should appear to be a clear yellow. If you purchase oil with brown particles, the oil is rancid and should be returned or thrown out.

Your **extra-virgin olive oil** should preferably be canned in either Italy or Spain. It's best to purchase oil canned, because light can reach the oil stored in a bottle and turn it rancid. Also remember that natural old-fashioned **peanut butter** is a great source of monounsaturated fats.

## SOURCES:

You can find flaxseed meal from brands such as Spectrum, which keeps it refrigerated while it is on the way to the store.

Fish oil capsules can be found at health food stores and drug stores.

## QUANTITY:

Consume fats in the way recommended by the diet charts on page 88.

## VITAMIN C

Vitamin C is a water-soluble vitamin that improves your immune system and assists in faster recovery from your workouts. It suppresses the amount of cortisol (a hormone that kills muscle and aids in the accumulation of fat) released by your body during a workout. This is the only Vitamin we recommend taken in mega dose quantities. Because it is a water-soluble vitamin, it will not be stored by the body. If taken an hour before a workout (1000 mg dose), research shows Vitamin C significantly reduces muscle soreness and speeds recovery.

**Important Note:** Ensure that your water intake during the day is adequate (bodyweight X 0.66 = ounces of water per day).  If you have a history of kidney stones, you should not take Vitamin C in these large quantities.  As always, when in doubt, consult your doctor.

## SOURCES:

Any health food store or drug store.

## QUANTITY:

We recommend a total of 3000 mg per day of Vitamin C. If your multiple vitamin pack already has 1000 mg, and you take this in the morning, then all you need is an extra 1000 mg at lunch and 1000 mg at dinner.

## CHROMIUM PICOLINATE

There are many claims surrounding Chromium Picolinate, and most of them are as yet unproven. However, we suggest its use from our own experience with this mineral. Some of its benefits surround its enhanced effect on insulin, upgrading insulin's capability to produce muscle and energy. An insulin-boosting vitamin could potentially assist you in gaining muscle and losing fat faster. Chromium can also keep blood sugar levels stable, thereby preventing insulin levels from going high enough to begin promoting fat storage. However, chromium only functions if a suitable diet is followed.

## SOURCES:

All chromium picolinate produced in the market is manufactured by a company called Nutrition 21; it is sold at stores like GNC, Eckerds, Walmart and Walgreens.

## QUANTITY:

200 mcg with the post-workout meal and with breakfast on days off.

## CREATINE MONOHYDRATE

### WHAT IS IT?

Creatine is a metabolite produced in the body composed of three amino acids: l-methionine, l-arginine, and l-glycine. Approximately 95% of the concentration is found in skeletal muscle in two forms: creatine phosphate and free chemically unbound creatine. The remaining 5% of the creatine stored in the body is found in the brain, heart, and testes. The body of a sedentary person metabolizes an average of 2 grams of creatine a day. Due to their high intensity training, bodybuilders metabolize higher amounts.

Creatine is generally found in red meats and to some extent in certain types of fish. However it would be hard to get the amount of creatine necessary for performance enhancement as even though 2.2 lbs of red meat or tuna contain approximately between 4 to 5 grams of creatine, the compound is destroyed with cooking. Therefore, the best way to get creatine is to take it in powder form.

### HOW DOES IT WORK?

While there is still much debate on how creatine exerts its performance-enhancing benefits, it is commonly accepted that most of its effects are due to two mechanisms:

- Intra-cellular water retention.
- Creatine's ability to enhance ATP production.

Basically, once the creatine is stored inside the muscle cell, it attracts the water surrounding such cell thereby enlarging it. This super-hydrated state of the cell causes nice side effects such as the increase of strength and it also gives the appearance of a fuller muscle. Some studies suggest that a super hydrated cell may also trigger protein synthesis and minimize catabolism.

In addition, creatine provides for faster recovery in between sets and increased tolerance to high-volume work. The way it does this is by enhancing the body's ability to produce Adenosine Triphosphate (ATP). ATP is the compound that your muscles use for fuel whenever they contract. ATP provides its energy by releasing one of its phosphate molecules (it has three phosphate molecules). After the release of one molecule, ATP becomes ADP (Adenosine Diphosphate) as it now only has two molecules. The problem is that after 10 seconds of contraction time the ATP fuel extinguishes and in order to support further muscle contraction, glycolisis (glycogen burning) has to kick in. That is fine and well except that as a byproduct of that mechanism lactic acid is produced.

Lactic acid is what causes the burning sensation at the end of the set. When too much lactic acid is produced, your muscle contractions stop, thereby forcing you to stop the set. However, by taking creatine, you can extend the 10 second limit of your ATP system as creatine provides ADP the phosphate molecule that it is missing (recall that creatine is stored in the muscle as creatine phosphate). By upgrading your body's ability to regenerate ATP, you can exercise longer and harder as you will minimize your lactic acid production and be able to take your sets to the next level with less fatigue. More volume, strength and recovery equals more muscle (assuming nutrition and rest are dialed in).

Creatine also seems to allow for better pumps during a workout. This may be due to the fact that it possibly improves glycogen synthesis. In addition, studies have shown that creatine helps lower cholesterol and triglyceride levels. The mechanisms by which it exerts such benefits remain unknown.

In our own experimentation with creatine, we have found that it provides all of the effects described above. As a way to prove to ourselves that these effects were just not a placebo effect, we finally convinced one of our training partners (who was extremely skeptical about the compound) to start using it. After two weeks he noticed that for some reason he was recovering faster inbetween sets, had a better tolerance to high volume work and his muscles were looking fuller. He did not understand why that was happening. We reminded him about the 5 grams of creatine that were being added to his post workout protein shake. While one subject does not provide the statistical leverage to claim that creatine will provide these effects, we are positive that provided your training, rest, and nutrition are in order, you will get results out of it.

## How to Use It

If you read the bottle, most companies recommend a loading phase of 20 grams for 5 days and 5-10 grams thereafter. While that is the commonly accepted way to use it, we have found no benefit to loading. As a matter of fact, our training partner only took 5 grams a day after the workout and started getting great results after only a couple of weeks. The reason for this is simple. There is only so much creatine that the body can store. Recall that the creatine is stored every time that you take it. So by taking it every day, eventually you will reach the upper levels that provide the performance enhancement. After you reach that level, you could get away with just taking it on your weight training days as it takes two weeks of no use for the body's creatine levels to get back to normal.

Another issue is cycling creatine. If creatine were a supplement that loses its effectiveness as time goes by, then we would recommend cycling. For example, it is beneficial to cycle fat burning supplements containing caffeine and ephedrine as the body's receptors begin to attenuate after two to three weeks of continual use. Once the body gets used to them, you need to either increase the dosage or stop their use so that the body begins to respond once again. However, that is not the way that creatine works.

Basically, creatine gets stored into your muscles and you get the effects mentioned above, period. It is really straightforward. As far as the initial weight gain that you may experience when you start taking it, whether you cycle it or not, you will get the same amount of initial weight gain as that extra weight is determined by the amount of intracellular fluid retention that your muscle cells can store (something that remains a static figure). The reason we say "the weight gain that you may experience" is because if once you start taking it you concurrently increase the volume of your workouts and remain at the same caloric intake level you may lose fat as you gain your added muscle volume. In this case, the scale might not register any weight gain (this is what happened to my training partner). However, the lack of "registered" initial weight gain by the scale does not mean that you are a "non-responder." To gauge creatine's efficacy, judge it by the muscle appearance effects and performance enhancement in the gym.

## Side Effects

The only adverse side effect that we have experienced in many years of continual use is the gastric upset at the very beginning. After a couple of weeks or so our systems adapted to absorbing the powder. Other than that, we have not observed any other side effects. Keep in mind, however, that the liver and kidneys have to process this compound. Therefore, we would not recommend it for someone with kidney or liver problems. Also, even if you are completely healthy, ensure more than adequate hydration levels (bodyweight x 0.66 = total ounces of water to drink per day) and if you drink coffee, add an extra 16 ounces of water for every cup that you drink over the day.

A side effect that we have read happened but are unable to quantify is that your body's production of creatine shuts down. However, after cessation of use, according to all of the literature, your body's production kicks in again. No adverse effects have been documented due to the creatine shutdown created by the body.

## WHAT HAPPENS IF I STOP TAKING IT?

After two weeks, your creatine levels return to normal. You will feel weaker for about three weeks due to the fact that your ATP system is no longer enhanced. You'll also lose your enhanced recovery capabilities. In this sense, and only in this sense, creatine is kind of like steroids. The difference is that creatine can be taken safely all of the time (personal opinion) while with steroids that isn't true.

However, in creatine's defense, we can also say that creatine is no different than weight training. What happens if you stop going to the gym? Will you look the same three months later?

Seriously speaking, however, since you already were lifting heavier weights while using the compound, your nervous system will remember those weights and you will be able to get back to them after three to six weeks. However, we suggest you lower the volume when you first stop taking it.

## CREATINE AND CAFFEINE INTAKE

Years ago there were some studies suggesting that the effects of creatine were cancelled if you also had caffeine. For people like ourselves that most of the time keep caffeine at bay this does not pose any problems. However, this is not the case for people on fat-burning formulas that contain caffeine. Our recommendation is that you take the caffeine (or the fat-burning supplement) at a time separate from your creatine intake (i.e. take your creatine after the workout with your protein shake and take your fat burner before the workout). Also, ensure that you follow the hydration guidelines described above.

## CARBOHYDRATE LADEN CREATINE

Due to studies demonstrating that the body's uptake of creatine is greater when you take it with carbs, most companies have been creating products that contain creatine and high levels of sugar. Our advice to you: save your money. Buy the powder form instead, as you will get much more servings of the pure compound. As long as you take it after the workout with a protein/carbohydrate-rich shake we guarantee that your body will absorb the creatine with the utmost efficiency.

## CONCLUSIONS

In our view, the greatest advantage that creatine gives you (besides the cosmetic effect of bigger looking and fuller muscles) is that it enables you to handle more volume and recover faster in between sets by upgrading the body's capabilities to produce ATP, thereby decreasing the production of lactic acid. Therefore, in our opinion, people who will get the most benefit from creatine are those who follow a high-volume workout with short rest in between sets. Remember that the more work that you can cram into an hour, the more you'll grow (provided good cycling of volume and intensity as we have discussed in previous articles).

Again, even though we believe that creatine is a safe supplement, don't take our word for it if you have doubts. Do your own research and objectively review the data. If you feel creatine may be good for you, then just follow the recommendations laid out in this chapter. Provided your overall training and nutrition strategy are good, we guarantee that you will see results.

Be careful to stick to reputable brands only, with a strong track record. The brands we personally use are Prolab, EAS, Chamption Nutrition, Lebrada, Beverly International, Met-Rx, and iSatori. If your brand is not on this list, it's not that it isn't reputable; these are only the brands we have personally tried.

## GLUTAMINE

L-Glutamine is the most abundant amino acid in muscle cells. It is released from the muscle during times of stress (such as hard weight training workouts) and dieting. This amino acid not only has been shown to be a great anti-catabolic agent (protects the muscle from the catabolic activities of the hormone cortisol), a contributor to muscle cell volume, and to have immune system enhancing properties, it also helps in the following ways:

- Regulation of protein synthesis (this is one of the ways in which steroids exert their muscle building effects).
- Accelerating glycogen synthesis after a workout.
- Sparing the use of the glycogen stored in the muscle cell (recall that the glycogen stored in the muscle cell is what gives the cell the healthy volume and firmness that you seek).
- Faster recuperation from weight training workouts.

### HOW TO USE IT

Due to its anti-catabolic properties and the fact that it accelerates glycogen synthesis after a workout, glutamine is best taken with a protein shake 20-30 minutes after a workout. On days that you don't work out, just take it with your last protein shake of the day. While there is much debate among experts regarding dosage, we always like to remain on the conservative side. Therefore, we feel that 3 grams is a sufficient dosage. Besides, recall that there is limited space within a muscle cell to store the glutamine, so taking higher dosages will not give you better results.

As far as cycling this supplement, there is no evidence that suggests cycling would improve its efficacy.

### SIDE EFFECTS

We have experienced a slight stomach discomfort during the first week of use (taking the straight powder form). Other than that, we did not experience any other side effects while using the compound and we have not found any literature that links its use to anything bad. As usual, we recommend that you start with a low dosage (such as only 1 gram a day) in order to assess your tolerance. From there you can build up to the recommended dosage of 3 grams.

## CONCLUSION

By looking at the effects that this supplement can provide, along with the fact that it can be purchased for a very cheap price, we wonder why more athletes don't use it. This is especially important during dieting, as a way to protect the muscle from being cannibalized by the effects of cortisol. On a final note, please remember that, like any supplement, you need to stick to high quality brands. Good brands of Glutamine are Prolab, EAS, Champion Nutrition, Beverly International, Met-Rx, and Labrada.

## MORE INFORMATION

If you are interested in more supplements, we suggest you read our additional Appendixes on this subject. We discuss a lot of testosterone-boosting supplements that could make all the difference in your training. Good luck and let's get to it!

# Chapter 5
# Rest & Recovery

For immediate Body Sculpting Bible support & coaching directly from James & Hugo, please visit www.BodySculptingBible.com

**5**

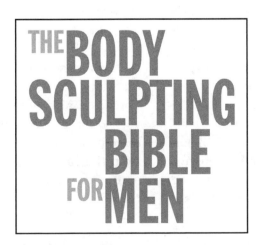

How much did you sleep last night; 5, 6, maybe 7 hours? Did you know that getting less than 6 hours a night can seriously affect your coordination, reaction time and judgment; not to mention your health?

Though the goal is to get in great shape, many of us are silently killing ourselves. With all of the stimulants now available such as high-octane coffee, ephedrine, "natural" fat burners and the like, why would we need sleep when we can simply get a "boost?" A recent segment on CNN discovered that "people who drove after being awake for 17 to 19 hours performed worse than those with a blood alcohol level of .05 percent. That's the legal limit for drunk driving in most western European countries, though most States in the U.S. set their blood alcohol limits at .1 percent and a few at .08 percent." The study revealed that 16 to 60 percent of all road accidents involved sleep deprivation.

Have you ever been in a situation where you needed to pull an "all-nighter" for school or work? We see it all the time; people bragging about not sleeping because they don't have enough time in a day. Not surprisingly, nearly half of all Americans have difficulty sleeping. A growing collection of research indicates that America's sleep problems have reached epidemic proportions and may be the country's number-one health problem. Would it change your mind if you knew that those who sleep fewer than 6 hours a night don't live as long as those who sleep seven hours or more?

Lack of sleep can be expensive: The National Commission on Sleep Disorders estimates that sleep deprivation costs $150 billion a year in higher stress and reduced workplace productivity. Yes, most of us truly enjoy staying up late, ready to dive into the night life. We are magnetized to late night movies and late night surfing on the internet, yet did you know that we are robbing ourselves of 338 hours–two full weeks–of rest per year?

New research indicates that rest and sleep may well be the third essential component of a long and healthy life, right up there with a good diet and regular exercise! "Society is being victimized by not getting enough sleep," says David Dinges, director of experimental psychiatry at the University of Pennsylvania School of Medicine. "Our productivity, our safety, our health are at risk." The findings are far from definitive but they strongly hint that long-term sleep debt could be a factor in the national epidemics of diabetes and obesity. Research is proving that sleep deprivation can weaken the immune system, leading to colds and other infections. There is even a bit of evidence proving how the increase in breast cancer, and perhaps other cancers, could have a link to decreased sleep.

## THE SLEEP CYCLE

When we deprive ourselves of sleep, we disrupt a delicate cycle.

**Phase One:** Phase one begins as soon as the sun sets, when the pineal gland starts to release melatonin, a hormone released in the absence of light and responsible for making us sleepy. When you lay down in your bed at this time, your muscles relax, heart rate and breathing slow down, and body temperature drops. The brain also relaxes but still remains alert. If you could look at the wave patterns being generated by the brain, you would see a change from the rapid beta waves of daytime to slower alpha waves. When the alpha waves disappear, replaced by theta waves, the sleeper has tumbled into the sensory void called stage one sleep. In this stage, the sleeper is unable to sense anything.

**Phase Two:** Phase two occurs a moment after phase one and in this stage the sleeper lays still for about 10 to 15 minutes.

**Phase Three:** After phase two is over, the sleeper falls into a deeper sleep. During this stage, the sleeper falls deeper into phase three which lasts about 5 to 15 minutes.

**Phase Four:** With a maximum of 15 minutes spent within the phase three cycle, the sleeper then falls into yet another relaxed stage called phase four, lasting a half hour or so. In stage four, the eyes move back and forth very quickly in what's called rapid eye movement, or REM. This is the point at which the first dream occurs. After this dream has ended, the sleeper goes back to phase two and starts the whole process over again. These processes repeat themselves about five times during the night.

Sleep research indicates that the average sleeper will sleep approximately 8 hours and 15 minutes when uninterrupted. During this research, there were no alarm clocks or disturbing noises to interrupt normal sleep patterns. 8 hours and 15 minutes is believed to be the ideal physiological amount of time that the body requires for proper sleep.

## MALADIES CAUSED BY SLEEP DEPRIVATION

The following are the maladies that, according to research, can be the result of consistent sleep deprivation:

**Impaired glucose tolerance:** Without sleep, the central nervous system becomes more active, inhibiting the pancreas from producing adequate insulin, the hormone the body needs to digest glucose. "In healthy young men with no risk factor, in one week, we had them in a pre-diabetic state," says researcher Van Cauter when referring to a study that he conducted on the effects of sleep deprivation.

**Possible link to obesity:** This is due to the fact that much growth hormone is secreted during the first round of deep sleep. As both men and women age, they naturally spend less time in deep sleep, which reduces growth hormone secretion. Lack of sleep at a younger age, however, could drive down growth hormone prematurely, accelerating the fat-gaining process. In addition, there is also research that indicates a lowering of the hormone testosterone as well as fat gain and muscle loss.

**Increased carbohydrate cravings:** Sleep deprivation negatively affects the production of a hormone called Leptin. This hormone is responsible for telling the body when it is full. However, with decreased production of this hormone, your body will crave calories (especially in the form of carbs) even though its requirements have been met. Not a good situation to be in for a dieter.

**Weakened immune system:** Research indicates that sleep deprivation adversely affects the white blood cell count in humans as well as the body's ability to fight infections.

**Increased risk of breast cancer:** Richard Stevens, a cancer researcher at the University of Connecticut Health Center, has speculated that there might be a connection between breast cancer and hormone cycles disrupted by late-night light. Melatonin, primarily secreted at night, may trigger a reduction in the body's production of estrogen. But light interferes with melatonin release (recall that the hormone is secreted in response to a lack of light), allowing estrogen levels to rise. Too much estrogen is known to promote the growth of breast cancers.

**Decreased alertness and ability to focus:** A recent study showed that people who were awake for up to 19 hours scored worse on performance tests and alertness scales than those with a blood-alcohol level of .08 percent–legally drunk in some states.

**Hardening of the arteries:** Some studies suggest that the stress imposed on the body due to lack of sleep causes a very sharp rise in cortisol levels. Such an imbalance can lead to hardening of the arteries, increasing the risk of heart attack. In addition, we also know that very high cortisol levels lead to muscle loss, increased fat storage, loss of bone mass, depression, hypertension, insulin resistance (the cells in the body lose the ability to accept insulin), and lower growth hormone and testosterone production.

**Depression and irritability:** Lack of sleep also causes depletion of neurotransmitters in the brain that are in charge of regulating mood. Because of this, sleep deprived people have a "shorter fuse" and also tend to get depressed more easily.

## ARE YOU SLEEP DEPRIVED?

It's easy to tell if you're sleep-deprived. If you can lie down in the middle of the day and fall asleep within 10 minutes, you are sleep deprived. Catching up is basic math. For every hour, or fraction, under 8 hours, you need an equal extra amount of time asleep soon after. But if you're hundreds of hours in debt, you may never pay it all off. According to recent research, 17 hours was all the catching up people could do, and it generally took three weeks. Most people probably need three times that amount of sleep!

In an earlier section, we discussed the problem of trying to get to sleep while simultaneously dealing with stress. You may refer back to page 41 to learn how to "turn off the stress light."

## SLEEPING PILLS

Beware of sleeping pills! They not only tend to be addicting but people who use them find that they tend to wake up groggy. As far as melatonin supplementation, scientists are divided in opinion but most agree that the 3-milligram dose available in health food stores is too high, especially as the supplement has never been tested for safety in humans. Since we are very cautious when it comes to hormones, we would rather have you follow the guidelines below in order to ensure a good night's sleep:

- **Avoid activities that involve deep concentration before going to sleep** as these activities will increase adrenaline levels and will prevent the brain from achieving the state of relaxation required to achieve sleep.
- **Avoid watching disturbing shows at night on TV** as this may also increase your adrenaline levels thereby preventing you from a good night's sleep.
- **Avoid eating a large meal at night** since the digestion process will prevent you from falling asleep.

Attempt to totally relax at the same time each night. By doing so you condition the body to relax itself once the specific time that you choose comes every day. Ensure that at this time no thoughts other than relaxation and falling asleep come to your head. You need to really learn how to block all thoughts concerning work or other life issues that may be trying to get in your head. Listening to soothing music set at a low volume with the lights off can help you relax and achieve the state necessary to go to sleep.

## CONCLUSION

You need 7-9 hours of sleep each night (8 being the ideal) in order for your body to run efficiently. Deprive your body of sleep and you'll have lousy fat loss and hinder your body's ability to increase lean muscle tone. Without enough sleep the body stops producing anabolic hormones (muscle producing/fat burning hormones; e.g. testosterone and growth hormone) and starts increasing the production of catabolic hormones (muscle destroying/fat depositing hormones e.g. cortisol). So, to make matters worse, you'll also lose muscle, which lowers your metabolism. In addition, you will lack the energy and focus to get through your workouts, which will surely lead to overtraining. To top it off, research indicates that lack of sleep creates cravings and binges in addition to hardening of the arteries, which leads to heart attacks. In short: turn off the TV, relax and hit the sack!

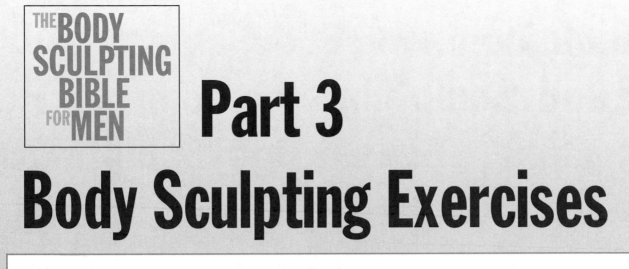

# Part 3
# Body Sculpting Exercises

Learning proper exercise technique is the backbone of every fitness program. If you train improperly you will not stimulate the intended muscle, and will risk major injury as well as receive little or no results. When you learn to use proper exercise technique you will receive twice the results in half the time, guaranteed! We see people in the gym day in and day out who have no idea how to properly train their muscles. Some of them are professional bodybuilders, some are professional athletes, and some are even certified fitness trainers. Unfortunately, the ones who really suffer the most are people like you who rely on these role models for wisdom and guidance. We will show you the proper exercise technique to use for optimal results. Just remember to utilize your newfound knowledge. Like the old saying, "Feed a man a fish and he'll eat for a day, teach a man to fish and he'll eat for a lifetime." We expect the same of you. We don't want you to read this book once and then forget everything you've learned. We want you to learn and utilize that knowledge to achieve astounding results.

Applying proper exercise form and technique is, without doubt, the most important component of any fitness program. Without it, many, many setbacks will occur. First, the musculature you intend to exercise will not be stimulated as efficiently as possible. Exercise should not be focused around just lifting barbells and weights. It shouldn't just be about how much you can lift. Optimum fitness is about the quality of exercise, the quality of your form and how you maintain that form, especially during heavier lifting. Proper exercise technique coupled with the Zone-Tone principle will bring you the most astonishing results with the minimum amount of sets. Why? Because as we have already discussed, one properly executed set is equivalent to five sets of "just going through the motions" type of exercise. It comes down to this: If you want to get the most out of your workout, keep the intensity high without sacrificing proper form. Neglecting to focus on proper form equals no results, while practicing perfect form equals incredible results quickly!

**TIP:** Throughout this section, you will see questions answered about exercises that can cause pain and discomfort. Please remember that doing or not doing a specific exercise is not going to stop body sculpting results. Yes, the Squat is the best exercise for your legs-but if you have a bad low back, don't do it. If you can't do a specific exercise because it hurts you, there is always another one that will give you the same results. The primary reason to weight train should always be to improve your health and help you look and feel great. If you perform an exercise that you know will ultimately hurt you, we guarantee you'll be feeling really bad when you're laid up in bed. Follow your instincts and play it safe.

# Chapter 6
## Legs

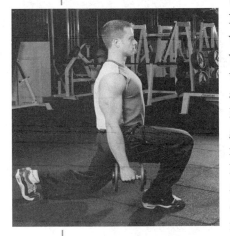

We decided to start the exercise description part of this book by discussing leg exercises. There are many reasons for this.

First of all, many guys just want to go to the gym and workout their upper bodies. These guys claim that their legs are "fine." This attitude is OK if what you want to do is end up looking like a light bulb with two pencils for legs. Don't you guys know that the best bodies have tight looking legs accompanied with a nice firm behind? Besides, do you realize how much upper body growth you are missing out on if you decide not to work out the legs? Hard leg exercises, like the squat, stimulate more testosterone and growth hormone than any other exercises out there. Besides, there are very few lifts that require the use of all of the muscles in the body the way that the back squat does.

Now that you realize how important leg exercises are, you're ready to learn how to perform the king of all exercises: the Barbell Squat.

For immediate Body Sculpting Bible support & coaching directly from James & Hugo, please visit www.BodySculptingBible.com

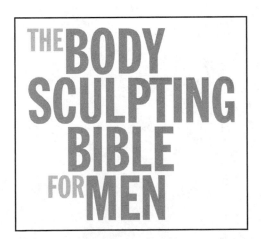

6

# Foot Stances and Quadriceps and Hamstring Development

To better target different areas of your legs, most specifically your quadriceps and your hamstrings, you need to pay attention to the stance in which you are standing. There are three main stances for each position (on the ground, and on a machine):

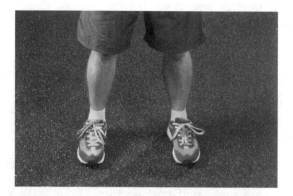

**Shoulder-width stance** with toes pointed slightly out: This stance works best for stimulating overall thigh development.

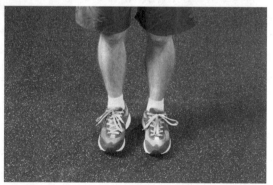

**Close stance** with toes pointed straight ahead: This stance works best for stimulating growth of the outer quadricep, better known as the vastus lateralis.

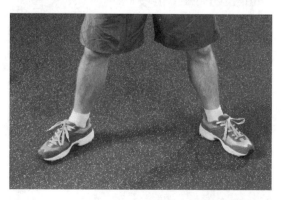

**Wide stance** with toes pointed out at least 45 degrees: This stance targets both the vastus medialis, which is the inside head of the quadriceps near the knee, and the inner thigh or adductor muscles.

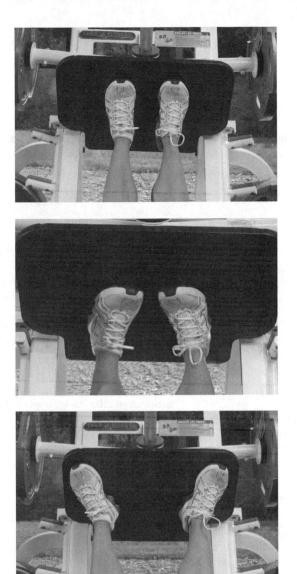

**Toes straight:** Good for overall development.

**Toes in:** Good for maximizing outer quadriceps and inner hamstring stimulation.

**Toes out:** Good for maximizing inner quad and outer hamstring stimulation.

It is important to mention that every time a quadriceps exercise is performed, it is imperative to push mainly with the toes, as that will emphasize quadriceps recruitment.

For hamstring exercises, you should push mainly with the heels, as that will emphasize hamstring/glute recruitment. In addition, there is only one main stance you should be concerned with for recruiting your hamstring, and that is the wide stance (toes pointed out at least 45 degrees).

# Barbell Squat

One of the best exercises you can do to build strong, ripped legs is the squat. This exercise is also known to provide beneficial results to the whole body because you use several body muscles to synergistically join forces and execute the lift.

It will primarily help develop the quadriceps muscles, and secondarily stimulate the hamstring muscles, the gluteal muscles, and the calves. However, it also will incorporate virtually all the body's major muscle groups in one way or another.

## PROPER ALIGNMENT

❶ Place a bar on either a squat safety rack or in a power cage, making sure you have the safety bars set just about even with the height of your thighs when they are parallel to the floor.

❷ Walk up to the bar and place your shoulders comfortably underneath it, making sure that the bar rests on the trapezoid muscles and not on the first and second cervical vertebrae. A shoulder pad is good to use. You can find them at most sporting good stores, or simply use a rolled up towel!

❸ Position your hands on the bar with a double shoulder width grip.

❹ Before lifting up the bar, either take a ready stance, making sure your body is properly aligned or, as we recommend, slowly step backwards with the weight already on your shoulders. This allows more room for the movement. If you are nervous about stepping backwards with the weight, you can always use the first option; or maybe you should re-evaluate how much weight you will be lifting. Whenever you feel nervous, be smart and consider either going a little lighter or having a qualified spotter assist you with the lift. Also, please don't just take someone's word for being a good spotter. Either ask reliable sources for someone who is qualified, or look around for someone whom you observe as a good spotter.

❺ Always align your body, starting from the bottom and moving to the top:

First, align your feet, making sure they are about shoulder width apart with a slight outward angle.

Next, slightly bend your knees to reduce undue stress from the lower back area.

Position your knees so that they are pointing directly in front of you.

Slightly contract the muscles of your lower back and the muscles of your abdominal section. This will ensure that you stay in proper alignment throughout the movement.

Stick out your chest while simultaneously squeezing your shoulder blades together. This helps to set the upper body in its proper position.

Finally, keep your head level at all times. Make sure your head and your eyes do not drop down or wander upward excessively as this is an easy way to lose your balance and fall.

We would rather you look slightly above level rather than below as looking below level can greatly affect your equilibrium and jeopardize your safety.

## TECHNIQUE AND FORM

Once you think you have properly aligned yourself, repeat the alignment steps starting from the bottom and moving up. Once you have secured your alignment, prepare to inhale as you begin your descent. As you execute the movement, keep the following points in mind:

❶ As you are squatting downward, it is very important that at no time throughout the movement do your knees go forward beyond your toes. This puts way too much pressure on the knees, and can seriously damage them. Here is a technique that will help keep this from happening: As you begin your descent, mimic the motion and alignment of sitting in a chair. Make sure you keep your back as straight as possible. This motion will naturally help you to utilize the proper form.

❷ Make sure you don't let your thighs go below parallel as you could injure your lower back and knees.

# Barbell Squat

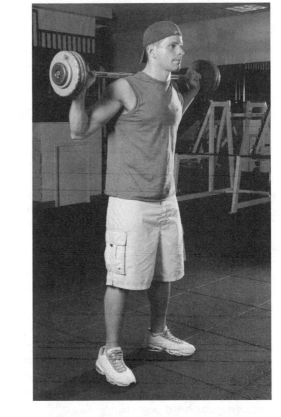

❸ As you reach parallel or just above it, begin to exhale and press off your feet, distributing the weight through the heel while pressing upward. You must concentrate on keeping and holding proper alignment throughout the movement.

❹ As you reach the top of the movement, make sure you do not lock out your knees since this will put too much stress on the knee joint. If at any time during the movement you should feel or notice yourself getting sloppy or not retaining the proper alignment, stop immediately! Never jeopardize your safety with bad form.

❺ When you've done the desired amount of reps, walk the bar back into the rack and place it down.

---

**FAQ:**

*I have a bad back and I've heard that you can seriously injure your back performing this exercise.*

**ANSWER:**

Squats are one of the greatest compound movements you can do for your entire body. When performed correctly, it will bring you great results. When done improperly, the squat will give you, well, squat! Here's the distinction: many people are injured when they try this with incorrect form or go overboard. Going overboard includes using too heavy of a weight, and not taking enough time or taking too much rest time between sets.

Recent research found that back injuries are often the result of low back muscular endurance, in other words, the back's ability to hold and maintain a muscular contraction. To beef up your lower back's muscular endurance, perform exercises that concentrate on your balance and coordination, like the Lunge, Abdominal Crunch on the Ball, and other rotational exercises.

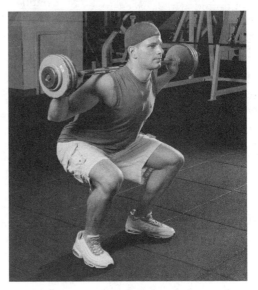

# Dumbbell Squat

This exercise emphasizes the same muscles as the barbell squat. Performing the exercise with dumbbells, however, places less stress on the lower back. Use this variation if all you have available is a pair of dumbbells or if you have had lower back injuries.

## PROPER ALIGNMENT

❶ Hold a dumbbell in each hand with arms extended down and palms facing your body.

❷ Align your body from the bottom up by first taking a shoulder-width stance.

❸ Slightly bend your knees and avoid locking them during this exercise.

❹ Contract your abdominal muscles to help support and sustain your posture during the exercise.

❺ Stick your chest out and simultaneously bring your shoulder blades back, keeping them there throughout the movement.

❻ Keep your head level at all times, making sure your head or your eyes do not drop down, or excessively wander upward. This is an easy way to lose your balance and fall. It is preferable to look slightly above level rather than below because looking below level can greatly affect your equilibrium and jeopardize your safety.

❼ If you feel unstable, you may put small 2 1/2 pound plates under each heel for stability.

## TECHNIQUE AND FORM

❶ When you think you have properly aligned yourself, repeat the alignment steps starting from the bottom and moving up. Once you have secured your alignment, prepare to inhale as you begin your descent.

❷ As you are squatting downward, it is very important that at no time throughout the movement your knees go forward beyond your toes. This puts way too much pressure on the knees and can seriously damage them. Here is a technique that will help prevent this from happening: As you begin your descent, mimic the motion and alignment of sitting in a chair. Make sure you keep your back as straight as possible. This motion will naturally help you to utilize the proper form.

❸ Make sure you don't let your thighs go below parallel as you could injure your lower back; and this can also push the knees past the toes, once again leading to injury.

❹ As you reach parallel or just above it, begin to exhale and press off your feet, distributing the weight through the heel while pressing upward. Concentrate on keeping and holding proper alignment throughout the movement.

❺ As you reach the top of the movement, make sure you do not lock out your knees since it will put too

much stress on the knee joint. If at any time during the movement you should feel or notice yourself getting sloppy or not retaining the proper alignment, stop immediately! Never jeopardize your safety with bad form!

❻ When you've done your desired amount of reps, simply squat down once again and place the dumbbells on the floor or place them back on the dumbbell rack. Never bend over to either pick up or place the dumbbells down. Doing this can injure your lower back area.

# Dumbbell Squat

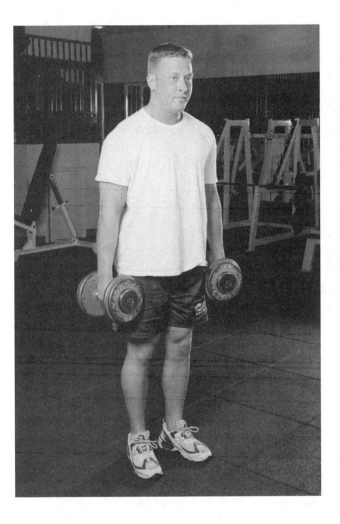
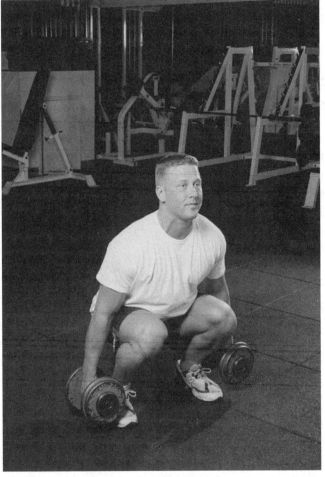

**FAQ:**

*Because I don't have barbell on my back, can I assume that the dumbbell squat will not bother my aching lower back?*

**ANSWER:**

Whether you're doing squats with a barbell or a dumbbell, your back will be affected. Your objective must be to maintain proper form, anatomical alignment, and technique, from the beginning until the end of the exercise. If you get sloppy with any of these three elements, you risk the chance of injuring your lower back. The squat can be a very safe and effective exercise, so long as you are cautious enough to make it work.

# Ballet Squat

This exercise is to be performed the same way as the barbell or dumbbell versions described previously, with the exception that your foot stance will be wider than shoulder-width. This variation will yield a stronger emphasis on the inner quads. Some guys are afraid that a wide stance will give them a big butt and hips. This is not true. A wide-stance squat can actually help shape the quadriceps and the inner thighs. You must make sure though that you don't have too wide a stance. An overly wide stance can cause knee problems and possibly generate some rather painful groin pulls. A good stance is about 1-1/2 times shoulder-width, with the toes pointed outward at a minimum of 25-30 degrees. No matter how wide your stance, your ankles should always remain in line with your knees. A good indication that a stance is too wide is when the ankles are outside of the knees in the bottom position of a squat. While you are discovering the width of stance best suited for you, don't worry about the amount of weight to use. Instead concentrate on your overall technique and form with your adjusted stance.

## PROPER ALIGNMENT

❶ Hold a dumbbell in each hand with arms extended down and palms facing your body or a barbell on your back with your arms holding the barbell in place.

❷ Align your body from the bottom up by first taking a shoulder-width stance.

❸ Slightly bend your knees and avoid locking out your knees anytime during this exercise.

❹ Contract your abdominal muscles to help support and sustain your posture during exercise.

❺ Stick your chest out and simultaneously bring your shoulder blades back, keeping them there throughout the movement.

❻ Keep your head level at all times. Make sure your head and your eyes do not drop down or wander upward excessively as this is an easy way to lose your balance and fall. We would rather you look slightly above level, rather than below, as looking below level can greatly affect your equilibrium and jeopardize your safety.

❼ If you feel unstable, you may put small 2 1/2 pound plates under each heel for stability.

## TECHNIQUE AND FORM

❶ When you think you have properly aligned yourself, repeat the alignment steps, starting from the bottom and moving up. Once you have secured your alignment, prepare to inhale as you begin your descent.

❷ As you are squatting downward, it is very important that at no time throughout the movement your knees go forward beyond your toes. This puts way too much pressure on the knees, and can seriously damage them. Here is a technique that will help keep this from happening: As you begin your descent, mimic the motion and alignment of sitting in a chair. Make sure you keep your back as straight as possible. This motion will naturally help you to utilize the proper form.

❸ Make sure you don't let your thighs go below parallel since you could injure your lower back; this can also push the knees past the toes, once again leading to injury.

❹ As you reach parallel or just above it, begin to exhale and press off your feet, distributing the weight throughout the heel while pressing upward. You must concentrate on keeping and holding proper alignment throughout the movement.

❺ As you reach the top of the movement, make sure you do not lock out your knees since it will put to much stress on the knee joint. If at any time during the movement you should feel or notice yourself getting sloppy or not retaining the proper alignment, stop immediately! Never jeopardize your safety with bad form!

❻ When you've done your desired amount of reps, simply walk the bar back to the rack. Or, if using dumbbells, squat down once again and place them on the floor or back on the dumbbell rack. Never bend over to either pick up or place the dumbbells down. Doing this can most definitely injure your lower back area.

# Ballet Squat

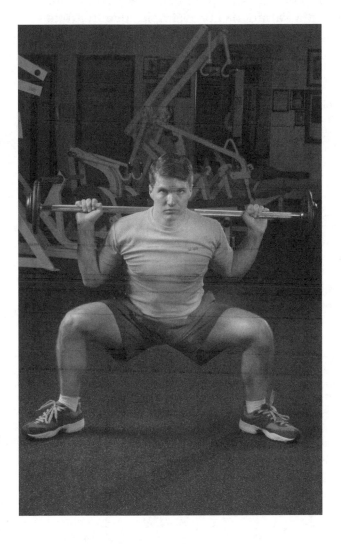
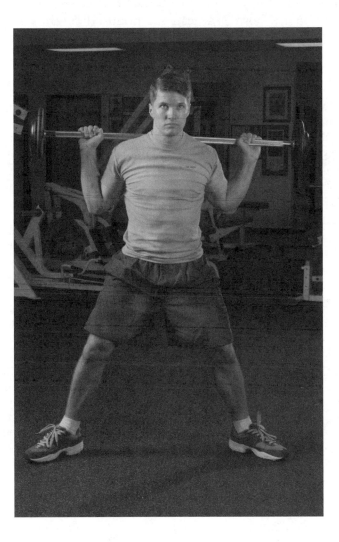

# Sissy Squat

This exercise is a great way to squat, using your own bodyweight as resistance. You can perform this practically anywhere, and it's especially useful when you're on the road. You shouldn't try this exercise if you suffer from knee problems, however, as it stresses the knee. Once you've got the basics down, target your quads differently by trying a variation. For example, use just one arm for support, and use the opposite arm to hold a plate on top of your chest.

## PROPER ALIGNMENT

**1** Make sure that there is nothing behind you so if you lose your balance and fall nothing will hit you.

**2** Stand upright with feet shoulder-width apart and heels raised an inch or two off the floor.

**3** Hold onto a stationary object such as one of the beams of a squat rack.

**4** If you are new to the exercise, it's a good idea to use two arms for support-so you'll need two beams of the squat rack in front of you.

## TECHNIQUE AND FORM

**1** Using your arms to hold yourself, bend at the knees and slowly lower your torso toward the ground by bringing your pelvis and knees forward.

**2** Inhale as you go down and stop when your buttocks almost touch your heels. Hold the stretch position for a second. Ensure that your hamstrings touch the calves at the bottom of the movement. This emphasizes the stretch!

**3** After the hold, use your thigh muscles to bring your torso back up to the starting position and exhale as you go up.

**4** Perform the determined number of repetitions after coming all the way up to the starting position and pausing momentarily at the top of the movement. This makes sure you do not bounce up and down (which places more stress on your knees) and it also ensures the squat is done with perfect form.

# Sissy Squat

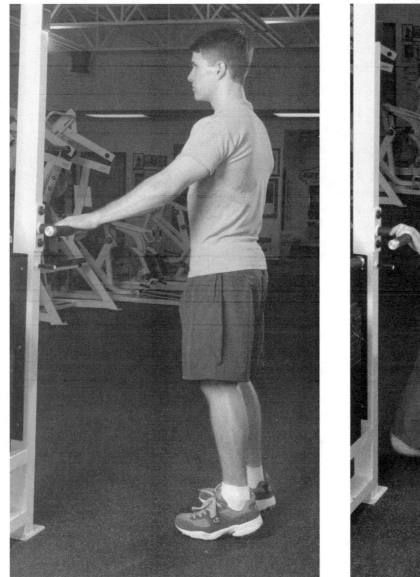 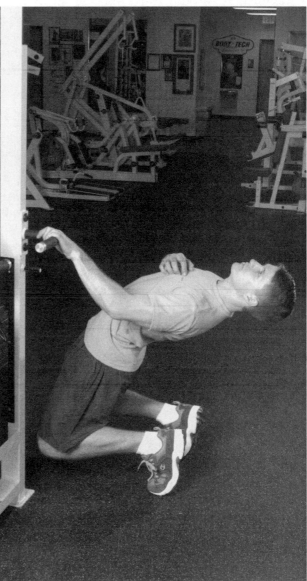

# Hack Squat

While free weights (like dumbbells and barbells) will help to target your body in motion, machines are also a great addition to your workout routine. The best thing about machines is that they isolate a body part, making it very safe to use them when recovering from an injury in an unrelated spot. Of course, if this is the case, you should consult your doctor before attempting any exercises. Form is still crucial when using machines. It's a myth that you automatically are in the correct form when seated at a machine. Be careful to position yourself correctly. Try varying your foot position to target different parts of your quads.

## PROPER ALIGNMENT

❶ Place the back of your torso against the hack squat machine back pad. Make sure your head is up at all times and your back remains against the pad.

❷ Position your shoulders under the shoulder pads provided on the machine.

❸ Put your legs in a shoulder-width stance with your feet on the platform, toes pointed slightly out.

❹ Place your arms on the side handles of the machine above your shoulders and disengage the safety bars.

❺ Your legs should be straight without locking your knees.

## TECHNIQUE AND FORM

❶ Begin to slowly lower the unit by bending your knees. Inhale and continue down until your thighs are parallel to the floor. The fronts of the knees should make an imaginary straight line with the toes that is perpendicular to the thighs.

❷ During the movement, your back will move along the pad (but the pad will stay in one place).

❸ Exhale and begin to raise the unit by pushing the platform with your toes, straightening your legs, and returning to the starting position.

❹ Remember to pause slightly at the top of the movement, making sure that your lowering is as measured as possible, in order to remain in perfect form.

# Hack Squat

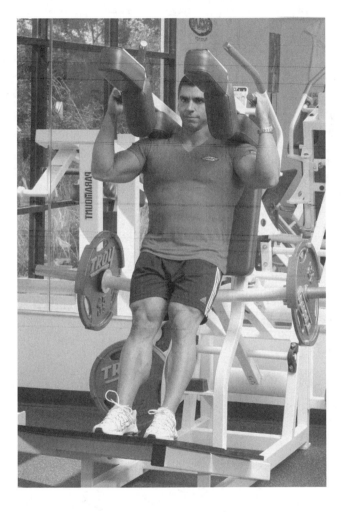 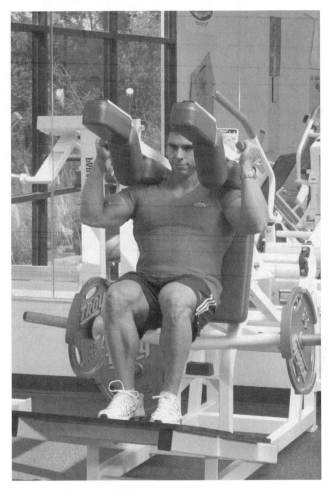

# Front Squat

If you are new to this exercise, use less weight. The squat is very safe, but only if performed properly, and this particular squat may be best suited for advanced athletes. If you have back problems, substitute the dumbbell squat variation or a leg press for the front squats. If you do perform this exercise, maintain perfect form and never slouch forward because this can cause injury. Try varying your stance to target a different muscle group in your quadriceps.

While this exercise is best performed inside a squat rack for safety purposes, for the purposes of properly demonstrating the movement, a squat rack was not used.

## PROPER ALIGNMENT

❶ Set the bar on a squat rack that best matches your height. A small block can be placed under the heels to improve balance.

❷ Bring your arms up under the bar, keeping your elbows high and your upper arms slightly above parallel to the floor.

❸ Rest the bar on top of the deltoids and cross your arms while grasping the bar for full control.

❹ Lift the bar off the rack by pushing with your legs while straightening your torso.

❺ Step away from the rack and position your legs with a shoulder-width stance.

❻ Your toes should be pointing slightly out and your head should be up at all times to help keep your back straight.

## TECHNIQUE AND FORM

❶ Inhale and bend your knees slowly and continue down until your thighs are slightly parallel to the floor. The fronts of your knees should not be past your toes, or you will place undue stress on the knee and do the exercise incorrectly.

❷ Raise the bar again, exhale and push the floor with your toes to straighten your legs and return to the starting position.

❸ Pause for a second at the top of the movement before performing the rest of the repetitions required. This allows you to ensure you are not using momentum to continue from one repetition to the next.

# Front Squat

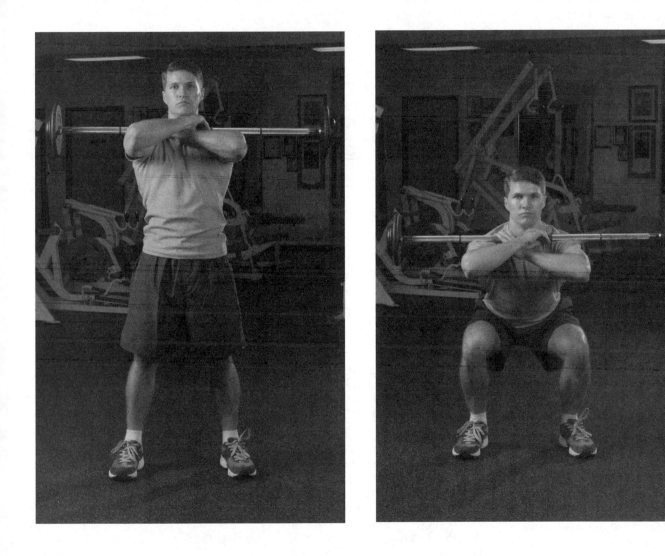

# Dumbbell Lunge

This exercise is an excellent movement for all of the muscles in the legs. It primarily stresses the buttocks, hamstrings and quads with a secondary emphasis on the calves. This movement can also be performed with a barbell on the back. The barbell variation, however, places more stress on the lower back. If you choose to use a barbell, use the same steps described below in order to perform the movement.

Lunges are a fantastic leg exercise for both men and women. Due to the fact that only one leg is used at a time, lunges require a balancing act. In order to maintain balance the body needs to recruit as many auxiliary fibers as possible. What this means to you is more muscle stimulation per repetition. In addition, lunges can be used to stimulate the hamstrings muscles or the quadriceps muscles by varying how far away you place your foot. If when you step forward you place your foot closer to your body, you will primarily stimulate the quadriceps. If when you step forward you place your foot farther away from your body, you will primarily stimulate the hamstrings. (Note: In no case, as you'll see in the exercise description, should your knee go past your toes.)

## PROPER ALIGNMENT

❶ Hold a dumbbell in each hand with arms extended down and palms facing your body.

❷ Align your body from the bottom up, first taking a stance with the feet together, and the toes pointing straight ahead.

❸ Keep your knees slightly bent to avoid any stress from locking the knee joint.

❹ Slightly contract the abdominal muscles.

❺ Stick the chest out while simultaneously bringing the shoulder blades back, keeping them there throughout the movement.

❻ Keep your head level at all times, making sure your head or your eyes do not drop down or excessively wander upward.

## TECHNIQUE AND FORM

❶ Step forward with your right foot.

❷ Bend at the knee making sure you descend slowly and in control.

❸ As your knee bends and your hips are lowering, lower yourself only until your left knee is about two inches from the ground and then stop.

❹ When you step forward at the beginning of the movement, make sure that the knee does not go past the toes when you are in the bent-knee position with your left knee two inches from the ground.

❺ Begin to reverse the movement by pressing off the right foot only. You may naturally want to use the left knee to assist in pushing back up, but do not let this happen. The objective is to fully isolate the right leg muscles and use the left leg only as a balancing tool, sort of like the rudder on a boat.

❻ Make sure you do not use momentum as you push off with the right leg to return. This will totally inhibit the stimulation of the leg muscles.

❼ Return to the start position but do not rest. Switch legs and repeat the same movement, making sure to maintain the alignment and posture throughout the movement.

---

**FAQ:**

*Isn't the lunge nothing more than a fancy second-rate exercise?*

**ANSWER:**

When done correctly, lunges are actually one of the absolute best leg exercises you can do to both build and strengthen all of your leg muscles.

# Dumbbell Lunge

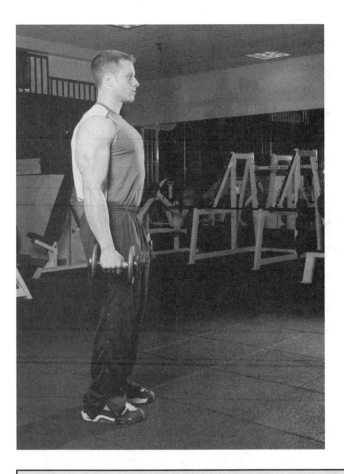
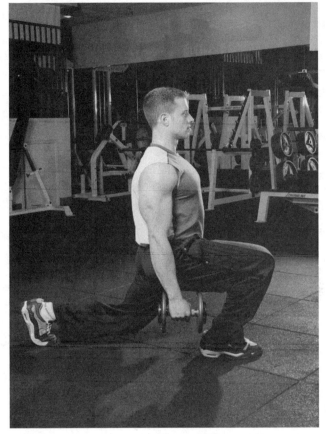

**FAQ:**

*If squats can be dangerous, what about lunges?*

**ANSWER:**

Any exercise can be dangerous if you don't pay attention to proper form, anatomical alignment, and exercise technique. With squats, because both feet are planted on the ground, both areas of the lower back become vulnerable. Also, because the lower back muscles (Errector Spinae) are working to hold your lumbar curve, they can become considerably exhausted during the exercise.

Lunges, on the other hand, work one leg at a time. This independent work also affects the lower back muscles-but differently than the squat. In other words, while one leg is working, the other side of your body is actually being guarded from exhaustion. Remember, muscular endurance is just how long a muscle can endure under tension. With squats, it's all or nothing. With lunges, you can pace yourself.

Lunges also really emphasize the negative (lengthening) phase of the exercise. The range of motion required to perform a lunge correctly is also usually much greater than with squats. Make sure to step in slowly with the lunge; going too quickly can be very dangerous to your lower back, knees, and many other areas of the body.

# Leg Press

The leg press machine is a great exercise for the legs. It can be used in place of the traditional barbell squat for people who suffer from lower back pain, as a rehabilitation exercise (especially if only using one leg at a time) or to just supplement your leg routine.

There are two ways to perform this exercise: one leg at a time or both legs at the same time. In this book we will discuss the more common two-legged version. However, the execution for the exercise remains the same for both versions.

**VARIATION:** The leg press can also be performed on a plate-loaded machine.

## PROPER ALIGNMENT

❶ Sit on the machine with your back on the padded support and align your feet evenly on the platform. The height placement of your feet on the platform will zone in on different areas of the quadriceps. The higher your foot placement on the platform the less intense the quad contraction and the less knee involvement.

The lower your foot placement on the platform, the more intense the quad contraction will be; but you will put a lot of stress and shear force on the knees.

❷ Make sure that your back and head are kept flush against the back pad and that you are seated securely.

❸ Take hold of the release lever handles and disengage the lock pins.

## TECHNIQUE AND FORM

❶ Immediately take hold of the secured handles, which are usually located to the sides of you. If the handles are placed in an awkward position, you can also take hold of the seat edge. This can help take some stress off the lower back.

❷ With the feet spaced evenly apart and flat upon the platform, slowly lower the sled towards you.

❸ Once again, do not grip the handles too tightly.

❹ Let the sled come down to a point just before your thighs would touch your chest. Depending on your condition, you might not want to bring the sled this low. Monitor your individual situation. Too many trainees don't allow the sled to go deep enough to sustain any type of quad muscle involvement, and they'll pack on the weights. Lighten the weight and tone!

❺ When you have reached the bottom portion of the exercise, return back to the starting position by slowly pushing the platform evenly with both feet. Do not lock your knees! This could injure your knees and will also take the resistance off of the quads, distributing it directly to the knee joints.

---

*FAQ:*

*If I have a lower back injury, is the leg press a good choice for a leg exercise? I assume this is the case because it's a seated exercise.*

*ANSWER:*

Actually, the leg press can be much more harmful than any other leg exercise, when you have an injured lower back. This doesn't have to be the case, so you must follow some advice to avoid further injury. One of the best exercises you can do on the leg press, if you are concerned with your lower back, is the one-legged press. When you're working just one leg at a time, it prevents you from lifting your back from its correct position. While one leg is working, the other is planted and supporting correct form. You must be careful, though-don't go too heavy. Make sure to stay steady during the movement; any jerking can disrupt your form and possibly injure your lower back.

# Leg Press

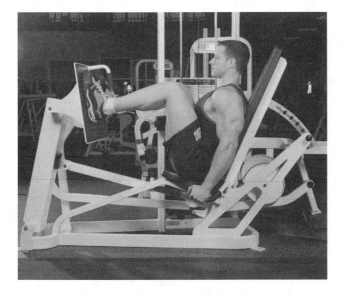 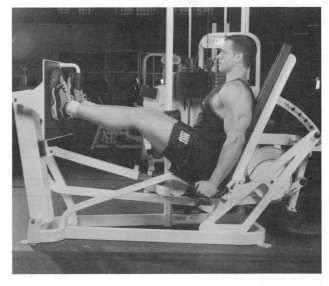

## VARIATION

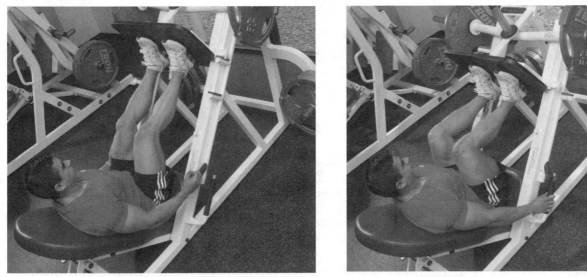

# Leg Extension

The leg extension is an excellent isolation exercise that really targets the quadricep muscles located on the front of the thigh. It also helps strengthen the knee, which is a commonly injured area. The leg extension is recommended by most physical therapists as a good tool for knee rehabilitation. The key to the effectiveness and safety of this exercise is to choose a machine whose starting position allows your toes to be right in front of your knees and to focus on contracting the thigh muscle (as opposed to lifting heavy) as you lift the weight. Focusing on lifting heavy weights will cause knee damage, especially if you are using a machine in which your toes start behind your knees (in this case the upper leg and the lower leg will be at an angle that is below 90-degrees).

There are two ways to perform this exercise: one leg at a time (in which case you will not be able to use as much weight) or both legs at the same time. In this book, we will discuss the more common two-legged version. However, the execution for the exercise remains the same for both versions.

## PROPER ALIGNMENT

❶ Seat yourself on the machine and position the back pad so that you are sitting totally upright.

❷ The back of your knees must be pressed flush against the front of the seat, which will help you avoid a potential knee injury caused by allowing the knee to hang over the seat without support. Doing this will give the needed support to your knees. You also want to make sure that the axis of the knees are in line with the machine axis, helping to set up the proper alignment (biomechanics) of the knee and direct the maximum resistance to the quadriceps. In addition, as discussed previously, ensure that the starting position allows the toes to be in front of the knees and that the upper leg and lower leg create a 90-degree angle.

❸ Adjust the shin roller pad against the lowest point of the shin to help optimize the shin as a lever and the knee as the fulcrum. This will again help to direct the majority of the resistance to the thigh muscles.

Before you begin the exercise, lightly grip the handles provided or grab the front of the seat on each side of your legs.

## TECHNIQUE AND FORM

❶ Begin the exercise with your legs totally relaxed and your shins behind the roller pad positioned at the bottom.

❷ Isometrically contract the quad muscles and slowly begin to lift the weight by lifting the roller pad with the shins.

❸ As you extend upward, stay in control by allowing the quad muscles to lift the weight. Do not use momentum or leverage. This is a very easy exercise to cheat on by using quick bursts of momentum at the bottom of the movement, or by leaning back and using leverage to lift the weight.

❹ As you reach the point of full extension, when the part of your leg below your knee is extended and as close as possible to being in a direct line with your upper thigh, focus only on fully contracting the quad

muscles. Sometimes people have the tendency to go through the exercise motions without consciously contracting the muscles that are supposed to be lifting the weight. As long as you make a great effort to squeeze or contract the quad muscle fully at the top of full extension, you will be taking full advantage of the exercise.

❺ Make sure that once you get to the fully extended position of the exercise, you don't just let the leg drop but slowly return back to the beginning of the movement.

❻ As you reach the bottom, do not rest! Slowly and smoothly lift the roller pad with your shins back to full extension. Always make sure that you are going through the full range of motion for these exercises as doing so will provide the maximum muscular development.

# Leg Extension

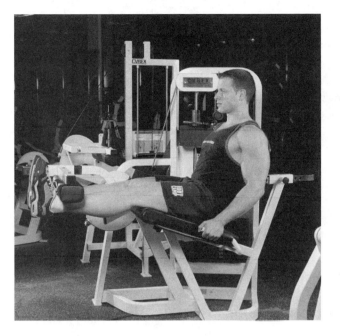 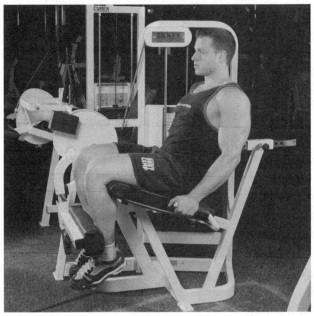

**FAQ:**

*I've seen people using lots of momentum when they do this exercise. Should I move as much weight as possible, even if I don't feel my quads being stimulated?*

**ANSWER:**

The purpose for doing any exercise is to stimulate the muscles you are working. In other words, if you don't feel the muscle really contract (especially at the top of the movement), and you instead feel your joints taking the brunt of the exercise, you are doing more harm than good to your body.

The point of this exercise is to put full emphasis on the front of your thighs (quadriceps). If you don't feel these muscles working, you're either going too heavy or you may not be a good fit for that machine. Some are built for a different shape of body. Make certain that your lower back is supported by the back pad and that the backs of your knees lie flush against the seat pad. Adjust the shin pad so that it is between the top of your foot and your shin.

If that doesn't work, try another leg extension machine and go just heavy enough so that it is a challenge, but not where you need momentum and joint support to move the weight. You should not be using momentum. If you are, it's too heavy.

# Lying Leg Curl

The lying leg curl is an exercise that focuses on the hamstrings located on the back of the upper leg. It also affects the gluteal muscles and the muscles of the lower back (erector spinae). Again, form over weight is crucial! It is very easy to pull a hamstring if you are using heavy weights and jerking the weights!

There are two ways to perform this exercise: one leg at a time or both legs at the same time. In this book we will discuss the more common two-legged version. However, the execution for the exercise remains the same for both versions.

## PROPER ALIGNMENT

There are several machines for training the hamstring muscles, but we recommend the lying leg curl machine. If you prefer, you may use the seated leg curl machine instead. No matter which machine you choose, the alignment will basically be the same.

❶ Position yourself on the machine and, as always, begin the alignment of your body starting with your feet.

❷ Lock your pelvis into place by contracting your abdominal muscles.

❸ Try to focus only on the hamstring muscles.

❹ When you're lying down, relax your upper body. (Allowing your body to stay tense during the exercise will only negatively affect hamstring stimulation.) If you like, you can hold on to the set of handles, which are usually supplied. Just make sure you do so with a very light grip. Squeezing too hard can change the focus of resistance in the hamstring muscles, causing this exercise to be less beneficial. Holding too tight can also cause leverage to do the work for you instead of working the muscle. Remember, don't sell yourself short trying to find the easy way of exer-

cising. You are here to work, not to make things easy. Besides, work is what produces results, not the alternative.

❺ Relax your neck and head. If you choose the seated leg curl machine, you should follow the same form; that is, space your feet evenly.

❻ Keep your knees pointed directly in front of you throughout the movement.

❼ Contract your abdominal muscles and relax your upper body, neck and head.

## TECHNIQUE AND FORM

❶ As you begin the movement, contract the hamstrings before actually moving as this will help to focus the resistance on the hamstring muscles and better stimulate the those muscles.

❷ Drive your heels to your butt, while pointing (this is very important) your toes toward your knees ("flexing your feet"). It will be the same whether sitting or lying down. Pointing your toes towards your knees helps to better isolate the hamstring muscles. Refer to pictures on showing the relaxed feet and the flexed feet positions.

❸ When you reach your butt, try to hold that position for a count of two seconds. This will help increase the intensity of the exercise; and once again, better stimulate the hamstring muscles. As you descend, do so with a slow, controlled movement. When you reach the starting position, without rest, slowly and smoothly change directions, moving upward once again. Following these guidelines will ensure your safety and greater results.

---

**FAQ:**

*This is the only exercise I've been doing for my hamstrings. Is it enough?*

**ANSWER:**

You should be doing a variety of exercises that stimulate the hamstrings. While the Lying Leg Curl Machine is a great isolation exercise, there are plenty of other exercises, which will incorporate parts of the hamstrings and help to fully develop this muscle. They include, but are not limited to: Stiff-Legged Deadlift, Standing Leg Curl, Seated Leg Curl, Glute-Ham Raises, and Step-Ups.

# Lying Leg Curl

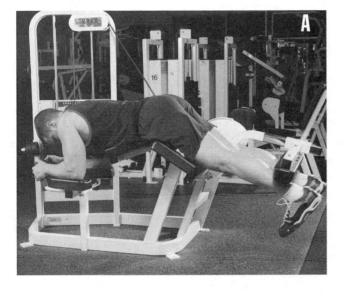

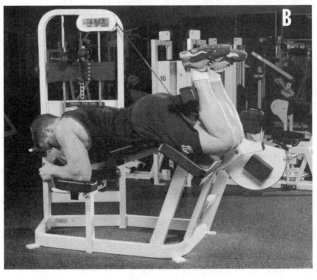

**RELAXED**

**FLEXED**

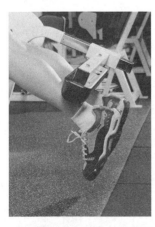

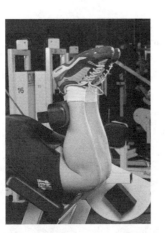

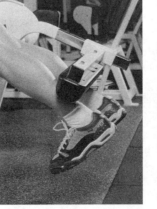

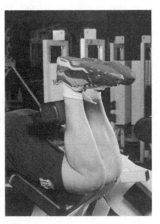

# Seated Leg Curl

This variation of the leg curl is great for simply adding variety to your hamstring training and also for preventing problems in some injury-prone areas such as the lower back. If you suffer from lower back problems and have access to this machine, feel free to use it. However, like any machine, the key is to focus on the form and not add weight haphazardly. Any machine will injure you if you use too much weight with improper form.

## PROPER ALIGNMENT

**1** Position yourself on the seated leg curl machine with your shins placed against the roller pads.

**2** Make sure to align your knees with the axis of the rotating pivot joint of the machine.

**3** Position the back pad forward or backward for the proper alignment of your knees with the axis.

**4** Loosely place your hands on the handles that are provided on the side of the machine.

**5** Keep your head relaxed and your back flat against the back pad at all times during the exercise.

## TECHNIQUE AND FORM

**1** Keeping your legs locked in place from your knee to your hip, bend your knees and curl the bottom portion of your legs down as far as you can go.

**2** Hold for a brief second while simultaneously contracting (flexing) your hamstrings.

**3** Slowly return to the starting position in a slow, controlled manner.

**4** You may hold onto the handles located on the side of the seat to keep your body locked in place during the exercise-just don't squeeze the handles too hard as it may take away from the focus on the hamstrings.

**5** Keep your head straight and avoid looking down during the exercise. Keeping your head in a neutral position will help maintain your overall balance.

**6** Don't let your back round. Keeping it straight will help take pressure off your lower back.

# Seated Leg Curl

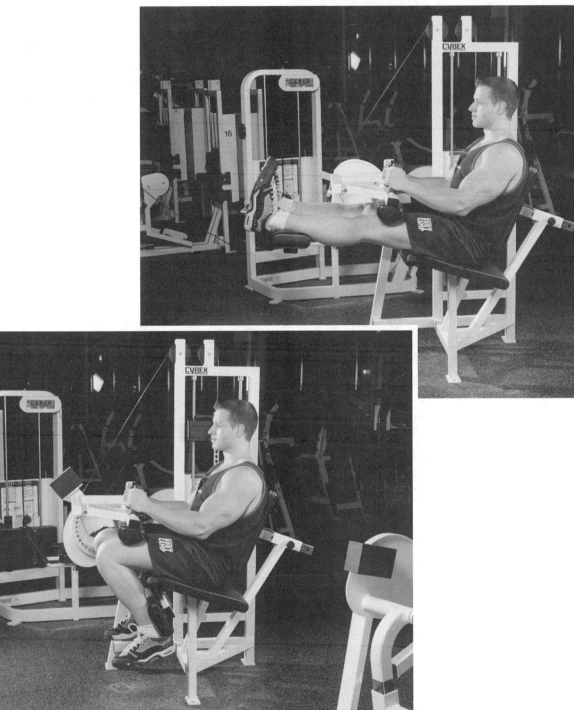

# Standing Leg Curl

This variation of the leg curl is a great way to both isolate the hamstring muscles and to focus on possible imbalances between the two legs. It is basically the equivalent of performing a barbell curl but for the leg biceps instead. You can do a great variation of this exercise at home by simply strapping on some ankle weights and holding onto a stationary object for stability. You can also use elastic cables strapped to a stationary object on one end and to your ankle on the other end. Use this exercise in lieu of the stiff legged deadlifts if you suffer from lower back problems.

## PROPER ALIGNMENT

**1** Stand next to the lever arm of the machine so that it is to the right of your leg.

**2** Hook your right heel under the roller pad attached to the lever arm.

**3** The type of machine you have access to will either allow you to kneel upon the knee rest with your left leg or stand with your left leg on a platform, which will keep your body elevated for your right leg to clear the platform when performing the exercise movement.

## TECHNIQUE AND FORM

**1** Keeping your upper leg from your knee to your hip securely in place, curl your right leg up as high as it will go, using your hamstring muscle.

**2** At the top, contract your hamstring muscle as hard as you can and hold for one second.

**3** Slowly return to the bottom in a controlled and smooth motion.

**4** Perform the determined reps for one leg, switch legs and do the same number of reps for the other leg.

**5** Make sure not to jerk or allow momentum to assist you with the exercise.

# Standing Leg Curl

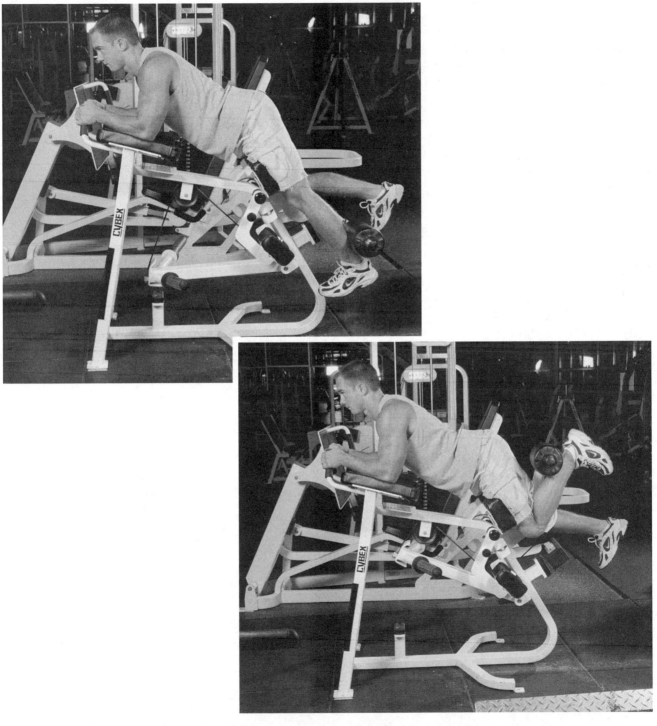

# Stiff-Legged Deadlift

The stiff-legged deadlift is a very good exercise for the hamstring muscles (located between your butt and knees) and the lower back "erector" muscles provided that:

You concentrate on perfect form and avoid using heavy weights.

You do not suffer from lower back problems.

You avoid going to total muscle failure.

You can do this exercise either with a barbell or while holding two dumbbells. If you have a lower back injury, we advise that you don't do this exercise. Although it is a fantastic exercise to help strengthen the lower back, if you already have a lower back injury, it can do more harm than good. If this is the case, use the standing leg curl exercise (with either a machine, ankle weights or elastic cables) instead.

**VARIATION:** Try this exercise with a barbell to best support your wrists.

## PROPER ALIGNMENT

❶ First, choose a weight for your barbell or dumbbells, making sure that the weight is light enough to practice perfect form.

❷ Position your feet shoulder-width apart, pointing straight ahead at all times during the movement.

❸ Position your hands on the barbell with a grip wider than your feet position. Your hands positioned slightly outside your foot stance should be adequate.

❹ Stand up straight and hold the barbell across your thighs or the dumbbells at your side with your palms facing toward your legs.

❺ The object here is to keep your legs completely straight, staying locked at the knee joints and bending forward at the waist. It is very, very important to make sure you keep your back completely straight while bending forward. We recommend that as you bend down, you keep your head and eyes looking straight ahead and level. If you look down at the ground, you will be very likely to hyper-flex your spine and cause a lower back injury.

## TECHNIQUE AND FORM

Before you begin the exercise and throughout the execution, you must direct all of your focus to the hamstring muscles of the rear thigh, to help activate them even more. "Put your mind in the muscle!" When you return to the starting top position of the exercise, focus on the erector muscles of the lower back by slightly arching the spine and sticking the chest out, contracting those lower back muscles.

❶ With your body straight, legs locked and arms hanging down, begin the exercise by bending over at the waist.

❷ Remember to look straight ahead as you bend over. Your eyes must be looking level with your body as you reach parallel to the floor.

❸ As you bend over, concentrate on the hamstring muscles of the thigh and make sure your back is maintained in a straight position as you lower yourself.

❹ As you reach a point when your torso is parallel to the floor and the bar or dumbbells are fairly close to touching the floor, slowly and without rest begin lifting your body back up from the waist, concentrating on focusing all of the work to the hamstring muscles of the thigh. Do not use any momentum during this movement, especially at this position! You will really feel the hamstring muscles contract in the lower position as you slowly change directions and begin your way upward.

❺ Keep your head and eyes looking straight ahead as you return to the standing position.

❻ As you return to the start position, really contract your hamstring muscles, but don't stop there. As you stand straight up, stick your chest way out and slightly arch your spine while you contract the muscles of the lower back.

❼ Hold that position for only one second, then slowly and smoothly begin lowering your body again, maintaining the same exact form as when you began the exercise.

# Stiff-Legged Deadlift

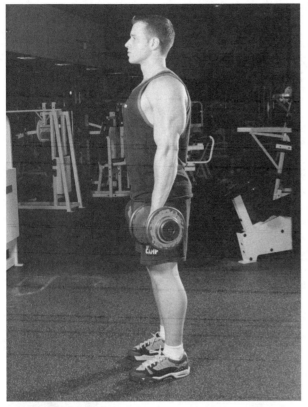

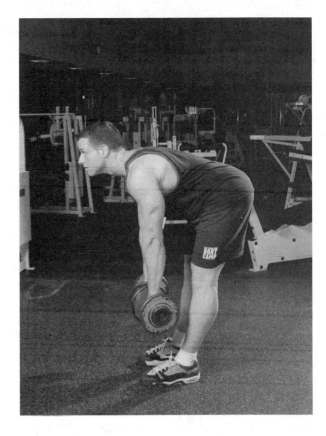

## VARIATION

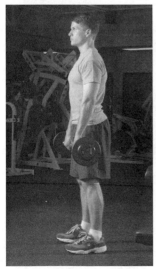

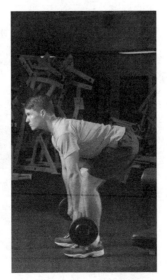

**FAQ:**

*I see many people doing this exercise and they are looking down at the ground while doing it.*

**ANSWER:**

Looking at the ground while doing this or any exercise in a similar stance (for example, squats, lunges, deadlifts, etc.), can be detrimental to your safety and could even "hamstring" your results. Looking down at the ground while doing this exercise rounds out your lower back and puts your lower back muscles in a very vulnerable state. When you round the low back instead of maintaining a lumbar curve, you have a very good chance of straining the lower back muscles.

# Step-Up

There are a couple of variations to this basic exercise. You can try performing all repetitions on one leg at a time, as well as using a barbell instead of dumbbells. Once again, using a barbell instead of dumbbells protects your wrists from twisting and thus injury.

## PROPER ALIGNMENT

❶ Choose a weight appropriate to your skill level. If you are just starting out, try this exercise with just your body weight.

❷ Position your feet shoulder-width apart, pointing your toes forward. You will be approximately half a foot behind an elevated platform like a step or flat 10 pound weights on the ground.

❸ Hold the dumbbells at your sides, palms facing each other.

❹ Stand up straight, your knees straight but not locked, with your chest out, shoulders back, and eyes forward.

## TECHNIQUE AND FORM

❶ Begin the movement by placing your right foot on the elevated platform, making sure that your heel and toes make solid contact, and neither are off the edge.

❷ Step up fully onto the platform by extending the hip and the knee of your right leg.

❸ Use the heel to lift the rest of you body up and place the foot of the left leg on the platform as well. Exhale as you push up.

❹ Inhale and step down with your left leg by flexing the hip and knee of the right leg.

❺ Return to the original standing position by placing the right foot next to the left foot.

❻ Repeat this exercise, alternating legs, until you have performed the number of repetitions required.

# Step-Up

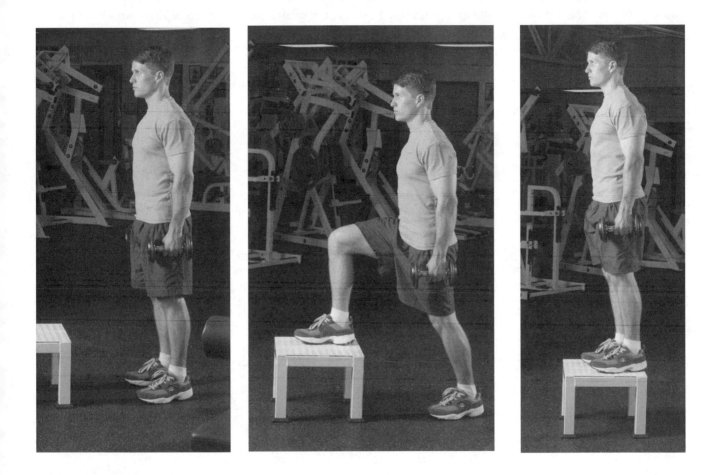

# Glute-Ham Raise

The Glute-Ham Raise is a great way to work your hamstrings, although it can be dangerous if you are a beginner. It's crucial to have a spotter if you are new to this exercise. It can also be hard on your lower back, so be careful if you have injuries. To make this easier, have your spotter assist you in getting to the upright position. If you are looking for a way to add to your resistance, add weight by holding a plate to your chest.

## PROPER ALIGNMENT

**1** You will need to use a pull-down machine for this exercise. First, adjust the padded supports of the machine as far down as possible.

**2** Kneel upright on the seat of the machine, facing away from it. Use a partner's support if necessary.

**3** Place your ankles between the padded supports and your feet flat against the platform where typically your thighs would sit. There should be a 90 degree angle created by the upper and lower leg.

**4** Hold your arms down by your sides, and keep your shoulders back and your chest up.

## TECHNIQUE AND FORM

**1** Bring your torso forward slowly. You should be thrusting your hips forward and straightening your knees slightly.

**2** As the torso comes down, inhale.

**3** Only your knees should be bending. Make sure you are not bending at the waist.

**4** As you exhale, pull your body upright by flexing at the knees until you are back in the original position.

**5** Pause slightly at the top of the movement, then resume with the next repetition.

# Glute-Ham Raise

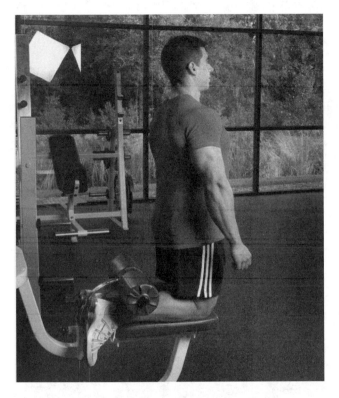 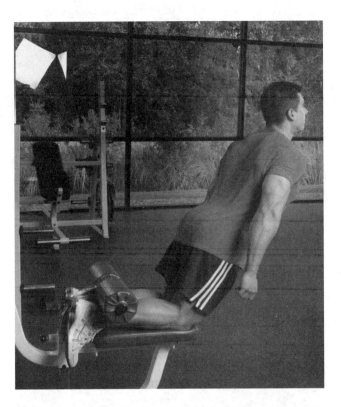

# Calf Raise

The calf muscles may be thought of as just a small part of the large spectrum of body parts, but having good calf development can mean the difference between having a great body versus having an asymmetrical, weak-looking one. The calves are one of the most eye-catching areas of the body, and are often associated with how fit a person really is. The calves, abdominals and shoulder muscles are three areas of the body that seem to work with each other. If one of the three is out of balance with the others, it can have a terrible effect on the overall appearance of your body. On the other hand, if all three body parts are in sync with each other, your body will look like a symmetrical whole.

The calf muscles are very stubborn and they won't respond to training unless you train them correctly. Besides needing different angles of training with proper technique and form, they need a lot of weight and repetitions in order to grow. If you think about how much work your calves do every day with just your normal routine (walking, running, sitting down, standing up, etc.), and take into account that these activities are done with your full body weight; you can see why your calf muscles would require special training to grow. The calf muscles have adapted to the rigors of everyday life. You must introduce them to training that they are not used to—heavy weight with high repetitions! This will shock them, and they will now be forced to adapt to the new training by growing!

In this program, we will discuss four exercises that will help you tremendously in reshaping your calf muscles. The standing calf raise, calf press and donkey calf raise will primarily help develop mass in the bulk of the muscle (gastrocnemius muscle) and secondarily stimulate the soleus muscles (lower and outer portions of the calf); and the seated calf raise will primarily target the soleus muscles. Of crucial importance when performing calf exercises is to focus on stretching the muscle at the bottom of the movement and contracting the muscle at the top. Typically, when we train calves, we like to spend a second in the stretched (bottom) position and a second or two in the contracted (top) position.

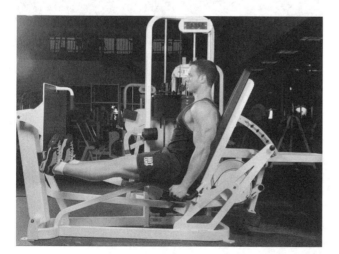 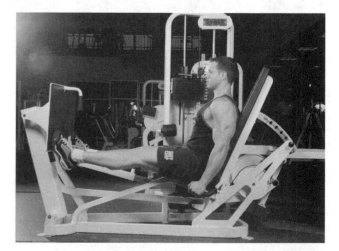

## STANDING CALF RAISE

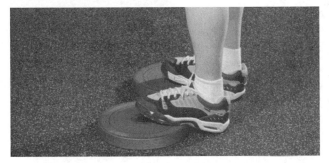

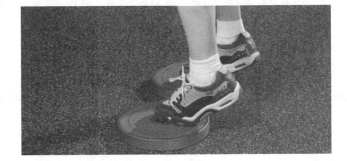

## CALF PRESS

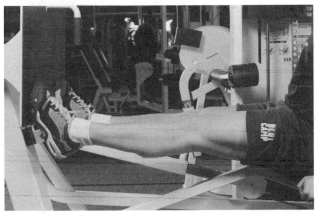

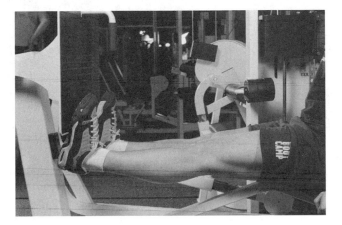

## SEATED CALF RAISE

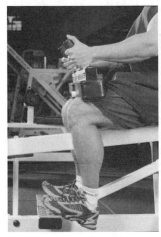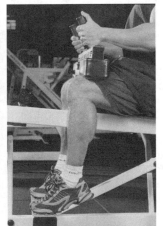

## DONKEY CALF RAISE

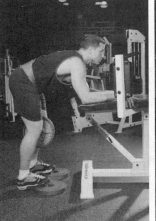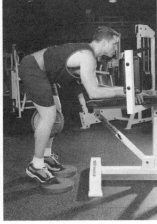

# Standing Calf Raise

**(Using A Machine, Barbell Or Dumbbells)**

The standing calf raise machine is a great tool for building quality calves. If you don't have access to a calf raise machine, you may use a pair of dumbbells instead to hold at your sides. Of course, you'll want to get yourself a pair of dumbbells that you can add extra weight to.

There are two ways to perform this exercise: one leg at a time (holding yourself to a stationary object if using dumbbells) or both legs at the same time. For this exercise, you can use dumbbells, barbells or a machine. In this book we will discuss the more common two-legged version in a machine. However, the execution for the exercise remains the same for all versions.

**VARIATION:** A variation of the Standing Calf Raise is using just one leg. For this, you should make sure to have a fixed object nearby as support, like the beam of a squat rack. Simply work one leg at a time by holding the other behind you, bending its knee.

If your gym mops frequently, please make sure to dry the area or machine pad before doing calf raises. You could be seriously injured if your feet slip off the platform.

## PROPER ALIGNMENT

### For the machine:

❶ Set the weight to a resistance you can handle while practicing perfect form.

❷ Step on the platform and take hold of the grip bars on the sides of the shoulder harness.

❸ With your feet pointing straight ahead, place your toes and the balls of your feet on the platform.

❹ Set the shoulder pads so they will be slightly lower than your shoulders while you are in this position.

❺ Bend at the knees and position your shoulders underneath the shoulder pads comfortably.

❻ Stand up straight so that your shoulders lift the shoulder pads, which will lift the weight plates up.

❼ Keep your knees pointing straight ahead and keep them bent very slightly during the exercise. The bent-knee position can help stretch the calves in the lower position and will save your lower back in the upper position.

❽ Make sure to keep your body straight during the exercise. Be careful not to bend at the waist during any portion of the movement or hyperextend your back at the top of the movement. Doing either of these can injure your back.

❾ Stick your chest out and keep your shoulders squared at all times during the exercise.

❿ Keep your head straight and level and look straight ahead at all times.

### For dumbbells:

❶ First, pick up the dumbbells and stand in front of a platform, which should be about 1 inch high.

❷ Step onto the platform and position your feet a couple of inches apart.

❸ Bring the dumbbells to the sides of your body, with your palms facing each other.

❹ Place your toes and the balls of your feet on the platform.

❺ Keep your knees pointing straight ahead and keep them bent very slightly during the exercise as the bent knee position can help stretch the calves in the lower position and will save your lower back in the upper position.

❻ You must make sure to keep your body straight during the exercise. Be careful not to bend at the waist during any portion of the movement or hyperextend your back at the top of the movement. Doing either of these can injure your back.

❼ Stick your chest out and keep your shoulders squared at all times during the exercise.

❽ Keep your head straight and level and look straight ahead at all times.

## TECHNIQUE AND FORM

The technique and form will be the same for both the standing machine and the standing dumbbell raise.

❶ Keeping your body as straight as possible, lower your heels toward the floor and slowly bring the calves to a full stretch.

❷ Hold this position for a count of 1 second.

❸ From this position, without momentum, push off the balls of your feet and come up on to your tiptoes, pushing as high off the toes as possible. Contract the calves as hard as you possibly can and con-

# Standing Calf Raise

centrate all of your efforts on doing so. Hold this position for a 1 second count.

**4** Slowly begin lowering your body to the stretch position, making sure you make the calf muscles endure the negative portion of the resistance.

**5** As you reach the bottom position, with the heels pointing to the floor, make sure you do not allow your heels to drop too fast. Go slow and focus on the stretching of the calf muscles.

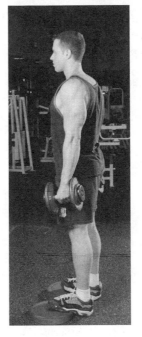
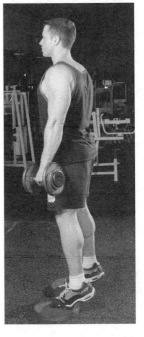

## VARIATION

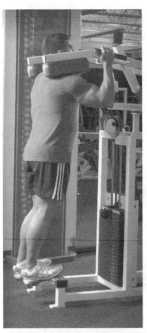
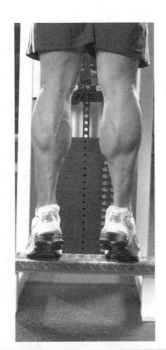

## VARIATION

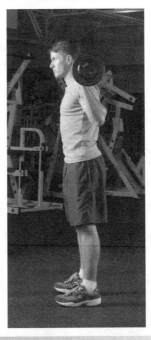
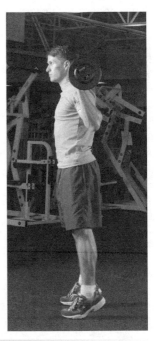

# Seated Machine Calf Raise

This exercise primarily targets the soleus muscles underneath the gastrocnemius. This movement is an excellent tool for shaping the calves.

## PROPER ALIGNMENT

**1** Choose a weight with which you can practice perfect form. The object is to use good form rather than just trying to lift a gargantuan amount of weight.

**2** Sit down and position your feet on the platform.

**3** With your feet pointing straight ahead, place your toes and the balls of your feet on the platform.

**4** Place the padded support on top of your thighs. Make sure that the pad fits snugly against the thigh close to the knee rather than high on top of the thigh.

**5** Position your hands on the sides of the thigh pad.

**6** Keep your torso straight and do not lean forward or backwards during the exercise.

**7** Keep your head straight and level and look straight ahead at all times.

## TECHNIQUE AND FORM

**1** Once you are in position and ready to begin the exercise, lower your heels toward the floor and slowly bring the calves to a full stretch.

**2** Hold this position for a count of 1-2 seconds.

**3** From this position, without momentum, push off the balls of your feet and come up onto your tiptoes, pushing as high off the toes as possible. Contract the calves as hard as you possibly can and concentrate all of your efforts on doing so. Hold this position for a 1-2 second count.

**4** Slowly begin lowering your body back once again to the stretch position, making sure you make the calf muscles endure the negative portion of the resistance.

**5** As you reach the bottom position, with the heels pointing to the floor, make sure you do not allow your heels to drop too fast. Go slow and focus on the stretching of the calf muscles.

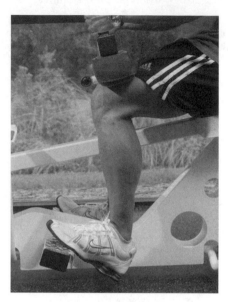

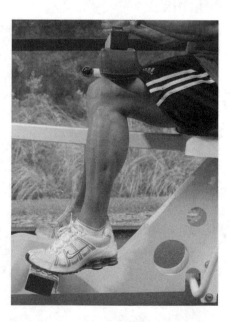

# Seated Machine Calf Raise

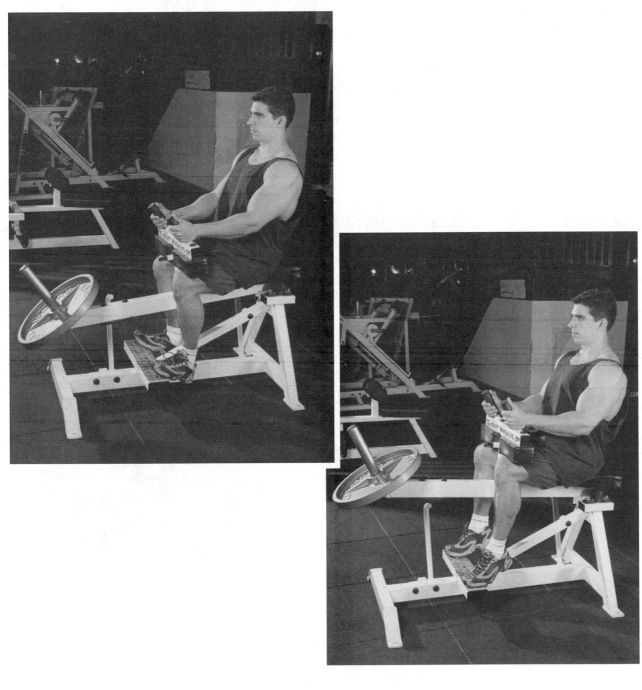

# Donkey Calf Raise

This is a great exercise for the calves because it helps to develop the entire calf musculature. You have the option of performing this exercise in a few different ways. One way is with the use of a specially designed machine called the donkey calf press. Another way, which might seem a bit odd, is by using the assistance of another person who actually sits on you!

Most gyms will have a piece of fitness gear called the "Dip Belt." It is a leather belt with an attached chain that allows you to add weight plates. Look at the picture below to see how it looks and how it is used. Instead of using a machine or the assistant, you simply strap the belt to your waist, add weight and begin. Follow the same steps listed below with the exception of #4 To purchase a dip belt, refer to the resource page in the back of the book and visit our web sites for all of your fitness gear needs.

**PROPER ALIGNMENT**

❶ Take a firm grip on a bar or the rail of a staircase.

❷ Bend over at the hips, so that your torso is parallel to the floor.

❸ Place a 4-5 inch platform or piece of wood beneath your feet.

❹ Have your assistant sit upon the lumbar region of your lower back, making sure that it is secure. They must be sure not to move around or one of you could be seriously injured.

**TECHNIQUE AND FORM**

❶ Make sure that you are secure and in stable alignment.

❷ Begin by pressing up onto the tips of your toes, focusing on the entire calf area.

❸ Press up as high as you can and briefly hold the contraction.

❹ Slowly lower yourself, bringing the heels down towards the ground for a deep stretch. Do not go too deep; gauge yourself.

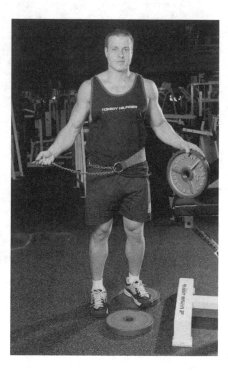

# Donkey Calf Raise

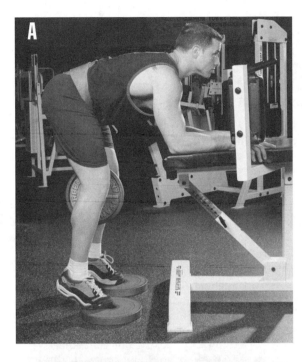

A

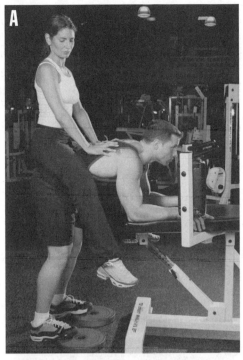

A

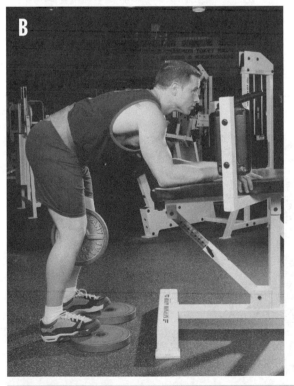

B

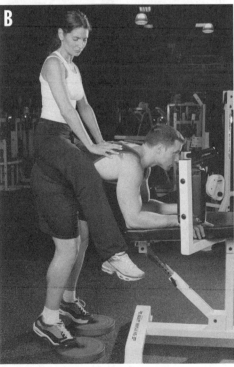

B

# Calf Press

This particular exercise zones in on the gastrocnemius muscles of the calves. It is performed on the same machine where you do your leg presses. This is an excellent alternative to standing calf raises for people that have lower back injuries.

There are two ways to perform this exercise: one leg at a time or both legs at the same time. In this book we will discuss the more common two-legged version. However, the execution for the exercise remains the same for both versions.

**VARIATION:** The calf press may also be accomplished on a plate-loaded machine.

### PROPER ALIGNMENT

❶ Step on to the platform of the machine and place your feet about 3-5 inches apart.

❷ Load the machine with the desired resistance.

❸ Position your feet on the platform so only the upper edge of your foot rests on the platform. The other half will hang off the platform.

❹ Take hold of the handles, usually located to the sides of the machine.

❺ Try to keep the legs straight during the exercise, with your knees slightly bent.

### TECHNIQUE AND FORM

❶ Maintaining your form, raise up onto the tips of your toes as high as you can and hold.

❷ Focus on contracting the calf muscles at this point. It is one thing to just do the movement, it is another to intensely participate in it!

❸ Slowly lower yourself, bringing the heels towards you for a deep stretch. Do not go too deep.

> **FAQ:**
>
> *When I perform the Calf Press, should I keep my knees locked out?*
>
> **ANSWER:**
>
> Locking out your knees can not only damage your knees, but actually takes away from stimulating your calf muscles. You may think that locking out your knees helps you to fully contract the calves, but you will actually be able to get a better range of motion by keeping a slight bend in both knees.

## VARIATION

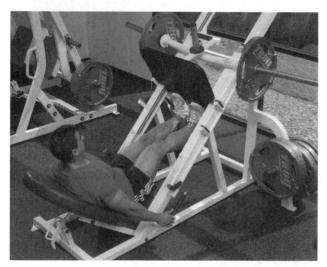
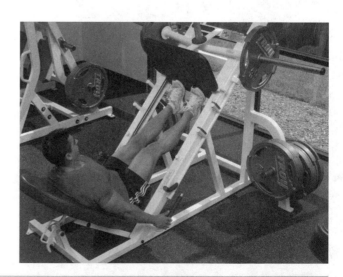

# Calf Press

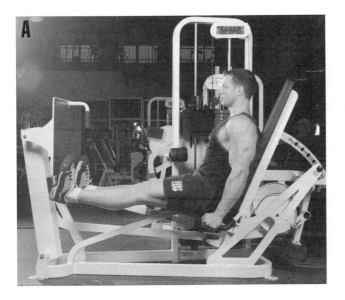

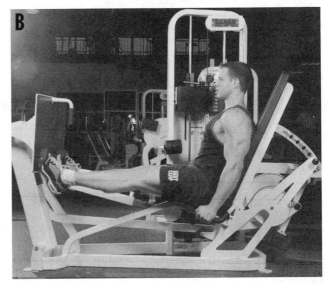

**CLOSE UP**

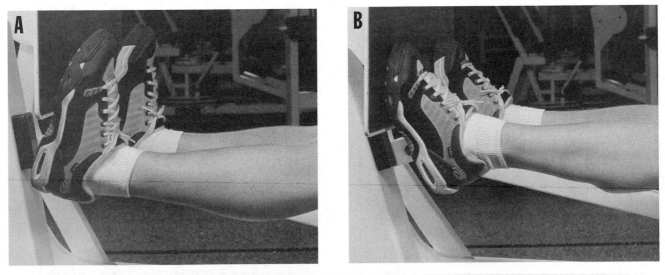

# Tibia Raise

This exercise works the front of your calves, and depends on your body weight as resistance. If you're interested in making it more difficult and need to add resistance, you can hold a dumbbell between your feet (squeezing your feet together to grip the dumbbell securely).

## PROPER ALIGNMENT

❶ Pull a calf block or other type of raised platform up to a fixed object that can support your weight (like a squat rack).

❷ Step up onto the calf block, placing your heels on the forward edge. Your feet should be facing straight ahead, with toes pointing down and your legs slightly less than shoulder-width apart.

❸ Reach out with one arm to hold onto the fixed object to keep your torso in balance. You should not be using the object to take away from the resistance of the exercise.

## TECHNIQUE AND FORM

❶ Lower your toes until they are at a comfortable position with your heel solidly on the calf block.

❷ Now exhale, and raise your toes towards you. Point them up as high as possible.

❸ Hold one second in the contracted position.

❹ Inhale while lowering your toes back to the original position.

❺ Pause for a moment at the bottom of the movement, then repeat for the recommended number of repetitions.

# Tibia Raise

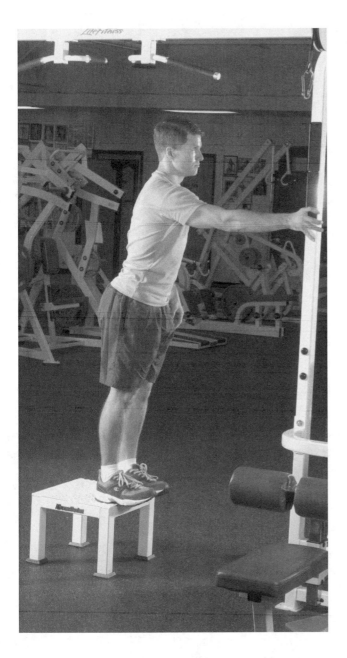

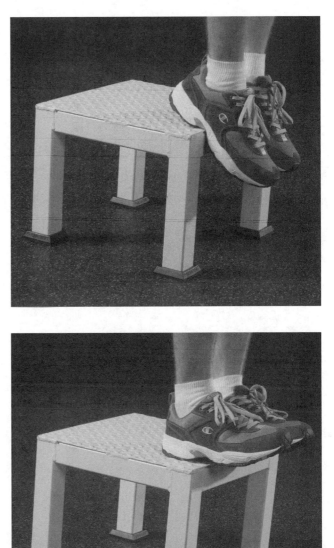

# Chapter 7
# Back

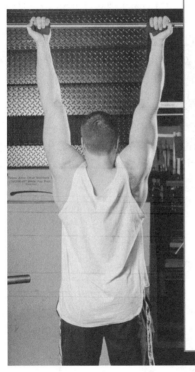

The back is composed of several different muscles. They are the second most neglected muscles by guys (the first being legs) since most people figure that which cannot be seen from the front cannot be important. However, we are here to tell you that not only can a well developed back be seen from the front (as lats do get wider), but it also creates a powerful V-shaped look that will turn heads. Besides, the wider and thicker your back is, the smaller your waist looks.

We will focus on the very best exercises for full development of the back region. Pay attention to the proper alignment, technique, and form principles as this will help to ensure your success.

For immediate Body Sculpting Bible support & coaching directly from James & Hugo, please visit www.BodySculptingBible.com

**7**

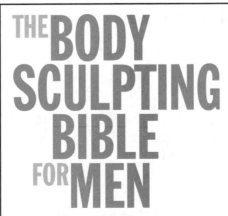

## A WORD ABOUT EXERCISES THAT UTILIZE VARIOUS HAND POSITIONS AND HOW EACH VARIATION CAN AFFECT DIFFERENT MUSCLE GROUPS.

Although many people do not enjoy reading information full of jargon, sometimes we need to learn important facts that in turn will produce the results we wish for. Do not underestimate the power of the information contained below.

Most people do not realize just how powerful a slight variation in your handgrip and hand position on the exercise bar can be. This variation of your hand placement can stimulate completely different areas of muscle concentration.

Whether you choose a wide-grip or narrow-grip, an overhand-grip or an underhand-grip, the area of muscle concentration will in some way be different. The enormous variety of exercise bar attachments available to us further enables us to attach many diversely shaped attachment bars to a pulley cable system. (If you are unaware of the large assortments of attachment bars available to you and how each works, refer to the web site resource page in the back of this book for further information).

You can perform exercise movements that are almost identical to one another, but the difference in exercise bars, hand placement, grip position and the mechanics of the body, will result in stimulating many different muscle groups.

Just as you may not have been able to pull yourself up with the wide-grip pull-up exercise, you might also have difficulty doing a narrow-grip pull-up. If you look at the differences between the wide-grip pull-up and the narrow-grip pull-up, you will notice that the wide-grip pull-up utilizes a wide and overhand grip placement. The narrow-grip pull-up utilizes a narrow and underhand grip placement. Now take a moment and think about which muscles are primarily working when you perform a wide-grip

pull-up or a wide-grip pull-down. Because of the overhand-grip you take with these particular exercises, muscles such as the forearm muscles (extensor muscles), shoulder muscles (deltoids), and the back muscles (latissimus dorsi and erector spinae) will take a majority of the work efforts necessary to carry out these movements.

During the underhand narrow-grip pull-up, because of your underhand grip placement, the biceps muscles take the majority role of prime muscles involved during exercise execution. Although your focus should be to keep the biceps from becoming involved too much during this exercise and to instead concentrate on stimulation of the back muscles, it can be extremely difficult, if not impossible to completely avoid the participation of the biceps muscles.

This discussion should begin to help you realize the enormous benefits of practicing the mind/muscle connection and muscle control techniques found within the Zone-Tone method.

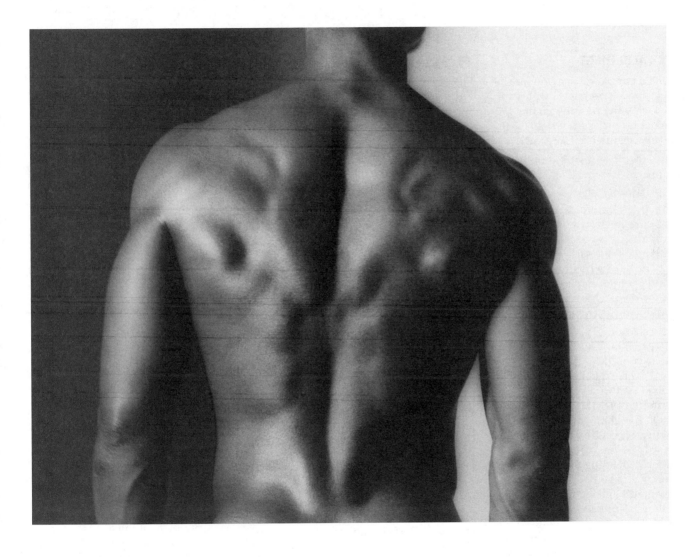

# Bent-Over Barbell Row

The bent-over barbell row places primary emphasis on the mid back muscles and the latissimus dorsi with a secondary emphasis on the on the lower back, rear deltoids, and biceps. If you follow correct training protocol, you will soon be able to move up in weight. People with lower back problems are better off using the dumbbell version.

## PROPER ALIGNMENT

❶ Place a bar in front of you on the ground, or on a rack level with your hips. Placing the bar any higher will just make it harder for you to lift it when the weights are increased.

❷ Align your feet about shoulder-width apart.

❸ Make sure your knees are pointing directly in front of you throughout the movement. (Do you notice the similarities in postural and alignment positions for all exercises so far? They are all relatively the same since nothing really changes except for the positions of the body, depending on the exercises performed.)

❹ Bend over at the hips, making sure that your lower back is not slumped over. To make sure of this, squeeze or contract your abdominal section while slightly arching your low back, mimicking again yourself sitting in a chair. Do not bend over all the way as this can injure the lower back. Bending at the hips to a position where your upper arm (triceps) can still follow directly towards the ceiling is sufficient for back muscle stimulation. If you stand too upright, this positioning will not sufficiently activate the back muscles. You must be bent over to a degree where the elbows will naturally remain close to the body. At the same time, the back of the arms (triceps) follow a row-like movement, directly towards the ceiling.

❺ Pick up the bar using either a palms-down or a palms-up type of grip. The palms-down grip is recommended for beginners as with this grip there tends to be less biceps involvement. Advanced trainees can benefit from a palms-up grip as it stresses the "lats" in a more direct manner. Also, at the advanced level, trainees know how to keep the biceps from getting as involved throughout the performance of the exercise.

❻ Stick out your chest while slightly squeezing your shoulder blades together. This will position and keep your body in the proper alignment throughout the movement. Holding these alignment positions throughout the exercise will help make sure that stimulation remains in the back muscles.

❼ Keep your head up and looking straight ahead throughout the movement. This will help you keep your balance and make it easier to maintain the described position.

With a few practice sessions, you will be able to perform the exercises with ease. We have noticed that once most clients learn to correctly execute exercises they often make dramatic progress within the first few days of beginning the program.

## TECHNIQUE AND FORM

As you pick up the bar, think about what muscles you are about to exercise. The latissimus dorsi, also known as the "lats," are located on the outermost side of the back and are a good point of focus.

❶ Align your body in the correct postural alignment.

❷ Let the bar hang down.

❸ Keep the elbows slightly wider than shoulder width.

❹ Slightly squeeze the shoulder blades together.

❺ Begin rowing the elbows up toward the ceiling, allowing the back of the arms (triceps) to lead the motion.

❻ Drive the elbows and back of the arms upward until the barbell is touching your lower belly and you are able to fully contract the back muscles. Imagine that there is an egg in the middle of your back. Your objective for each repetition, when the bar is being pulled to your belly, is to crack the egg with your back muscles.

❼ Try to squeeze and hold that position for a 2-second count, focusing on an intense contraction of the back muscles. When you consciously squeeze the muscles at the top of the movement, you are simultaneously learning to isolate those specific muscles. When you apply this technique to an exercise, you are actually optimizing your training

# Bent-Over Barbell Row

sessions through the increased muscle recruitment.

**8** Begin your descent with a slow and controlled movement.

**9** As you reach the bottom, slowly and smoothly begin the movement upward again without resting. Make sure that no momentum is involved while changing over from the bottom position to the upward movement.

Once again, when your form starts to get sloppy, STOP! Either reduce the weight or take a rest in preparation for the next set.

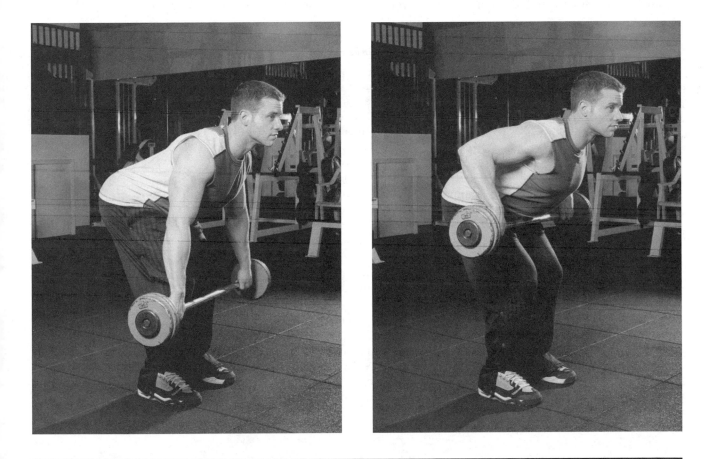

---

**FAQ:**

*I sometimes see people bent over to a degree where their torso is completely parallel to the floor. Is this safe?*

**ANSWER:**

No. When you bend over that much, you are more likely to injure your lower back. It is very important to maintain a lumbar curve in your lower back during this type of exercise. If you bend to where your torso is parallel to the floor, it is not going to make the exercise any more effective and is far more dangerous.

# Bent-Knee Deadlift

This exercise should be taken very seriously. If you have any type of back problems, substitute a rowing motion instead. If you have a healthy back and feel comfortable performing this exercise, also ensure proper form and never slouch as this can cause back injury. Be very cautious when adding weight—when in doubt, use less weight instead of more. Always ensure that you can handle the load. It is very effective but additional weight can make this exercise very dangerous to the lower back because of slight changes in form.

Dumbbells can also be used with this exercise, but you may find using the barbell to be easier because it is easier to find the correct rhythm of the exercise when using the barbell.

## PROPER ALIGNMENT

❶ Stand facing a loaded barbell.

❷ Keep your back as straight as possible, bend your knees, and bend forward, grasping the bar with a medium (shoulder-width), overhand grip (palms facing down).

❸ Make sure your knees are pointing straight ahead for the entire movement. Your head and eyes should be pointing straight ahead for the duration of the exercise as well.

## TECHNIQUE AND FORM

❶ While holding the bar, start the lift by pushing your legs while getting your torso to the upright position. You should be exhaling throughout the movement.

❷ In the upright position, stick your chest out and contract your back and abs by bringing your shoulder blades back. Think of how soldiers look when they are at attention.

❸ Inhale and return slowly to the starting position by bending at the knees and leaning the torso forward at the waist. Make sure to keep your back straight.

❹ When the weights on the bar touch the floor, you are back in the starting position and ready to do another repetition. Perform the desired number of repetitions smoothly and without using momentum.

# Bent-Knee Deadlift

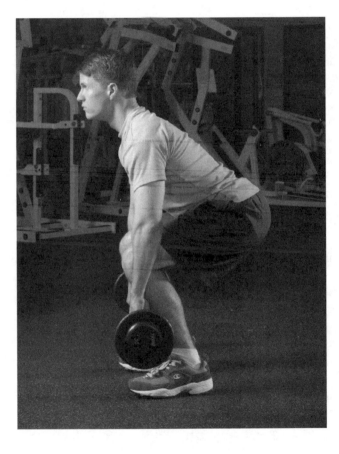

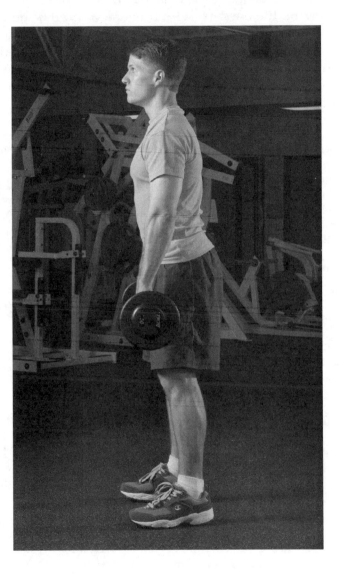

# Dumbbell One-Arm Row

The dumbbell row emphasizes the same set of muscles as the bent over barbell row version with an added benefit of less lower back involvement. In addition, this exercise allows you to focus more on the back muscles because you will be doing one side at a time.

There are two ways to perform this exercise: one arm at a time or both arms at the same time (in which case the exercise will be identical to barbell rows except for the fact that the palms of the hands will be facing your torso). In this book we will discuss the more common one-arm version. This exercise variation is great if you have back problems or are concerned that you have not yet mastered the bent-over row exercise yet.

## PROPER ALIGNMENT

This exercise is very similar to the bent-over row. You will be exercising the same muscle group, the back muscles; however, with the dumbbell row your position will be different and you will be exercising one limb at a time as opposed to two.

❶ To start, pick up a dumbbell that is light enough to focus primarily on form. Many people find that practicing perfect form with a light weight is much easier than practicing with no weight. The reason for this is because the resistance helps you to feel the desired muscle being exercised, making it easier to isolate and stimulate that muscle. This is another example of the "mind-to-muscle" connection.

❷ Find a bench and set the dumbbell at the right side of it.

❸ Position your right foot on the floor while positioning your left knee on the bench. Your left hand should be positioned slightly in front of your body on the bench. Lean slightly into your left hand to help support your bodyweight. Here you will be training the right side of your back.

❹ Pick up the dumbbell with your right hand while remembering to support your bodyweight with your left hand.

❺ Your back should be parallel to the floor. The back should be flat as you lean over from the hips and you should be looking straight ahead to help maintain balance and form. Do not look down or up during the exercise.

## TECHNIQUE AND FORM

As you pick up the dumbbell, think about what muscle you are about to exercise; the right side of the back called the latissimus dorsi, or the "lats."

❶ Align your body in the exercise's correct postural alignment.

❷ Let the dumbbell hang down.

❸ Slightly lift the right shoulder blade, making sure that it maintains a level position.

❹ Begin rowing the right elbow up toward the ceiling, allowing the back of the arms (triceps) to lead the motion.

❺ Row the right elbow and back of the right arm up towards the ceiling, and row as far as you can until the back of the arm and elbow reach the level of the torso. Make sure that you are fully contracting the right

side of the back muscles. Imagine that there is an egg in the middle of your mid-back. Your objective, when the dumbbell is being rowed, is to squeeze the right side of the back muscles to the left and crack the egg with your back muscles.

❻ Try to squeeze and hold that position for a 2-second count, focusing on an intense contraction of the back muscles.

❼ Begin your descent with a slow and controlled movement.

❽ As you reach the bottom, slowly and smoothly begin the movement upward again without resting. Make sure that no momentum is involved when changing over from the bottom position back to the upward movement. Again, when your form starts to get sloppy, STOP! Either reduce the weight, or take a rest in preparation for the next set.

# Dumbbell One-Arm Row

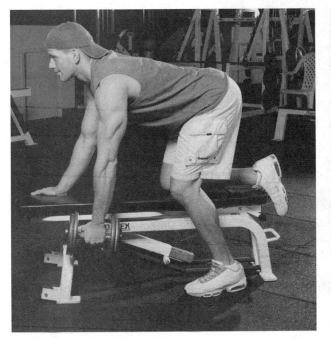 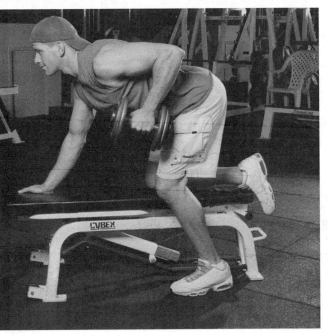

**FAQ:**

*I always see guys using big weights during this exercise. I want a powerful back. How heavy should I go?*

**ANSWER:**

Have you ever paid close attention to the people using those huge amounts of weight for this exercise? Often, the person is barely bent over and is using more momentum than a sling shot. The objective of this exercise is to stimulate the back muscles. Let the muscles you intend to stimulate do the work, not your ego! That will get you your big back.

# Two-Arm Row

This is a great exercise for your back, but improper form could lead to injury. This exercise is not recommended for people with back problems. Instead, try a seated low-pulley row with a V-bar. Make sure you maintain perfect form for this exercise and never slouch the back forward, as this can cause back injury. If you are new to this exercise, begin using a small amount of weight.

### PROPER ALIGNMENT

**1** Hold a dumbbell in each hand with your palms facing your torso.

**2** Your knees should be bent slightly, head up, and your shoulders back. The weights should hang with your arms perpendicular to the floor.

**3** Now, push your torso forward by bending at the waist, keeping your back straight until it is almost parallel to the floor.

### TECHNIQUE AND FORM

**1** While holding your torso stationary, exhale and lift the dumbbells to your ribs. Keep your elbows close to your body. You should not be using your forearms for anything but positioning.

**2** At the top of the contraction, squeeze your back muscles and hold for one second.

**3** Slowly lower the weights to the starting position, inhaling as you do so.

# Two-Arm Row

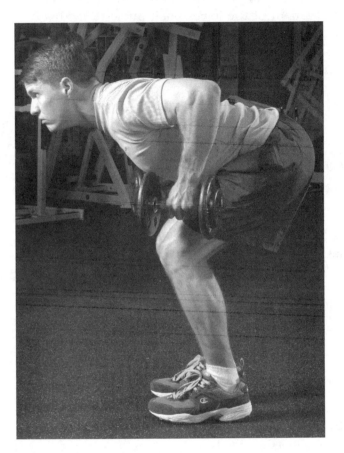
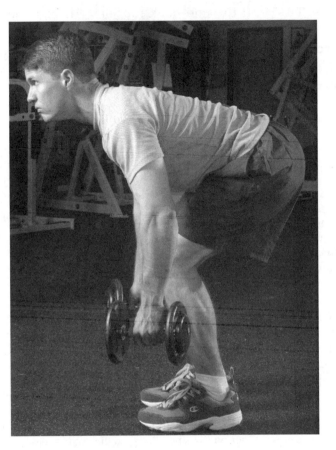

# Wide-Grip Pull-Up to Front

The pull-up is a very challenging back exercise. However, its ability to deliver quick results and functional upper body strength makes it well worth its weight in gold. Its main emphasis is on the "lats" and the mid-back muscles. There is no involvement of the lower back muscles in this exercise. Secondary muscles involved are the rear deltoids and the biceps.

**Note:** If you cannot pull your own body weight there are two things that you can do. If your gym has Gravitron machines (machines that assist you in pulling your body weight) feel free to use those. If your health club is not equipped with such machines, then either have someone provide assistance by holding your legs or just use the pull-down machines. Then, when you get strong enough, feel free to start doing pull-ups.

## PROPER ALIGNMENT

The pull-up focuses on the natural resistance and mechanics of the body. Too many people perform this exercise incorrectly. They use too much momentum, do not use a full range of motion, or simply do not know the proper technique and form to follow for optimum results.

❶ To start, take hold of an overhead bar with an overhand grip.

❷ Align your body by spacing your hands about shoulder-width apart. It's important to realize that different hand spacing will sometimes focus on one muscle more than another. We recommend a grip 1 1/2 times your shoulder width since it will help keep the biceps from being stimulated and is a great position for back muscle stimulation.

❸ Contract your abdominal section, which helps to sustain your postural alignment throughout the movement.

❹ Stick your chest out while depressing your shoulders (downward), which will help isolate the intended musculature of the back.

❺ Throughout the movement, always keep your head and eyes looking up. Knowing that you must reach your target position at the top adds that extra push.

## TECHNIQUE AND FORM

❶ Holding onto the bar with an overhand grip 1 1/2 times your shoulder width, let your body hang while bending your knees and crossing your feet.

❷ Keep your elbows as wide as you can while you pull your body up.

❸ As you are pulling up, make sure your chest is sticking out as much as possible. Your shoulders should be depressed (downward) and as relaxed as possible.

❹ When you reach the top (which will be when you can no longer move upward while maintaining the proper alignment), consciously focus on squeezing and contracting the back muscles as hard as you can. Try to hold that contraction for at least 1-1/2 seconds, which will help to isolate the back muscles.

❺ As you begin your descent, slowly lower your body while mentally focusing on the back muscles being activated. When you feel yourself fatiguing or losing control on the way down, try to pull back up. You'll notice that as you get tired, even

your best attempt to pull yourself back up will not stop your descent. This technique will add some intensity and overall stimulation of the back muscles.

❻ For a full range of motion, let your arms straighten completely at the bottom of the movement. Most people only come down two-thirds of the way and leave out perhaps the most important portion of the exercise—the fully stretched position. Next, slowly and smoothly begin the transition upward once again without using any momentum.

# Wide-Grip Pull-Up to Front

## WIDE-GRIP PULL-UP WITH ASSISTANCE

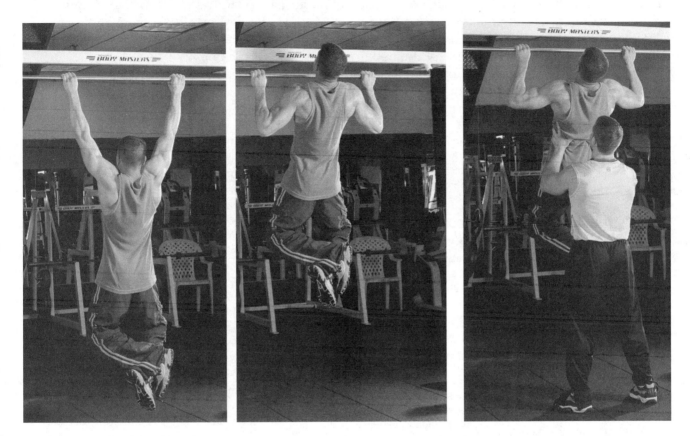

**FAQ:**

*In the exercise description, you mention depressing the shoulders downward. How do I do this and why?*

**ANSWER:**

Depressing the shoulders downward helps to take some of the initial stimulus away from the trapezoid, rhomboid, and teres muscles of the upper back. These muscles are naturally stimulated during a pull-up. When you lower your shoulders, you will help block the assistive muscles and force the lats to become the primary working muscles.

# Close-Grip Pull-Up

Some people think that similar looking exercises, such as this and the wide-grip pull-up, will affect the same musculature of the back. This couldn't be further from the truth. Wide-grip pull-ups focus on widening the muscles of the upper back and lats. Narrow-grip pull-ups focus more on widening the muscles of the lower lats and also on the serratus muscles (the little finger-like muscles) located on the lower outside of the pecs, near the front of the body.

Avoid making the biceps the primary muscles stimulated in this exercise by focusing on form and concentrating your mind on the back muscles.

## PROPER ALIGNMENT

❶ Choose your grip of choice, either the parallel close-grip bar or the underhand chin-up. No matter which grip you choose, both of the exercises will be done the same way.

❷ Take your grip and focus all of your attention on the lower lat muscles of the back.

❸ Hang from the bar with arms at full length. The object of this exercise is to angle your body backwards so that your chest is able to contact the parallel bars or chin-up bar for a greater muscle contraction in the lats.

❹ Bend your lower legs at the knees and cross your feet.

❺ Stick your chest out as far as possible and lean your head back.

❻ The key to isolation of the back muscles and negation of the biceps is to isometrically contract the lat muscles as you hang. The isometric contraction will help activate the lat muscles well before the exercise begins. This will help you to better control and force the lat muscles to become the major muscles being stimulated during the exercise. If you don't know how to isometrically contract the muscles, practice posing in the mirror without using any weights.

Once you isometrically contract the lats and have set yourself up into the proper alignment, you can begin the exercise.

## TECHNIQUE AND FORM

❶ First, with your lats already isometrically contracted and your body and head leaning back on an angle, begin slowly pulling your body upwards.

❷ As you are driving your way upward to the top of the movement, keep your elbows riding close to your body, rowing them back behind you. You should start to see how the back muscles become stimulated through exercise. The reason you are angled backwards here is so that the elbows can follow their natural arc across and behind the body.

❸ At the midway point, moving upward, you should really be feeling the lat muscles working and taking on the majority of your body's resistance. If you don't, stop and practice using light weight on a pull-down machine.

❹ As you reach the top of the movement, you should try to touch your chest on the bar, or at least come close to doing so.

❺ Your main objective in this upper position is to contract the lat muscles as hard as you possibly can and hold

that position for a count of 1-2 seconds.

❻ From this point, it is very important for you to slowly lower yourself from this position. The negative resistance you'll achieve while lowering your body is extremely valuable for overall muscle stimulation. Too many people, simply let their muscles go limp and drop immediately from the top position to the bottom position, completely wasting the valuable negative component of this exercise.

❼ As you reach the bottom position, let your arms hang completely straight, allowing for a full and complete stretch of the lats.

❽ In this position, without resting, once again isometrically contract the lat muscles. Remember, by activating the lat muscles first, you will help isolate them right from the beginning of the exercise.

❾ Align your body and head on an angle leaning backwards and begin pulling upward again in a smooth and fluid motion without using momentum.

# Close-Grip Pull-Up

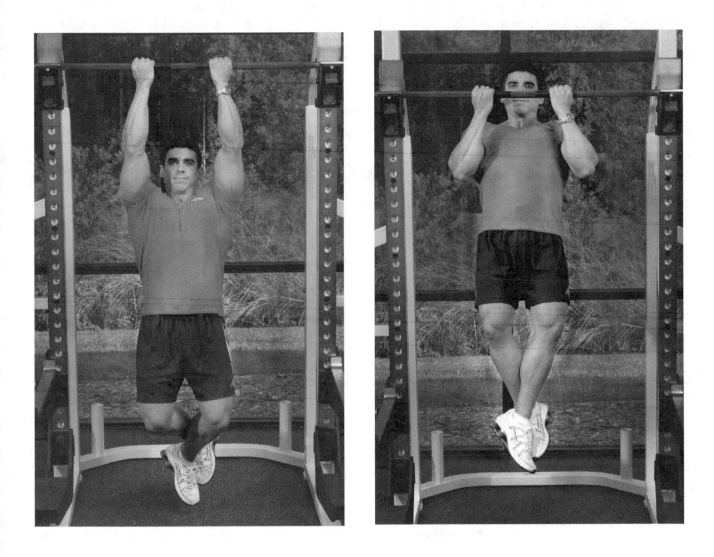

# Neutral-Grip Pull-Up

The pull-up is a difficult exercise that requires a lot of upper body strength. This version widens the lower lats and the small serratus muscles on the lower outside of the pecs. The pull-up can deliver fast results and functional upper body strength. It focuses on the natural resistance and mechanics of the body. It is easy to perform it incorrectly. Do not use momentum—it is necessary to perform a full range of motion in order to see results. Always use the proper technique and form.

If you do not have the strength to do this exercise, use a pull-up assist machine if available. These machines use weight to help you push your body up. Another option is to have a spotter hold your legs. If neither of these two options is available, then substitute a pull-down using the V-bar attachment.

If you are looking to add weight to this exercise, try using a weight belt.

## PROPER ALIGNMENT

❶ You will need to use a V-bar (the triangular bar with two handles used for the low pulley rows) and a pull-up bar. To begin, place the middle of the V-bar in the middle of the pull-up bar. The V-bar handles will be facing down-this way you can hang from the pull-up bar using the V-bar handles.

❷ Once you have secured the placement of the V-bar, hold onto the bar on each side and hang from it. Hold your body steady; keep your head and eyes looking up the entire movement. Knowing that you must reach your target position at the top adds that extra push.

❸ Stick your chest out and lean back slightly in order to better engage your lat muscles.

❹ Contract your abs-this helps you sustain your postural alignment throughout the movement.

## TECHNIQUE AND FORM

❶ Pull your torso up, using your lats, and contract your abs while leaning your head back slightly so that you do not hit your head on the chin-up bar and stick your chest out as much as possible. Your shoulders should be as relaxed and depressed as possible.

❷ Exhale and continue until your chest nearly touches the V-bar.

❸ Hold for a second or two in this contracted position, consciously focusing on squeezing and contracting the back muscles as much as possible. Holding the contraction helps to isolate the back muscles. Then slowly lower your body to the starting position as you inhale and focus on your back muscles being activated. When you feel yourself fatiguing or losing control on the way down, try to pull back up. You will notice that as you get tired, even your best attempt to pull yourself back up will not stop your descent. This will add to the overall intensity and stimulation of the back muscles.

❹ For a full range of motion, let your arms straighten completely at the bottom of the movement. The fully stretched position is perhaps the most important segment of the exercise. Lowering slowly and with control is essential. It enables you to reap the muscle-building benefits of the negative or eccentric phase of an exercise (the phase during which you elongate your working muscles).

❺ Without resting or using momentum, repeat this exercise slowly and smoothly for the recommended number of repetitions.

# Neutral-Grip Pull-Up

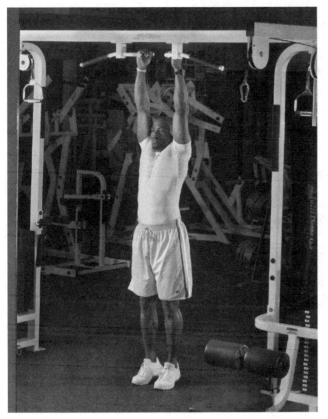 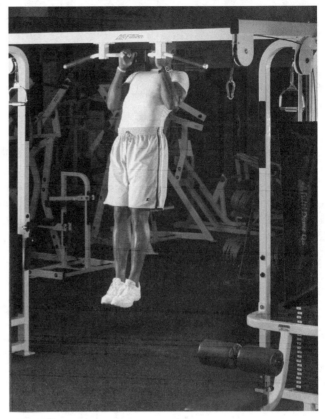

**FAQ:**

*I rarely ever see anyone doing pull-ups - Aren't pull-downs a more effective back exercise?*

**ANSWER:**

The reason why you probably don't see many people doing pull-ups in your gym is either your gym doesn't have pull-up bars or more likely, the exercise is too difficult for most people to do. This doesn't mean that because they are difficult, you should shy away from them. Yes, pull-ups take some practice to perfect, but once you get the hang of them, they can quickly become one of the most productive and challenging upper body exercises there are.

The only way you can progress at doing pull-ups is to practice. By practicing consistently and challenging yourself to always exceed the level and performance of your previous workout session, you will inevitably get to the point where pull-ups become easier and easier to do.

When you do get to that point where you can do 8 to 12 pull-ups, using a full range of motion and no momentum, then it will be time to further challenge yourself by adding additional weight (using a weight belt or weight plate held between your thighs.)

# Wide-Grip Pull-Down

If you are not able to pull up your own body weight, you can use the lat pull-down machine to help increase your strength. Although the pull-up is a much better exercise for back muscle development because it works with the body's natural mechanics and range of motion, the pull-down can help prime and get you ready for the pull-up. If you use this exercise, really concentrate on isolating and contracting those back muscles.

## PROPER ALIGNMENT

**1** Position the thigh support so that you are in a snug position with your feet placed flat on the floor.

**2** Choose your desired weight and take a grip equal to twice your shoulder width.

**3** Lean back slightly from the hips while contracting the abdominal muscles for support.

**4** As you prepare to pull down, stick your chest out while keeping your elbows wide.

**5** With a slight lean backwards at the hips, your chest pushed out and your elbows wide, you are ready to begin the exercise.

## TECHNIQUE AND FORM

**1** Once in position and focused on the muscles of the back, pull the bar down to your collar bone while maintaining your postural alignment.

**2** Make sure that you pull the bar down in a smooth, controlled manner, letting the muscles of the back do the work and not your biceps or momentum. If you don't know the difference between controlled form and momentum already, you will feel the difference in muscle stimulation when you use controlled form.

**3** As you reach the bottom of the movement, make sure to squeeze the back muscles for a count of 1 1/2 seconds with the bar close to or touching the collar bone.

**4** Slowly begin moving the bar upward and allow it to return to the start position.

**5** When you reach the top, do not rest! Immediately begin pulling down making sure you do so slowly while maintaining the correct form and postural alignment. Remember the time under tension principle of continued motion and no rest. You are here to work, not rest. You will accomplish a great deal more by keeping constant tension in the muscle throughout the entire set as opposed to resting at every transition of the top and bottom positions.

---

**FAQ:**

*In the pull-up exercise, you request that you depress the shoulders to help isolate the lats. Would it make sense to do that here, as well?*

**ANSWER:**

Yes! There are many things to remember and if you can remember to include the depression of the shoulders maneuver, in addition to the other variables of the pull-down exercise, it will only help to enhance the results.

# Wide-Grip Pull-Down

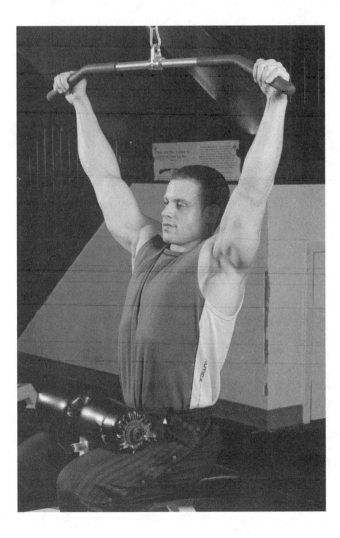
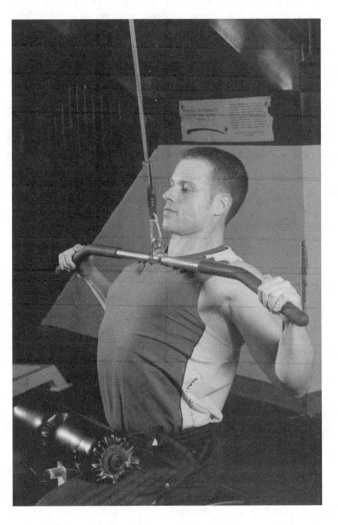

# Close-Grip Pull-Down with a V-Bar

During the narrow-grip pull-down exercise, the positioning of your hands will take a different hand position and grip placement when compared to the narrow-grip pull-up. The narrow-grip attachment in the pictures at right has two handles that are structured parallel to one another. When you take your hand position, the palms of your hand will be closely facing each other.

As you can clearly see, your whole arm position has now changed in comparison to the narrow underhand-grip pull-up. Notice how close the arms are to one another. You can see how the arms remain close to each other from the beginning of the exercise to the finish position. If you were to perform the narrow-grip exercise and immediately follow with the wide-grip pull-down exercise, you would feel a major difference in the muscles stimulated. This is evidence of how dramatic the variation in bar attachments and your hand placement can be in stimulating different muscles.

The same way you have the option of using the lat pull-down machine to help you if you are not able to do a wide-grip pull-up, you have the option of performing the narrow-grip pull-down exercise, if you cannot yet do a narrow-grip underhand pull-up.

**VARIATION:** One variation you can try is the Close-Grip Pull-Down. In this variation, you will install a wide bar instead of a v-bar, and grasp the bar with palms facing your torso and a narrower than shoulder-width grip.

## PROPER ALIGNMENT

❶ Position the thigh support so that you are in a snug position with your feet placed flat on the floor.

❷ Choose your desired weight and take your desired narrow grip that we discussed above.

❸ Lean back slightly from the hips while slightly contracting the abdominal muscles for support.

❹ As you prepare to pull down, stick your chest out while keeping your elbows narrow and close to your body.

❺ With a slight lean backwards at the hips, your chest pushed out and your elbows staying close to your body, you are ready to begin the exercise.

## TECHNIQUE AND FORM

❶ Once in position and focused on the muscles of the back, pull the bar down to your upper chest region, while maintaining your postural alignment.

❷ Make sure that you pull the bar down in a smooth, controlled manner, letting the muscles of the back do the work, while trying to avoid your biceps or momentum from becoming involved. If you don't know the difference between controlled form and momentum already, you will surely feel the difference in muscle stimulation when you use correct, controlled form.

❸ As you reach the bottom of the movement, make sure to squeeze the back muscles for a count of 1 1/2 seconds with the bar close to or touching the upper chest region.

❹ Slowly begin allowing the bar to move upward, returning back to the start position.

❺ When you reach the top, do not rest! Immediately begin pulling back down, making sure you do so slowly while maintaining the correct form and postural alignment. Remember the time under tension principle of continued motion and no rest. You are here to work, not rest. You will accomplish a great deal more by keeping constant tension on the muscles, throughout the entire set as opposed to resting at every transition of the top and bottom positions.

# Close-Grip Pull-Down with a V-Bar

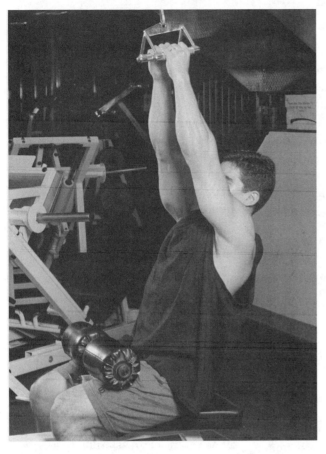

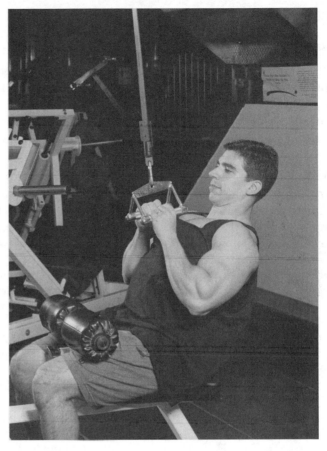

## VARIATION

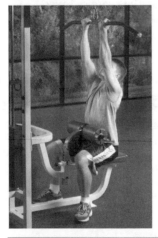
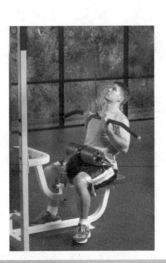

**FAQ:**

*When I do this exercise, it hurts my shoulders.*

***ANSWER:***

If you experience pain with any exercise, stop! It doesn't make any sense to continue doing an exercise if it is hurting you. Try variations of this exercise until you find a pain-free exercise. Some variations you can try include similar movements, hand grips, bar attachments, or machines. A simple modification can make all the difference in the world.

# Seated Low-Pulley Row

**(Lower Lats and Mid-Back Muscles)**
**Using a close-grip parallel attachment**

The low-pulley row is an exercise that most people perform incorrectly. They either lean too far forward in the beginning or too far backwards at the top, taking the stress off the lat muscles, or they use momentum instead of muscle to move the weight. You can choose a variety of different handles for this exercise. Each one hits a slightly different area of the back, providing a great variety for an exciting and never stale back routine. The description of technique and form below assumes that you will be using a close-grip parallel bar attachment.

## PROPER ALIGNMENT

**1** Once you attach the bar to the pulley system, take a seat on the machine bench.

**2** Choose a weight that will allow you to practice perfect form while also providing enough weight to stimulate the back muscles. Using too light a weight will keep you from feeling the desired muscle stimulation.

**3** Take hold of the bar, either leaning forward or having someone hand it to you.

**4** Sit straight up while you bend at the knees.

**5** Plant your feet evenly on each side of the platform and point them straight ahead.

**6** Slightly contract the abdominal muscles.

**7** Stick your chest out and retract the scapula and shoulder blades.

**8** Keep your elbows close to your body and hands down by your lower abdominals.

**9** Keep your head level and look straight ahead throughout the movement.

## TECHNIQUE AND FORM

**1** First, to avoid lower-back injury, make sure that your knees are bent and that you don't lean too far forward. A very slight lean forward is okay.

**2** With the arms fully stretched forward, retract the scapula from this position. This will pre-isolate the lat muscles of the back.

**3** Your objective will be to pull the bar back to your lower-to-mid abdominal section, making sure you adhere to the following steps.

**4** You will want to keep the elbows riding close to the body, helping to stimulate the back muscles. The farther you bring the arms away from the body, the less the desired muscles will be stimulated.

**5** As you begin pulling the bar toward your abdominal section, stick your chest out as far as it will go while you strive to sit straight up. Do not lean backwards.

**6** Concentrate completely on the lat muscles of the back so they do most of the work.

**7** When the bar reaches your abdominal section, squeeze the back muscles as hard as you possibly can. Picture having an egg planted square in the middle of your back. While the bar is touching your abdominal section, your main objective, while contracting the muscles of the back as hard as you can, will be to squeeze your shoulder blades together so hard that the egg breaks.

**8** Hold the contracted position for a count of two seconds.

**9** From the contracted position, slowly begin your return to the starting position with a slow and controlled movement.

**10** As you reach the starting position, slowly and smoothly begin pulling the bar towards you without resting. Maintain the same form as when you began the exercise, making sure that no momentum is involved while changing over from the contracted position to the starting position.

# Seated Low-Pulley Row

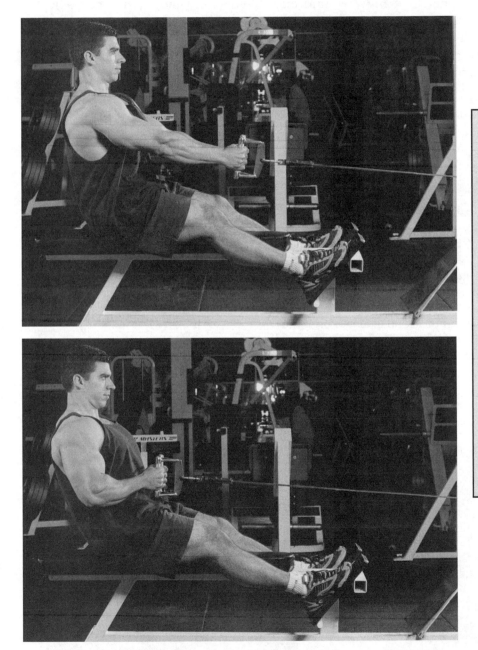

**FAQ:**

*When I do this exercise, it hurts my lower back.*

**ANSWER:**

This can be a tough exercise if you have a low back injury. This is especially true if you're going very heavy. The excessive weight will naturally pull you forward while your lower back muscles hold you in place. When you oppose the back muscles with the force of this pull, it can strain your lower back muscles. Your best bet is to maintain a strict lumbar curve in your lower back, keep your abdominals contracted to help secure your anatomical posture, don't bend forward at the hips, and avoid momentum at all costs. These four things will greatly diminish pain and strain to the lower back.

# Dumbbell Pullover

Although this exercise looks a little strange, it's great for the upper body. There are two variations: one that focuses mostly on the chest muscles and one that focuses mostly on the back muscles. In this section, we will be discussing the variation that focuses on the back. Please pay attention to the exercise description steps below to help differentiate between the two exercise variations. Not only will this exercise help to create a powerful and thick-looking back region, but it will also benefit the triceps muscles located in the back of your arms.

**VARIATION:** As a variation on this exercise, lie down on a bench, feet flat on the floor as in the Dumbbell Pullover. You will be using an EZ-Bar and a pronated grip to grasp the bar behind your head, lifting it over your chest. Throughout the movement, your elbows will be slightly bent.

**NOTE:** Pictured below is the incorrect way to perform the back Dumbbell Pullover. When you drop your middle, you are stimulating the wrong muscle!

### PROPER ALIGNMENT

**1** Lie with your body across a flat bench.

**2** Ensure that your neck and your upper back are the only body parts resting on the bench.

**3** Lift a dumbbell overhead and hold it at arm's length right in front of your face. (Please ensure that the dumbbells you are using have their weights properly secured).

### TECHNIQUE AND FORM

**1** Slowly lower the dumbbell over your head in an arc.

**2** Ensure that your hips are not being raised as you lower the weight.

**3** When you reach the fully stretched position, hold the stretch for a second and start raising the weight back up in an arc until you reach the starting position once again.

## CHEST

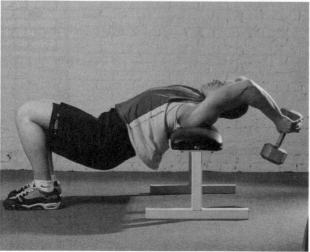
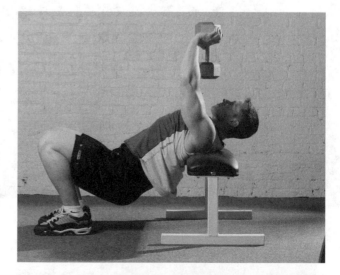

# Dumbbell Pullover

## BACK

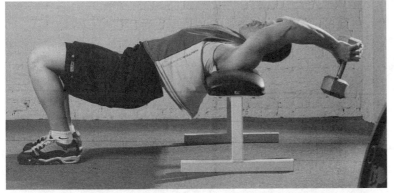

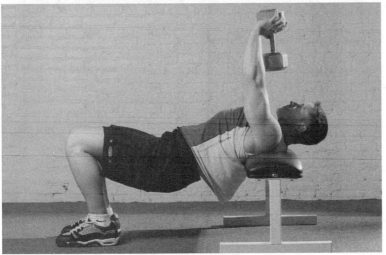

**FAQ:**

*In your exercise pictures, I see very little difference between the chest and back versions of this exercise. What are they?*

**ANSWER:**

With the chest variation, your objective is to sink the torso down as low as you can while simultaneously bringing your arms as low as possible, resulting in an exercise that functions from the shoulder joint only. For the back version, remember to keep those elbows locked in place and don't allow them to lower the dumbbell.

With the back variation, your objective is to keep the torso up and maintain that level throughout, while keeping your arms and elbows much straighter than in the chest variation.

## VARIATION

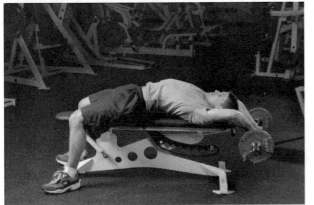

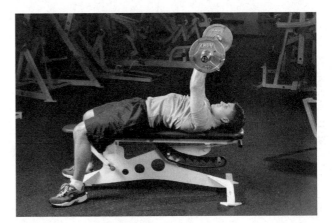

# Straight Arm Pull-Down

This is a great isolation exercise for the back as it allows you to work it without the involvement of secondary muscles such as the biceps. In addition, you get the bonus of working the abs indirectly as you will need to contract them in order to maintain the position required to perform the exercise.

## PROPER ALIGNMENT

**1** Stand in front of a pull-down bar with your arms extended in front of you holding onto the bar at shoulder width using a palms-down grip.

**2** In order to gain stability, bend your legs slightly at the knees, contract your abdominals and keep your weight at the heels.

**3** Keep the elbows slightly bent and the wrists in a locked position.

**4** Maintain a comfortable and forward tilt of the upper body in order to maintain stability throughout the movement.

## TECHNIQUE AND FORM

**1** Push the bar down toward the body in an arc, making sure that you are only moving from the shoulder joint and not extending at the elbow. There must be no movement at the elbow joint. It must be locked securely in place.

**2** Contract your lats as you lower the bar towards your thighs.

**3** As soon as the bar touches your thighs, hold the position for a second or two and then slowly go back to the starting position.

### FAQ:

*I've seen people using wider than a shoulder-width grip. Why?*

### ANSWER:

A shoulder-width grip usually makes for a great position to engage the back muscles, but what works for most might not work for you. If you don't think you are fully getting the benefit from the shoulder-width grip, by all means try another grip width. Try both narrower and wider grips and see what works best for you and your particular body mechanics.

# Straight Arm Pull-Down

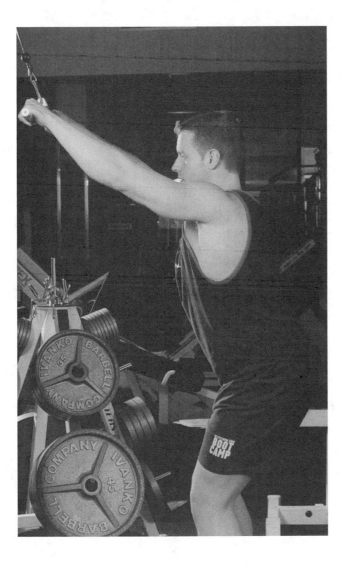
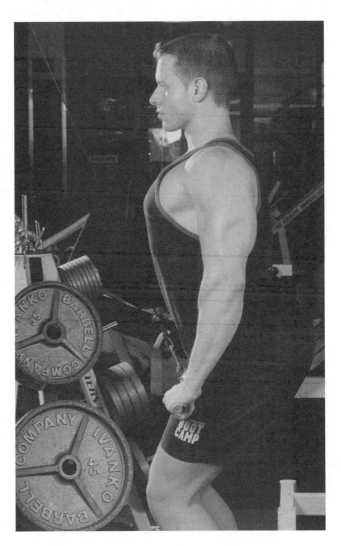

# Chapter 8
# Chest

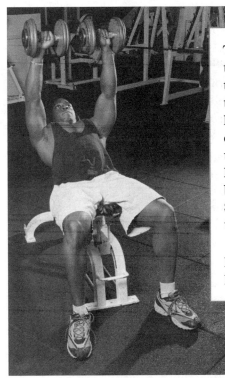

There are many misconceptions when it comes to men and chest training. While most guys think that the flat bench press is the exercise that will provide them with the big chest they are looking for, it is the incline bench press that will deliver the goods. When you develop a large upper chest, you create the optical illusion of having a gigantic looking chest. If you don't believe us then just look at pictures of Arnold Schwarzenegger and Lee Haney. You will notice that both have huge upper pecs.

For immediate Body Sculpting Bible support & coaching directly from James & Hugo, please visit www.BodySculptingBible.com

**8**

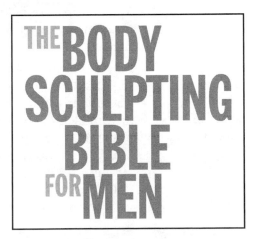

There are four areas of the chest that men should be emphasizing the most:

a)   Upper chest area with exercises such as the incline dumbbell press.

b)   Overall pec area with exercises such as the dumbbell press, chest dip and push-up.

c)   Outer chest upper area with exercises such as the incline dumbbell fly.

d)   Inner Upper Chest Area with exercises such as the incline cable crossovers.

We will mostly recommend dumbbells for the performance of chest exercises for several reasons:

•   They allow for both a greater range of motion and a deeper stretch at the bottom of the movements.

•   They allow for better isolation and muscle contraction at the top of the movements, helping to recruit more muscle fibers within the chest and surrounding musculature.

•   They are harder to control and hold than a barbell, helping to strengthen and develop the extremely important antagonistic and synergistic muscles of the chest and shoulders. Overall, the benefits you'll receive from using dumbbells outweigh the barbell by a long shot.

## PROPER ALIGNMENT

The postural alignment is basically the same for all of the following chest exercises. However, you will notice differences in some of the following positions, techniques and forms. The most important thing to remember is to always consciously focus and contract the muscles of the chest while maintaining the postural alignment and form during all of the exercises. This will help to stimulate the chest muscles during exercise.

The following sequence of movements will ensure that you learn how to properly lift a dumbbell off the ground and into position to start many of the exercises we describe. It will also demonstrate how to bring the dumbbells back to the start position of an exercise when you have completed it from a lying position. This is an invaluable technique to learn and can prevent many injuries from occurring.

1.   When you pick up dumbbells, make sure to bend at the knees while you lift the weight with your legs.

2.   Lift with your legs, not with your back! You can easily injure your lower back by bending over to pick up the weight.

3.   While standing, place the bottom plate of the dumbbells against your thighs and keep them there as you sit on the bench seat. You will find that by keeping the dumbbells against your thighs as you sit, it will allow you to easily manipulate them to the top of your thighs.

4.   Begin positioning your body into the correct postural alignment, starting from the bottom of your body and moving to the top.

5.   Space your feet about shoulder-width apart.

6.   Make sure your knees are pointing straight ahead throughout the movement.

7.   As you raise the dumbbells to the starting position on top of your thighs, do not try to muscle them up with your arm muscles. This will only drain your strength and can easily cause an injury. You need 100 percent of your strength for the exercise itself and cannot afford to waste it on something that you can easily avoid. To properly raise

the dumbbells from your thighs into exercise position, follow these guidelines; you will be using your leg muscles and momentum to help place you and the dumbbells into position. While sitting in an upright position, with the dumbbells on your thighs, thrust one leg up, leveraging one dumbbell up to around your chest level.

8. Immediately thrust the second dumbbell upward, while simultaneously allowing momentum and the dumbbells to guide you back into the lying position while your abdominal muscles help safely ease you into that position. The reason for lying back immediately when the second dumbbell is thrust upward is so you do not injure your shoulder joints or lower back from having to hold the dumbbells in that otherwise awkward position. Lying back immediately following the dumbbell's momentum while allowing the abdominal muscles to ease you into position will help ensure your safety and keep your strength at its peak for the exercise. This may sound difficult, but it's not. It is the safest and easiest way of getting the dumbbells into position (especially if you're using heavy dumbbells).

9. Once you've gotten the dumbbells up, lay back, until your back touches the bench.

10. The dumbbells should now be in position at the sides of your chest.

11. Again, make sure your feet are shoulder-width apart, and that they are flat on the ground at all times.

12. Make sure your knees are straight.

13. Your lower back should be flat against the bench at all times, with no excessive arc in the lower lumbar region (small of the back).

14. Make sure your back is flat against the bench, with the arms and elbows out to the sides and the forearms perpendicular to the floor. When you're correctly positioned, retract or squeeze the shoulder blades together. At first it may seem uncomfortable or odd, but do not underestimate the significance of this technique. You must learn to hold this position throughout the movement, and consistent practice will ensure this. By squeezing the shoulder blades together and keeping your entire back in constant contact with the bench, you will actually be taking the anterior shoulder out of the exercise. The chest muscles will now be the primary muscles lifting the weight.

15. Relax your head throughout the movement, and make sure you do not twist it or lift it from the bench while engaged in the exercise. Alignment is generally the same for all of the exercises.

---

**FAQ:**

*I see that you suggest manipulating the shoulders for an additional effect. What is the difference between the maneuver for the pull-up for the back and the pull-up for the chest?*

**ANSWER:**

The back pull-up requires you to depress your shoulders to block out the secondary working muscles. The chest pull-up requires that you now retract (or pull back) your shoulder blades (scapula). This helps to block the anterior (front) deltoids from being a primary working muscle during chest exercises. This particular maneuver can feel quite uncomfortable at first and you might feel frustrated that you won't be able to lift as much weight as you can when your shoulders handle much of the work.

Kick your ego out of the gym and realize that unless you're a power lifter, one of the main reasons you're here is to build a great looking physique. Building that beautiful physique is mostly about fully stimulating and isolating (as much as you can) the intended muscles-not about lifting as much as you can.

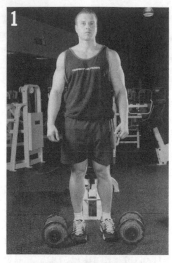

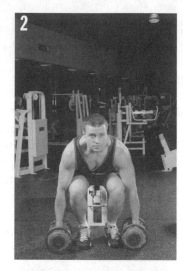

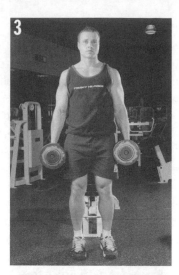

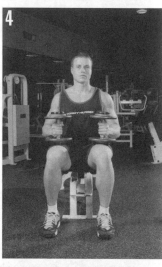

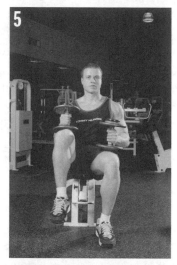

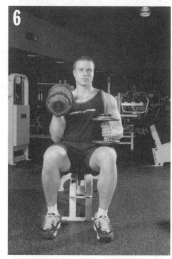

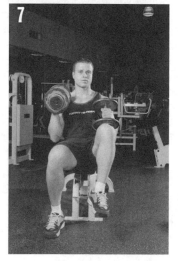

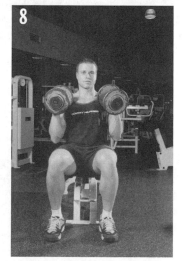

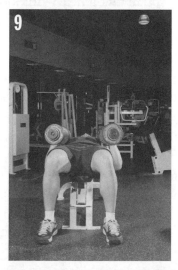

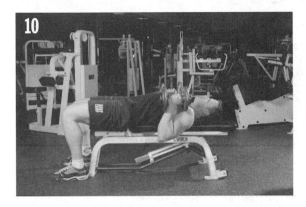

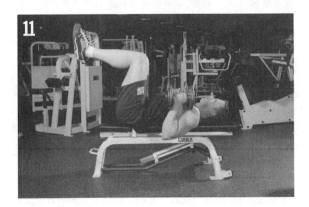

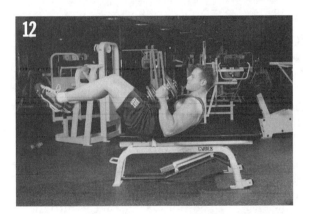

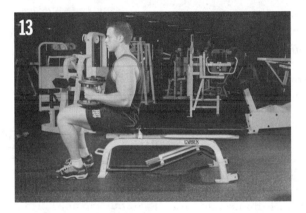

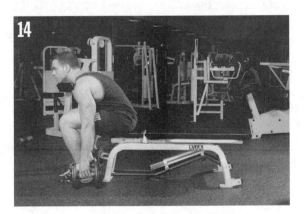

# Incline Dumbbell Press

This is an excellent exercise for the upper pectoral muscles. The dumbbells are more challenging than the barbells as they involve stabilizer muscles needed in order to keep the weights in balance. The exercise can be performed in two manners for variety: with palms facing away or palms facing each other. For both variations, the only difference is the position of the palms throughout the movement. However, the movement itself remains the same.

You will notice how you have the option of either touching the dumbbells at the top of the movement or keeping them separated when you reach the top of the movement. This is mostly preference and you will discover yours soon. Some people feel the ability to get a better muscular contraction in the chest muscles when they touch them at the top, while others feel like it is a waste of valuable time and strength. Try both and see what works better for you.

## TECHNIQUE AND FORM

❶ With the dumbbells on your thighs, thrust one leg up, leveraging one dumbbell up to about your chest level.

❷ Immediately thrust the second dumbbell upward while simultaneously allowing momentum and the dumbbells to guide you back into the angled, incline position. Use your abdominal muscles to help safely ease you into that position.

❸ As you are lying on the inclined bench, align your body as you were instructed above.

❹ Position the dumbbells out to the side of your chest, keeping your elbows wide and your forearms perpendicular to the floor throughout the exercise movement. Find a position that is wide enough to be comfortable and not so wide as to redirect the force to the shoulders. Some trainers believe that bringing the arms out excessively to the sides of the body will help to better isolate the chest muscles. This is a misconception that can actually inhibit chest development and worse, cause injury. The wider you go beyond a comfortable position, the more likely you are to redirect the force of the weight on to the shoulders rather than the pecs. Even worse, when you widen your arms excessively and then proceed to press a heavy or even moderate weight, you are actually causing the outer pectoral muscle to tear. Once again, bring your arms out to the side of your body to a point where they are still positioned wide, but not excessively!

❺ Because the incline dumbbell press positions you on an inclined angle, your shoulder muscles are more likely to move the weight than the chest muscles. To avoid this, not only will you want to retract the shoulder blades against the bench; but you must also depress or press the shoulders downward. This slight variation will take the shoulders out of the chest movement, allowing the chest to be the primary area worked during the exercise.

❻ With the chest in its elevated position, the elbows out and wide and the forearms perpendicular to the floor, press the dumbbells up toward the ceiling.

❼ As you reach the top of the exercise, you can either touch the dumbbells together or press them straight up like a bench press. You can play around with different positions at the top of the movement as you may get a better muscle contraction varying the dumbbell positions. Two people may use two different dumbbell variations in order to fully stimulate their chest muscles. The most important thing you are concerned with is getting the most intense contraction possible! There are a couple of different ways to do this. You can simply touch the dumbbells together and squeeze, or you can turn the dumbbells slightly inward at the top of the movement, allowing for a controlled and isolated contraction. Are you starting to see how you can apply the many new tools of this program to any and all facets of your training regimen?

❽ Begin lowering the weight while holding your proper postural alignment throughout the exercise.

❾ As your elbows and the back of your arms are lowered, bring the dumbbells to a level that is comfortable, making sure that the chest muscles hold the majority of the resistance. If you don't have any type of shoulder injuries or muscle

# Incline Dumbbell Press

impingement, you may allow the dumbbells to lower to a comfortable stretch where the dumbbells are parallel with your chest. Always make sure that you stay in control of the dumbbells and maintain this control throughout the exercise.

🔟 Once you reach the bottom position, slowly begin to press the dumbbells up again in a controlled, smooth and fluid motion without using any momentum.

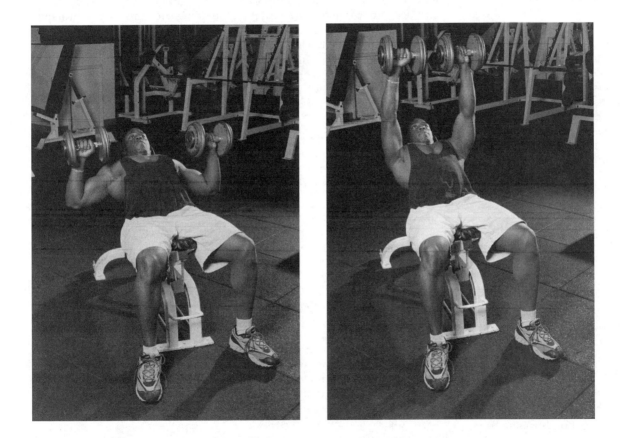

*FAQ:*

*Because I am now sitting on an incline versus a flat surface, does the shoulder maneuver still involve retraction of the shoulder blades?*

*ANSWER:*

Great question! Now that you are on an incline bench, simultaneously retract (bring straight back) and depress (pull down) your shoulders to help isolate the upper chest muscles as much as possible.

# Flat Dumbbell Press

This exercise primarily targets the muscles of the middle chest. As you will soon discover, the fact that you may be able to hoist very heavy weights with the barbell bench press does not necessarily mean that you will be able to do the same over here. At the end of this exercise, it is crucial that you use the techniques we present on how to handle the dumbbells as we have met many people that injure their shoulders from using incorrect techniques at the when they bring the dumbbells back to their starting position.

## TECHNIQUE AND FORM

This exercise requires you to use the same technique as the incline dumbbell press, but there will be some slight variations in your postural alignment. You will align your body the same way you did before, but now you will obviously be in a flat position. You'll want to focus more on retracting the shoulder blades rather than depressing them. Otherwise, follow the same technique and form for this exercise as you learned for the incline press.

❶ With the dumbbells on your thighs, thrust one leg up, leveraging one dumbbell up to about your chest level. Immediately thrust the second dumbbell upward while simultaneously allowing momentum and the dumbbells to guide you back into the lying, supine position (flat, with your body facing the ceiling). Use your abdominal muscles to safely ease you into that position.

❷ Lay back and align your body as you were instructed above.

❸ Position the dumbbells to the outside of your chest, keeping the elbows wide and the forearms perpendicular to the floor throughout the exercise movement.

❹ Because your shoulder muscles are more likely to move the weight than your chest muscles, you must retract the shoulder blades against the flat bench. This slight variation will take the shoulders out of the chest movement, allowing the chest to be the primary area working during the exercise.

❺ With the chest in its elevated position, the elbows out and wide and the forearms perpendicular to the floor, press the dumbbells up toward the ceiling.

❻ As you reach the top of the exercise, you can either touch the dumbbells together (as shown on image C) or press them straight up (as shown on image B) like a bench press. You can play around with different positions at the top of the movement as you may get a better muscle contraction varying the dumbbell positions. Two people may use two different dumbbell variations in order to fully stimulate their chest muscles. The most important thing you are concerned with is getting the most intense contraction possible! There are a couple of different ways to do this. You can simply touch the dumbbells together and squeeze, or you can turn the dumbbells slightly inward at the top of the movement, allowing for a more controlled and isolated contraction.

❼ Begin lowering the weight while holding your proper postural alignment throughout the exercise.

❽ As your elbows and the back of your arms reach parallel or bench level, slowly begin to press the dumbbells up again in a controlled, smooth, fluid motion, without using any momentum.

# Flat Dumbbell Press

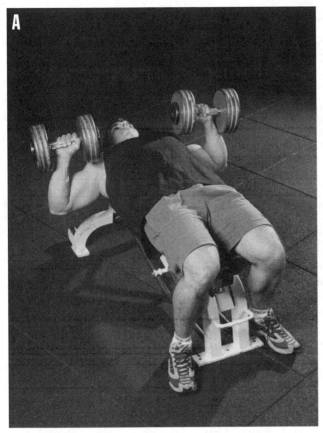

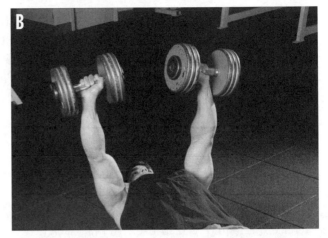

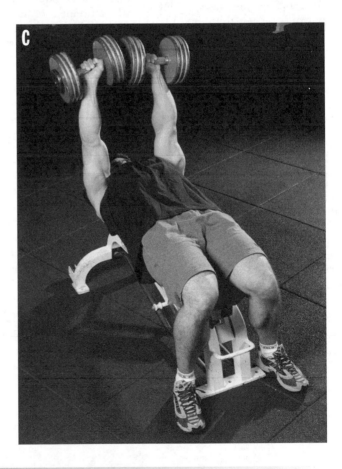

# Flat Dumbbell Fly

This exercise is truly a great one. It might seem a bit hard to master, but once you do, it will be a pleasure to perform. It might look as if this exercise is identical to the dumbbell bench press, but it is not. With the dumbbell press, you are extending at the elbow joint and utilizing something called horizontal adduction—a movement together—of the shoulder joints. The dumbbell fly must only incorporate the shoulder joints movement and not the elbow joints extension. The elbows must be locked into place to allow the true magic to begin. The flat dumbbell fly focuses on the mid-chest muscles.

## TECHNIQUE AND FORM

For this exercise, your postural alignment will be very similar to the other two chest exercises. However, this exercise will require you to use a different technique and form. With this exercise you will retract the shoulder blades just as you did in the flat and incline dumbbell press, but the angle of the movement is changed. Instead of using the combination of horizontal shoulder adduction (when the shoulders move inward), and elbow extension (when the elbows themselves flex and extend during pressing) as you would in the pressing movements above, for this exercise you'll lock the elbow joint in place. You will set up the arms just as you would for the flat dumbbell press with the arms wide and forearms perpendicular to the floor, but having the elbow locked will prevent any elbow extension or flexion. This technique will exclude the triceps from being involved in the exercise while focusing the resistance completely within the chest muscles.

❶ You'll want to align your body exactly as you did with the flat dumbbell press, but now you will have the palms of your hands facing each other instead of facing the wall in front of you.

❷ This time you'll be using a visualization technique while engaged in the movement of the exercise. As you begin to squeeze the dumbbells towards each other, you will be following an arc-shaped movement. As you follow this arc, I want you to picture yourself hugging a tree. In other words, make believe there is a tree between you and the dumbbells; you will be mimicking the exact motion of hugging it. This visualization technique will help keep you in the correct position to follow the arc movement. All of this will ensure that your chest muscles receive the most intense stimulation and contraction possible.

❸ As you reach the top of the movement, be sure to consciously contract the chest muscles as hard as you possibly can for maximum muscle stimulation!

❹ Begin lowering the weight while holding the proper alignment, technique and form throughout the movement. As you reach the bottom of the movement, be sure not to let the back of the arms go too far below the level of the flat bench as this could cause injury to the shoulders' rotator cuff. When you do reach the bottom of the movement, slowly begin squeezing the dumbbells upward in an arc again with a smooth, controlled, fluid motion, making sure that you avoid using momentum!

# Flat Dumbbell Fly

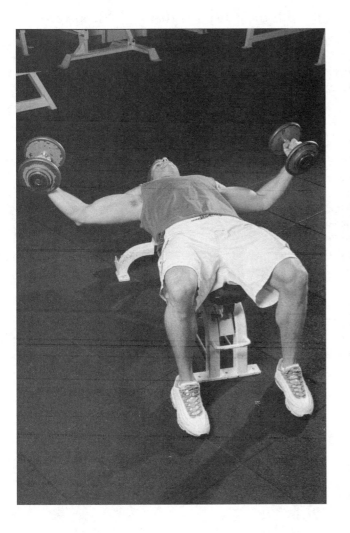
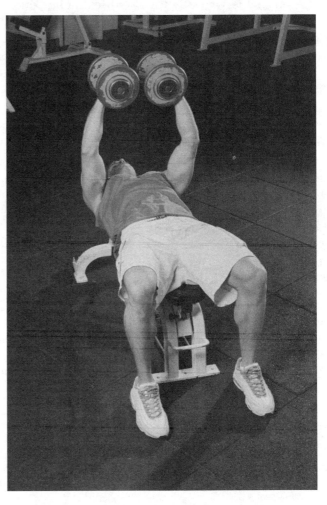

**FAQ:**

*How does the chest maneuver work with this exercise?*

**ANSWER:**

Because your anterior deltoids are in direct alignment with the line of movement, it is pretty difficult to take them out of this movement. The positive thing about this exercise is the fact that the triceps are not involved. When you take the triceps out of the movement, it becomes a very powerful way of helping to isolate stimulation in the chest muscles.

# Incline Dumbbell Fly

This exercise is virtually identical to the flat dumbbell fly with the exception that it will focus on the upper chest muscles. Remember that no matter what anyone tells you, it is impossible to avoid hitting muscles located in the same muscle groups. For example, if you are focusing on you lower abdominal muscles, you will inevitably be stimulating the upper abdominal muscles as well. It is great to zone in on the exact muscles you desire to train, but don't be surprised when other parts of the same muscle group are also feeling the work.

## PROPER ALIGNMENT

**1** Sit back on an incline bench with your feet wider than shoulder-width apart and flat on the floor.

**2** Make sure your shoulders are flat against the pad and your chest is out.

**3** Using your thighs to help you get the dumbbells up to your arms, clean the dumbbells one at a time and hold them at shoulder-width. Your backs of your hands will be facing behind you.

**4** Bend your elbows slightly to prevent stress at the biceps tendon.

## TECHNIQUE AND FORM

**1** Inhale while you lower your arms together in a wide arc. You should go until you feel a stretch on your chest. Your elbow joint will remain stationary, as the movement occurs solely at the shoulder joint.

**2** Pause for a moment at the bottom of the movement.

**3** Now, exhaling as you do so, return your arms to the starting position using the same arc of movement.

**4** Hold the upright position for a second and repeat for the desired number of repetitions.

# Incline Dumbbell Fly

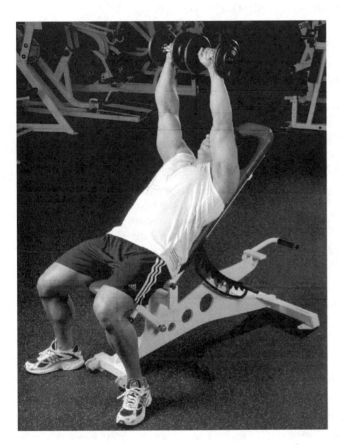 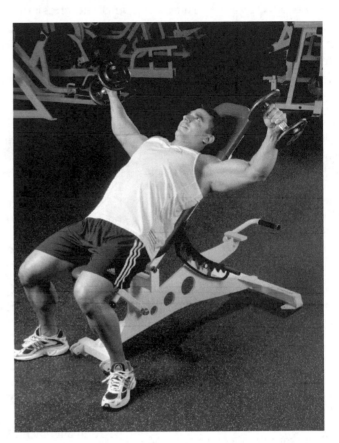

# Chest Dip

**(Using a parallel dip station)**

The chest dip is a great muscle-enhancing exercise that focuses on the lower chest and serratus muscles. Between dips and close grip chins you hit all upper body muscles! There is a major difference between the triceps dip and the chest dip. When we discuss the triceps dip later, we tell you to keep your entire body in a pin straight line, which helps to focus the majority of resistance on your triceps muscles. With the chest dip, we are only concerned with affecting the muscles of the chest. If you cannot do a dip, you might want to try using a weight assistant machine such as the Gravitron, which counter balances a portion of your body weight.

## PROPER ALIGNMENT

With this exercise, you'll want to bend at the knees, lock your feet and bend forward as you lower yourself. You must stay bent over to keep the focus of resistance in the chest muscles. These three steps will help transfer most of the resistance to the chest muscles and avoid triceps muscle recruitment. To do this, you will need a dip station or machine. If you are working out in your home, I suggest you purchase an inexpensive dip unit from one of the sports-related retail chains or a wholesale fitness supply store. In a wholesale store, you can usually negotiate a lower price and the quality of the apparatus is usually much better. Look in your local yellow pages for the store nearest you.

❶ Place your hands on the parallel bars as you position yourself for postural alignment.

❷ The best way to align yourself is to raise up onto the dip bars by locking out your arm. You will then align your body, starting with your head and moving down to your feet.

❸ While suspended in the top position of the exercise, your head will at first be level and looking straight ahead. You may find that bending your head slightly forward as you lower yourself will help you lean forward for increased muscle stimulation in the chest. You must constantly focus all of your attention on the chest muscles during this exercise as this will help increase their involvement, and keep you in the proper alignment.

❹ Bend your legs at the knees and hook your feet over one another. This will help keep your back arched forward for the ultimate involvement of the chest muscles. Your arms and elbows will ride away from your body as you lower yourself and when pushing upward to the lockout position. This will help keep the triceps muscles from becoming involved in the exercise.

## TECHNIQUE AND FORM

❶ Make sure that you have correct postural alignment. Begin the exercise once you are in position with your arms locked out (only in the beginning and end positions) and your body suspended from the floor.

❷ As you lower yourself from the lockout position immediately begin to lean forward. The farther you lean forward, the more your chest muscles will work.

❸ Lower yourself slowly while resisting your bodyweight all the way to the bottom position.

❹ Keep the elbows and arms away from your body, helping to better isolate the chest muscles and avoid recruiting the triceps muscles.

❺ Lower yourself until the backs of your arms are parallel or slightly beyond parallel with the floor. Remember, you should never go so low that you feel any chest or shoulder pain, or you could seriously injure yourself. Go to a point where you are comfortable and increase a little more the next session if needed.

❻ When you reach the bottom position, do not rest! Slowly, with a smooth transition, begin to press your body upward without using any momentum. Make sure that you maintain your postural alignment.

❼ As you begin pressing upward, make sure that all of your focus is once again directed to your chest muscles. This alone will help stimulate the triceps through increased muscle control. As you near the top of the motion, your goal is not to lock out the joint but to contract and squeeze the chest muscles as hard as you possibly can for a 1 second count. It is important for the chest muscles to hold you in this position rather than lock out with the triceps or the elbow joints.

# Chest Dip

**8** Remember that there should be no rest at the top of the exercise after the contraction period. From that lock out position, once again slowly lower yourself as you resist the weight of your body back to the bottom position. If you get to a point where your body weight is too light for the exercise, you may use a dip belt to hook some additional weight to your body, thus increasing the resistance. Please make sure that if you add weight, you do so in small incremental stages.

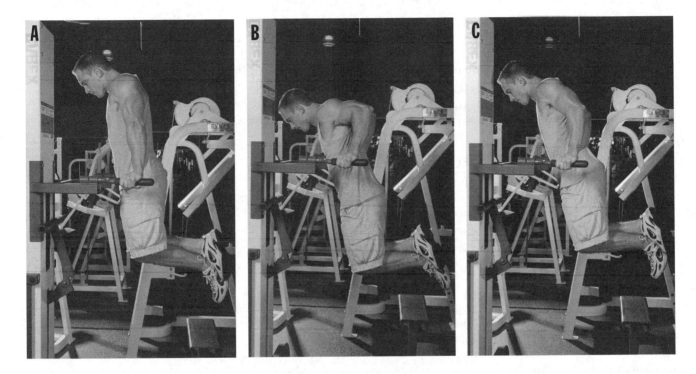

**FAQ:**

*When I do chest dips, I feel a lot of pressure and pain in my shoulders. Why?*

**ANSWER:**

The chest dip can be a very powerful and productive exercise. You do, however, need to make sure that you protect yourself from injury. Keep a few things in mind when doing the chest dip. Don't go too heavy, unless you know your muscles, joints, and connective tissue can handle it. Although you may be very strong and feel that your flexibility it great, you still may not be as strong as necessary to do this exercise at its full capacity. Don't go too low in your descent. To a degree, going low is great for training the chest through its full range of motion, but going too low defeats that purpose as eventually the chest will minimally be involved and the brunt of the stimulus will be directed to the shoulder.

# Incline Cable Crossover

Incline cable crossovers are very similar to the dumbbell fly, but there is a major advantage when you perform the incline cable crossover exercise. Only in the beginning of the dumbbell fly exercise is the majority of the resistance placed upon the chest muscles. This soon changes when the dumbbells are brought vertical (arms and dumbbells extended over the chest). At this point, instead of the pecs being responsible for sustaining the resistance of the dumbbells, the elbow joints and shoulders are. The force of gravity disappears when the arms are brought to this vertical position. Cable crossovers don't have this disadvantage. In fact, the degree of resistance remains constant throughout the entire movement.

Performing incline cable crossovers provides even greater benefits than the results obtained from doing regular cable crossovers. Incline cable crossovers add to the development of the upper chest muscles, and give you the appearance of a much larger chest overall. This exercise develops the pectoralis major and minor.

## PROPER ALIGNMENT

**1** Set the pin to the desired resistance and attach the handles to the cables.

**2** Sit down on an incline bench, your feet flat on the floor.

**3** Take hold of the handles with an overhand grip and position yourself so that you are in the middle of the pulley machine (in order to position yourself in the middle of the machine, you must pull each of the handles closer to you, thus lifting both weight stacks simultaneously.)

**4** Make sure that both weight stacks are even on the right and left sides. Do not allow the weight stacks to become uneven, or you will create a muscle imbalance when you begin the exercise.

**5** With the handles in hand, and palms facing each other, bend your elbows slightly and lock them there throughout the exercise.

**6** You will begin this exercise in the extended position (arms opened up as if about to give a hug) as opposed to the dumbbell fly where you started in a flexed (contracted) position.

## TECHNIQUE AND FORM

**1** To begin the exercise, keep the arms slightly bent and contract the chest muscles.

**2** Bring the cables across and in front of the body until the two hand-grips touch at the level of or just above your upper chest.

**3** Make sure to contract the chest muscles as hard as possible in this position and hold for a one second count.

**4** Once the two hands almost touch and you have forcefully contracted the chest muscles, let the resistance of the weight stacks bring the arms back to the starting position in a slow controlled manner.

**5** Repeat the movement.

# Incline Cable Crossover

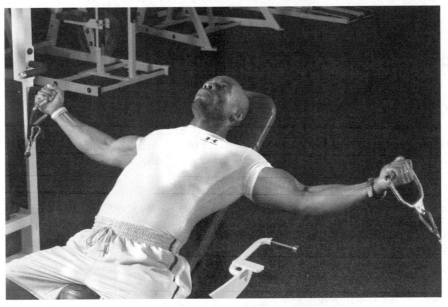

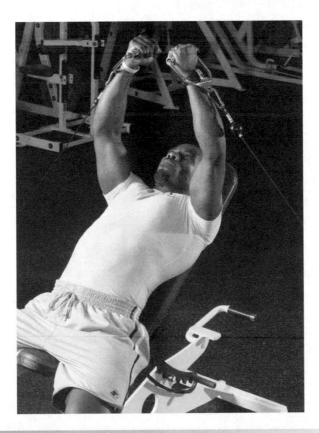

# Standing Cable Crossover

Much like the incline cable crossover, this exercise is superb in isolating your chest muscles. There are many different variations of this exercise, including varying the height from which the cable is connected, as well as varying the point where your arms meet.

## PROPER ALIGNMENT

**1** You will need to use a pulley machine for this exercise. Place the pulleys above your head, select the proper resistance, and hold the pulleys in each hand.

**2** Take a step forward from the imaginary straight line drawn between both pulleys while moving your arms straight out in front of you. Your torso will bend slightly from the waist.

**3** If it makes it easier for stability, place your feet into a shoulder-width stance. Otherwise, keep your knees together to better isolate the chest muscle.

**4** Bend your elbows slightly to prevent stress at the biceps tendon.

## TECHNIQUE AND FORM

**1** Inhale and extend your arms straight out to the sides in a wide arc until you feel a stretch on your chest. Throughout the movement, the arms and torso should remain still—movement should only occur at the shoulder joint.

**2** Using the same arc of motion, exhale and return your arms to the starting position. Pause for a second at the peak of the movement and repeat.

# Standing Cable Crossover

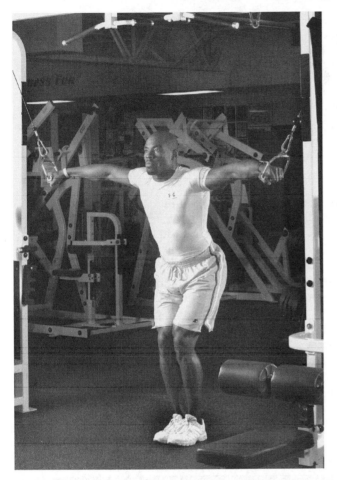 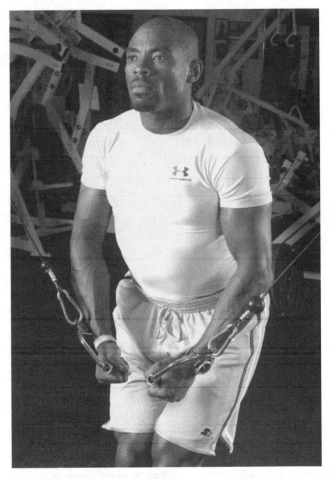

## VARIATION

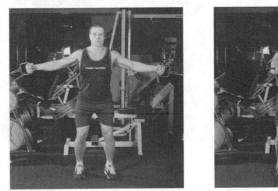

# Push-Up

The push-up has become a neglected exercise that hasn't received the acclaim it warrants. The push-up is a very powerful exercise for developing the chest muscles, triceps and anterior deltoid muscles. It allows the trainee to utilize the proper biomechanics, which can better help isolate the chest muscles. Push-ups work beautifully in a super-set protocol, helping to fully exhaust the chest muscles for total recruitment of the muscle fibers in the chest.

Please notice the variation of hand widths that you can play with here. The wider the hand width, the more focus on the outer chest muscles. The closer the hand widths, as shown in the diamond hand position on the next page, the more focus on the inner chest muscles and the triceps muscles of the arms.

### PROPER ALIGNMENT

❶ Align your body face down with your arms extended in an elevated position. Keep your elbows slightly bent.

❷ The hands will be flat on the floor directly underneath and a little wider than shoulder width.

❸ Keep the legs completely straight and your toes on the floor.

❹ Throughout the exercise, keep your head looking down in a neutral position.

### TECHNIQUE AND FORM

❶ With your body properly aligned, lower yourself to within one inch of the floor. Ensure that your elbows travel out away from your body. Push-ups performed with the elbows traveling close to your body mainly target the triceps muscles.

❷ Make sure to inhale through your nose on the way down and exhale through the mouth on your way up.

❸ Focus on your chest muscles (feel them working here) and push your body off the floor using your toes as a pivot point.

❹ Make sure to keep your back straight, stomach muscles tightened and your head in line with your body. Maintaining the proper alignment is crucial.

❺ When you reach the top of the movement, make sure to contract the chest muscles as hard as you can. Try to avoid hyper-extending the elbow joints!

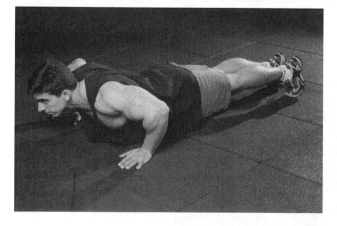
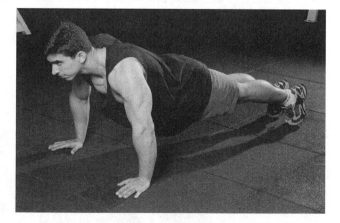

# Push-Up

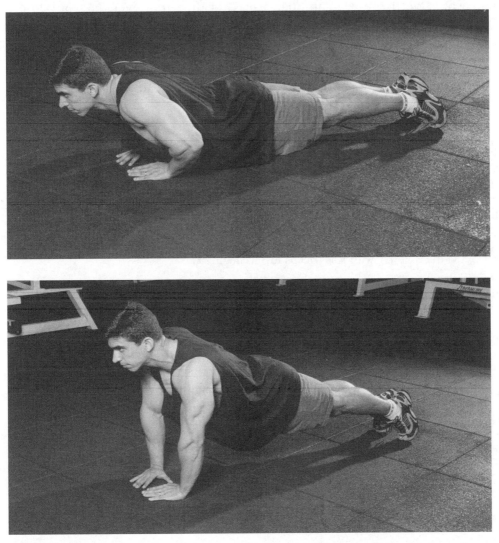

Narrow hand width will hit more of the inner chest and tricep muscles.

# Assisted Push-Up

If you need to, you may use this modified push-up exercise until you have gained enough strength to do the regular push-up. Take the same position and maintain the same form and technique as you would with the regular push-up. This time, however, let your knees stay in contact with the floor. You will find this exercise much easier because you will only be pushing up about half of your body weight. Follow the same procedure as the regular push-up.

If you can still not perform push-ups by using the modified position described above, then perform them standing up at an angle against the wall.

## TECHNIQUE AND FORM

❶ Take the same position and maintain the same form and technique as you would with the regular push-up. You will have a spotter stand behind you to help pull up your chest off of the floor. Make sure you are maintaining proper form and do not let the spotter support all of your weight.

❷ You will find this exercise much easier because you will only be pushing up about half of your body weight.

❸ Follow the same procedure as the regular push-up.

❹ If you still cannot perform push-ups by using the modified position described above, then perform them standing up at an angle against the wall, or in a regular position with your knees on the floor.

## MODIFICATIONS

Just as you can use various hand placement widths during the bench press exercise to focus in on specific areas of the chest, you can vary hand placement with the push-up.

• The wider your hand width, the more you'll zone in on the outer pecs with less triceps involvement.

• The closer the hand width, the more you'll zone in on the inner pecs with more triceps involvement.

• A medium hand width placement will be about 65 percent chest and 35 percent triceps.

# Assisted Push-Up

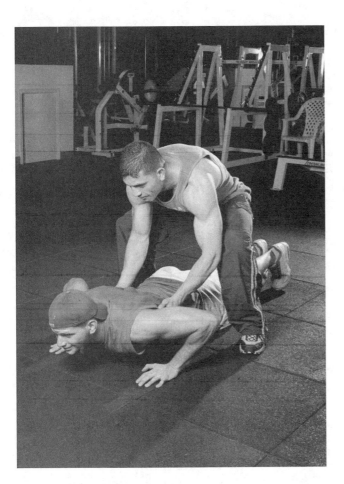 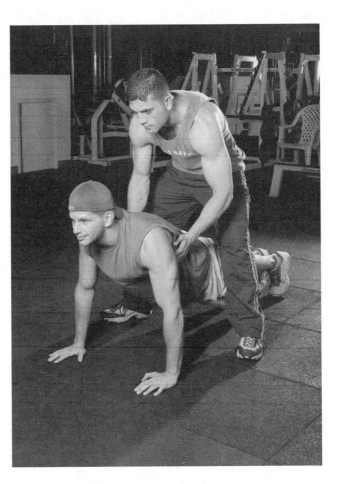

# Chapter 9
## Shoulders

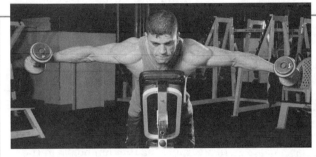

The shoulders are beautiful muscles when properly developed. They provide an appearance of width and also give the illusion of bigger arms. In order to achieve the three dimensional look that shoulders provide, all three heads (anterior, medial, and posterior) have to be developed.

The shoulders can be a very stubborn body part, especially if you don't know how to train them correctly. Even a slight variation in an exercise's proper form can mean the difference between no results and major results. Understand that most upper body exercises include the shoulders as a secondary muscle group, which could inhibit results for the shoulders because of over training. What it comes down to is this: if you don't learn how to train the shoulders correctly, you will not get the results you desire. If you learn what we teach here and implement the material into your shoulder training, you can definitely expect to receive the results you've desired.

For immediate Body Sculpting Bible support & coaching directly from James & Hugo, please visit www.BodySculptingBible.com

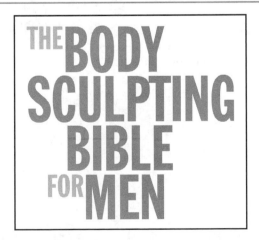

**9**

# Dumbbell Shoulder Press

The dumbbell shoulder press will focus on all of the muscles of the shoulder with primary emphasis on the front and side deltoids. In addition, the upper part of the movement will also involve the triceps muscles. Again, the balancing act that dumbbells require makes this a challenging exercise that will give you the best return on your effort.

## PROPER ALIGNMENT

❶ Set your bench setting to a 90-degree angle (fully upright position), unless of course you already have access to a 90-degree angle seat.

❷ Pick up your dumbbells and place them on your thighs.

❸ Align your body from the bottom up.

❹ Make sure that your feet are flat on the floor facing straight ahead throughout the exercise. Your knees should also be facing straight ahead.

❺ Make sure that your whole back is flush against the upright bench's back support. You must also concentrate on letting your chest relax. When you sit upright, it is natural for your chest to rise and move into the same upright position. This is bad because your chest muscles will end up becoming the primary muscles working during the exercise and will take the focus away from the shoulders. You want to focus on keeping your back straight against the back pad while completely relaxing your chest. This will help direct all of the stimulation onto shoulder muscles. If you see your chest rise or feel your chest muscles handling the majority of the work or helping to lift the weights, stop and correct yourself. You are either going too heavy or you just need to practice your form without weight. Once you are seated in a fully upright position with the dumbbells on your thighs,

thrust up one leg at a time. Let momentum help to lift the dumbbells into your starting position.

❻ Make sure that both dumbbells are held with your palms facing in front of you and level with the top of the shoulders.

❼ Relax your chest while keeping your back totally upright and your head and neck as relaxed as possible. Please note that you must never turn your head while doing any of these exercises. Position your body into proper alignment, keeping your head straight, and stay that way throughout the exercise. If you don't, you could end up seriously injured!

❽ Keep your elbows as wide as possible as if you were trying to touch your elbows behind your back.

❾ While keeping your upper arms horizontal to the floor, don't let the biceps and triceps sink below your shoulder height-this is the ideal level for a full range of motion for this exercise.

❿ Keep your upper arms in a perpendicular position while keeping your forearms pointed directly towards the ceiling at all times.

## TECHNIQUE AND FORM

❶ After you've set yourself up in proper alignment, slowly begin pressing the dumbbells up towards the ceiling in a smooth, controlled, fluid motion, making sure that you do not use any momentum. We advise that you do not touch the dumbbells at the top. Instead, press the weights in a straight-line overhead. Touching the dumbbells at the top of the movement may put some undue stress onto the rotator cuff muscles.

❷ When you reach the top of the movement, do not lock out the elbow joint. When you lock out the elbow joint, you distribute all of the weight from the shoulders to the elbow joint, thus interrupting muscle stimulation. This can hurt the elbow joint and limit shoulder muscle stimulation.

❸ Without resting, slowly bring the dumbbells back down, making sure that your arms are wide, your head is level and that you maintain an upright position with your chest relaxed.

# Dumbbell Shoulder Press

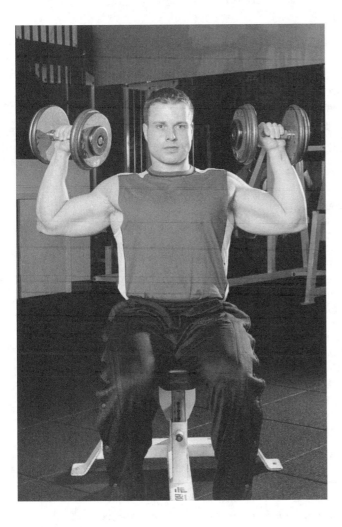
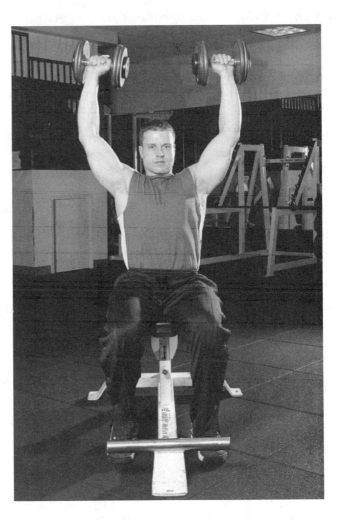

# Dumbbell Lateral Raise

The dumbbell lateral raise is a superb isolation exercise that primarily targets the side deltoid. When performed correctly, this exercise will add slabs of muscle to the medial head, providing you with extra inches of width. The key here is to leave the ego outside the gym: use a lower weight that allows you to concentrate on perfect form.

### PROPER ALIGNMENT

❶ Take a standing position with a shoulder-width stance. Align the body from the bottom up, beginning with the feet. Make sure the feet are pointing straight ahead.

❷ Keep the knees pointing straight ahead and slightly bent to help avoid any unnecessary back strain.

❸ Hold a dumbbell in each hand with arms down at your sides. Your palms should be pointed toward your body.

❹ It is important to remember that as you lift the dumbbells, your palms should be facing downward, so your shoulder muscles rather than the biceps muscles do the work.

### TECHNIQUE AND FORM

❶ Keeping your arms straight and at the sides of your body, lift the weights directly out to the sides until they reach the level of your cheeks.

❷ Hold the weights there for a one-second count.

❸ While maintaining your posture and body alignment, slowly lower the dumbbells in a controlled fashion back to the starting point. Make sure you pick a dumbbell weight that allows you to practice perfect form. If you pick a weight that is too heavy, momentum will force muscles other than the shoulders to do the work. Some people have the tendency to bend at the elbows, as incorrectly pictured to the right. Keeping the arms straight allows for better isolation of the medial deltoid.

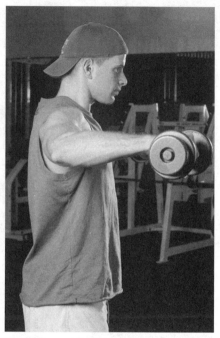

**Note:** Do not bend at the elbows as it is incorrectly demonstrated above.

---

*FAQ:*

*When I see people doing this exercise in my gym, they often bend their knees and then heave the weights up. What is this doing?*

*ANSWER:*

It's doing more harm than good. Using your knees to create momentum and lift the weights up and out to your sides does not benefit you at all. As you see in the exercise description picture, you lift the weight by focusing on lifting the elbows straight out to the sides of your body. Keeping the arms completely straight can be difficult and tough on the shoulder joints, which is why keeping a slight bend in your elbows will take some stress off of them.

# Dumbbell Lateral Raise

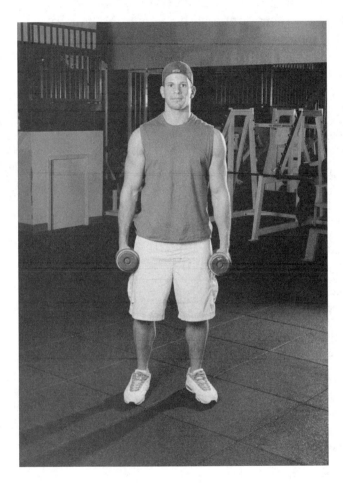
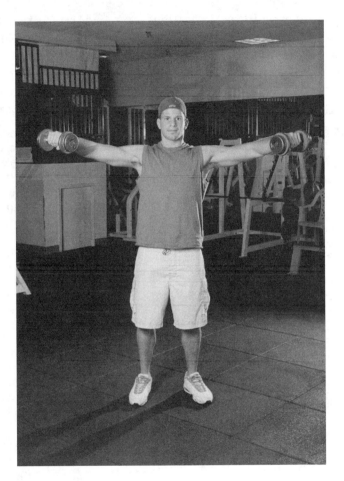

# Bent-Over Lateral Raise

This exercise develops the rear deltoids—the rear muscles of your shoulders—and helps to give your shoulders a three-dimensional appearance.

**VARIATION:** This exercise can also be done standing but those with lower back problems are better off performing this exercise seated. If you choose to stand, select a neutral position with a shoulder-width stance. Align your body from the bottom up, beginning with the feet. Make sure your feet are pointing straight ahead. Keep your knees pointing straight ahead and slightly bent to help avoid any unnecessary back strain. Hold a dumbbell in each hand. Look straight ahead. Bend over at your hips.

## PROPER ALIGNMENT

**1** Place a couple of dumbbells parallel to and in front of a flat bench.

**2** Sit on the end of the bench with your legs together and the dumbbells behind your calves.

**3** Bend at the waist while keeping your back straight in order to pick up the dumbbells. The palms of your hands should be facing each other as you pick them up.

**4** Make sure your abdominals are pulled in throughout this exercise.

## TECHNIQUE AND FORM

**1** Keeping your torso forward and stationary, and the arms slightly bent at the elbows, slowly and without momentum, lift the dumbbells straight out to the sides of the body until both arms are parallel to the floor—about shoulder height. Exhale as you lift the weights. Avoid swinging the torso or bringing the arms back, instead of to the side. This is very important for rear deltoid isolation. Your elbows should be leading the exercise. Many people doing this and similar exercises lead with the dumbbells and take all the focus off the shoulders. When you lead the movement with dumbbells, you will not optimally stimulate the desired rear deltoid muscle. Try to make sure to move the whole arm together.

**2** Contract the rear deltoid muscle as hard as you can, hold for one second at the top of the exercise (shoulder level or slightly higher), then slowly lower the dumbbells back to the starting position. Your rear deltoid muscles should still be working while lowering the weight.

**3** When you reach the starting position, do not rest. Slowly begin lifting the dumbbells out to each side of your body in a smooth, controlled, fluid motion, without using momentum. Repeat the recommended number of repetitions.

# Bent-Over Lateral Raise

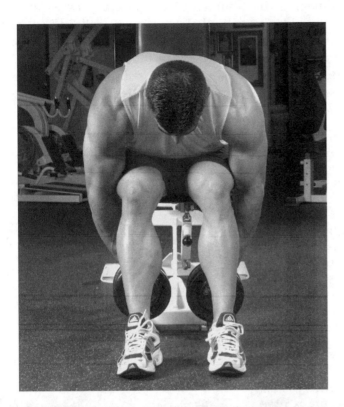

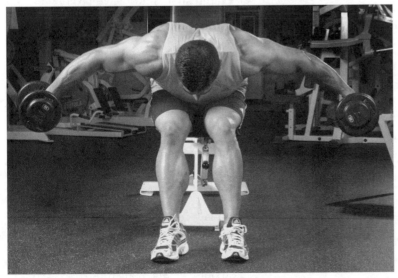

**VARIATION**

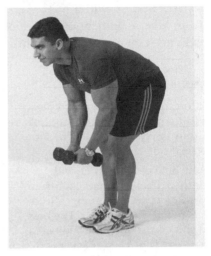

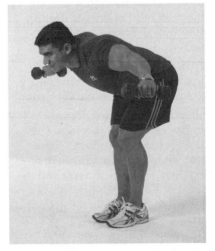

# Military Press

Unlike behind-the-neck presses, which risk damaging the rotator cuffs, military presses are a great exercise to develop all three heads of the shoulder or deltoid muscles. You will find that a narrower grip focuses more on the muscles of the medial and rear deltoids with an emphasis on the triceps. The wider you go, the more you'll incorporate the front and medial deltoids. Make sure to use a light enough weight to allow you a full range of motion; you should bring the bar down very close to your pec muscles, they will see unbelievable results from their efforts.

## PROPER ALIGNMENT

❶ Sit on the military seat and place your feet flat on the floor in front of you. Your knees should also be facing straight ahead.

❷ Take hold of the barbell with your grip of choice. Remember that grip variation will stimulate certain muscles more than others. The best thing you can do for your body is to assess your shoulder muscles and decide which portion of the three heads are in need of further development for overall muscle balance and symmetry.

❸ Sit all the way back in the seat, making sure that your back is straight and flat against the back pad.

❹ A mistake made when doing either this exercise or the dumbbell shoulder press is to stick the chest way out when pressing up. Do not do this! Remember, when you stick the chest out during the press, you take primary stimulation away from the shoulder muscles and direct it to the chest muscles. You want to relax the chest at all times during this exercise. If you see your chest rise or feel your chest muscles handling the majority of the work, stop and correct yourself. You may either be going too heavy, or you just need to practice your form without weight.

❺ As you hold the bar, make sure that your arms and elbows are as wide as possible (as if you were trying to touch your elbows behind your back).

❻ While keeping your upper arms horizontal to the floor, don't let the biceps and triceps region sink below shoulder height as this is the ideal level for a full range of motion for this exercise.

❼ Keep your forearms in a perpendicular position (keeping your forearms pointed directly towards the ceiling at all times).

❽ Make sure that your head and neck are as relaxed as possible throughout the entire exercise. Please note that you must never turn your head while doing any of these exercises. Position your body into the proper alignment, keeping your head straight, and stay that way throughout the exercise! If you don't, you could end up seriously injured.

## TECHNIQUE AND FORM

Before you begin the exercise, close your eyes and visualize yourself doing the movement. Focus on the shoulder muscles you are about to stimulate. Remember what we discussed about assessing your shoulder muscles and comparing the balance and symmetry of the muscles. This goes for all muscles. Pay close attention to the muscles that are lagging behind others and concentrate all of your energy to those areas during the exercise. If your muscles are already in balance and symmetric, focus on the muscle as a whole.

❶ You should now be in position to begin. First, pick up the bar and begin the exercise from the top position.

❷ With the arms and elbows wide and head level, slowly bring the bar down to an area slightly below the chin. The upper arms, from the elbow to the shoulder, should end up slightly below parallel to the floor, with your forearms perpendicular to the ceiling.

❸ When you reach the bottom of the movement, as your upper arms are lowered slightly below chin level, slowly begin pressing upward in a smooth, controlled, fluid motion, without resting. Make sure that you do not use any momentum.

# Military Press

**4** When you reach the top of the movement, do not lock out the elbow joint. When you lock out the elbow joint, you distribute all of the weight from the shoulders to the elbow joint, thus interrupting muscle stimulation. This can hurt the elbow joint and limit shoulder muscle stimulation.

**5** From this point, slowly begin to lower the bar in a smooth, controlled, fluid motion, without resting.

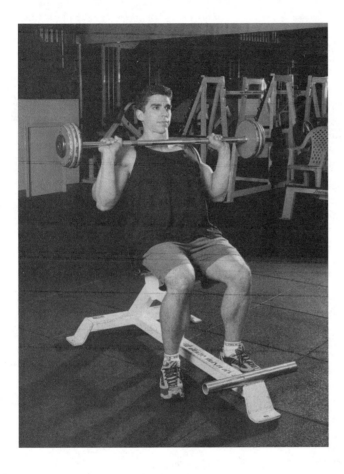

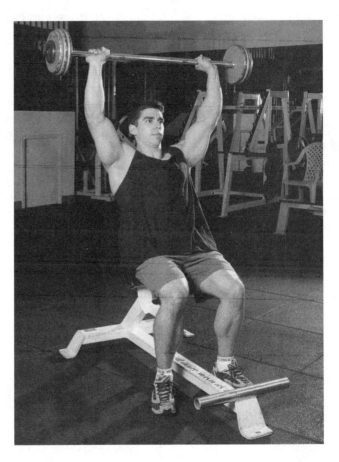

---

**FAQ:**

*Why do I constantly see so many people leaning back while doing this exercise?*

**ANSWER:**

Leaning back while doing the military press will bring your upper chest muscles into the movement. Because of this, it stops isolating the shoulder muscles. Many people do this because they are lifting too heavy a weight-or perhaps their shoulders became tired and they leaned back to get the weight up. If you have trouble staying upright during the military press, either go lighter, or plant your feet behind you to help to maintain your upright position.

# Front Raise

This exercise is great for working the shoulder muscles, as long as you keep yourself in perfect form and do not engage the chest muscles. There are several variations to experiment with, including performing with one hand alone, alternating hands, or using a barbell instead of dumbbells.

## PROPER ALIGNMENT

**1** Stand with a straight torso and the dumbbells resting in front of your thighs with the palms of your hands facing you. Align the body from the bottom up, beginning with the feet. Make sure the feet are pointing straight ahead.

**2** Keep your knees pointing straight ahead and slightly bent to prevent any unnecessary back strain.

**3** Remember that as you lift the dumbbells, your palms should be facing downward so that your shoulder muscles do the work, not your biceps muscles.

## TECHNIQUE AND FORM

**1** While standing still, lift the dumbbells straight to the front, with a slight bend to the elbow and the palms facing down.

**2** While exhaling, continue until your arms are parallel to the floor. Pause for a second at the top of the movement.

**3** Inhale and lower the dumbbells slowly in a controlled fashion to the starting position while maintaining your posture and body alignment. Make sure you choose a weight that allows you to practice perfect form. If you use a weight that is too heavy, momentum will force muscles other than the shoulders to do the work.

# Front Raise

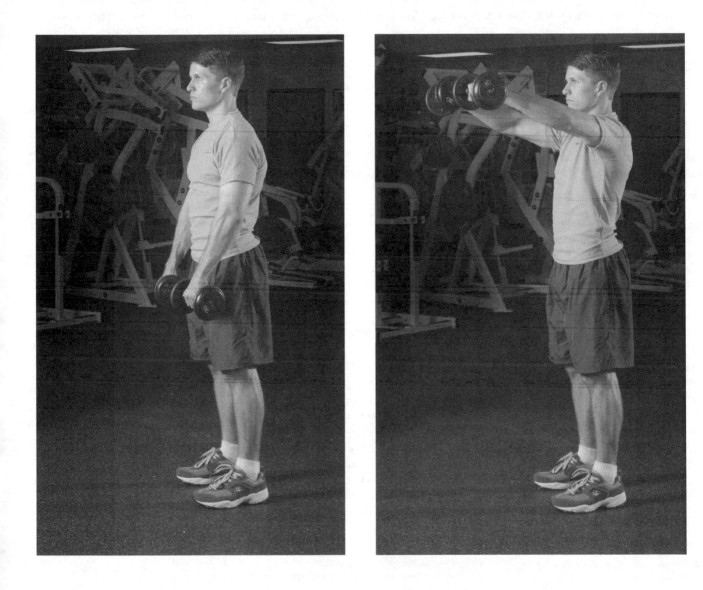

# Dumbbell Upright Row

**(Using A Cambered Bar Or Dumbbells)**

Upright rows are a great exercise to develop the tie-in muscles, aesthetically tying your shoulders and trapezius muscles together and also for the medial head. You must make certain that you use very strict form with this exercise, avoiding momentum at all times. The rotator cuff muscles of the shoulder are extremely delicate and prone to injuries that occur as a result of using poor form and excessive weight. The upright row exercise alone can stress the rotator cuff muscles. Because of this, it is imperative that you use a weight you can handle, and practice perfect form and technique with no momentum at all. We recommend that you practice the exercise using a cambered (E-Z Curl Bar) bar at first. This is usually much easier on the wrists and shoulders than a straight barbell. After you've mastered the perfect form methods, you can begin using two separate dumbbells for variety. We will now discuss the alignment phase of the exercise.

## PROPER ALIGNMENT

**1** Choose a weight for the cambered bar that is easy enough so you can focus only on your form. Once you have mastered the correct form, it will become second nature and you will find it easy to move up in weight, thereby being able to fully stimulate the shoulder muscles.

**2** Grasp the bar using a shoulder-width grip.

**3** Place your feet shoulder-width apart and point them straight ahead.

**4** Keep your knees slightly bent at all times during the movement to take stress off the lower back region. Also, keep the knees pointing straight ahead.

**5** Contract the abdominal muscles slightly to help keep your postural alignment.

**6** Keep your back straight and body still as you do the exercise.

**7** Relax the musculature of your chest and back.

**8** Keep your head level and look straight ahead at all times during the exercise.

**9** Hold the bar across your thighs and keep your palms facing toward your body.

**10** Begin focusing on the muscles of the shoulder including the trapezius muscles. Although you will be pulling the weight up with your hands, you must let the elbows lead the motion, keeping them high as you pull up.

## TECHNIQUE AND FORM

**1** Before you begin the exercise, close your eyes and once again visualize yourself actually doing the movement while focusing on the shoulder and trapezius muscles.

**2** With proper form and postural alignment, begin pulling the bar up slowly, concentrating on feeling the stimulation of the focused muscles.

**3** Pull the bar up, leading with your elbows, to a point where it comes close to your chin.

**4** The most important thing to do at this position of the exercise is to consciously focus on and physically contract the muscles of the trapezius.

**5** Hold the contraction here for a count of one to two seconds.

**6** With just enough time to contract the trap muscles, slowly begin lowering the bar while maintaining the same exact form and posture you did when pulling up.

**7** When you reach the bottom (start) position, slowly begin pulling the bar back to the top position of the exercise using a smooth, controlled, fluid motion. Make sure that you do not jerk or use momentum to lift the bar at any time during this exercise.

# Dumbbell Upright Row

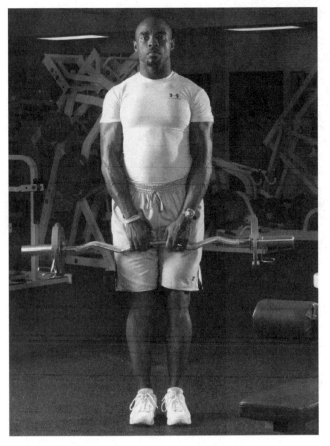

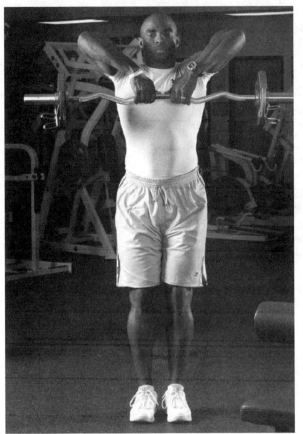

## VARIATION

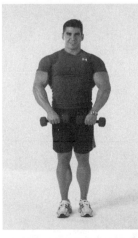

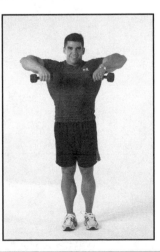

---

**FAQ:**

*When I do this exercise it sometimes hurts my shoulder joints and rotator cuff muscles. Why?*

**ANSWER:**

To avoid pain, try this: when you begin the movement with the bar lying on your upper thigh, as you pull it up, bring the bar about 4 to 6 inches away from your body. This distance will take some pressure off of the joints and the rotator cuff. It will be more challenging, so you may need to go a bit lighter.

# Bent-Arm Bent-Over Row

This exercise can also be done standing, but those with lower back problems are better off performing it seated.

## PROPER ALIGNMENT

**❶** Place a couple of dumbbells parallel to and in front of a flat bench.

**❷** Sit on the end of the bench with your legs together and the dumbbells behind your calves.

**❸** Bend at the waist while keeping your back straight in order to pick up the dumbbells. As you pick them up, the palms of your hands should be facing each other.

**❹** Bend at the elbows until there is a 90-degree angle between the forearm and upper arm.

## TECHNIQUE AND FORM

**❶** Keep your torso forward and stationary with arms bent at a 90-degree angle at the elbows, and lift the dumbbells straight to the side until both upper arms are parallel to the floor. The forearms should be pointed to the floor in this contracted position. Exhale as you lift the weights. Avoid swinging the torso or bringing the arms back rather than to the side.

**❷** After a one second contraction at the top, slowly lower the dumbbells back to the starting position.

**❸** Repeat for the recommended number of repetitions.

# Bent-Arm Bent-Over Row

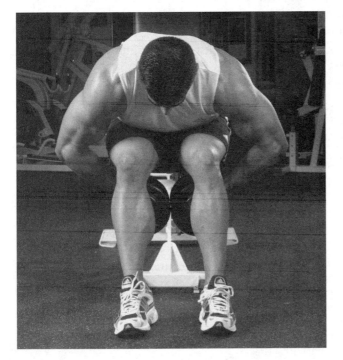 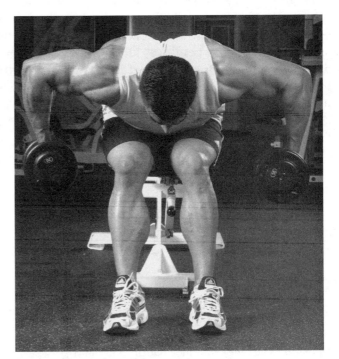

# Bent-Over Lateral Raise on Incline Bench

The bent-over lateral raise is a great exercise for developing the rear deltoid muscles of the shoulder, which, in our opinion, is one of the most neglected muscles in the body. By using this exercise to develop this muscle, you will give your shoulders a fantastic three-dimensional look.

There are three ways that you can do this exercise. We will describe one in depth and the other two briefly. The first version is the seated bent-over lateral raise in which you sit on the edge of the bench, bend at the waist with your head down and lift the dumbbells to each side of your body. The other version is the standing bent-over lateral raise, in which you stand in the same postural alignment as you did with the standing dumbbell lateral raise with the exception that this time, you bend over at the hips. Once again, you will be bending your knees while keeping your back straight and parallel to the floor as you lift the dumbbells to the sides of your body, leading the movement with your elbows (this is the version to be used by those of you with little equipment).

The exercise we will discuss now, however, is the best exercise for developing the rear deltoids. This exercise is the bent-over lateral raise done on an incline bench. It will give you the best of both of the exercises we first discussed, allowing you to stay very strict while keeping you almost parallel to the floor. In addition, this exercise eliminates any stress to the lower back.

## PROPER ALIGNMENT

❶ Choose two light dumbbells so that you may practice perfect form.

❷ Rest your entire torso, from your pelvic bone to your chest, on the incline bench's angled pad with your head and eyes looking straight ahead.

❸ Position your feet shoulder-width apart, pointing them straight ahead at all times during the exercise.

❹ Make sure that your knees are bent so there is no unnecessary lower back stress.

❺ Bring the dumbbells down to each side of your body with your palms facing each other.

❻ Make sure that you are positioned steadily on the bench incline.

❼ Bring your head up to the level of your torso, which must be close to or parallel to the floor. Look straight ahead.

❽ As you prepare to do the exercise, focus all of your attention and concentration on the rear deltoid muscles of the shoulder. Know where these muscles are located and how they feel when stimulated. This is why we suggest that you go light, so that you may isolate these muscles without incorporating others into the movement.

❾ As you lift the dumbbells to the sides of your body, your elbows will be leading the motion. Many people who do this and similar exercises lead the movement with the dumbbells and take all of the focus off the shoulders. When you lead the exercise movement with the dumbbells, you will not optimally stimulate the desired rear deltoid muscles.

## TECHNIQUE AND FORM

❶ Slowly and without momentum, begin lifting the dumbbells out to each side of your body.

❷ Try to move your whole arm together, or at least make sure that the elbows are leading the movement.

❸ Do not lift your torso as you lift. If you find that you are in fact lifting for momentum assistance, stop! Either lighten the weight or rest for one minute and do your next set. Don't just go through the motions only concerned with getting the weights up. Focus on isolation of the rear deltoid muscles, and make them work hard.

# Bent-Over Lateral Raise on Incline Bench

**4** Make sure that you lift the dumbbells straight out to your sides rather than behind you. This is very important for rear deltoid isolation.

**5** Maintain your postural alignment and bring the dumbbells up to level with your shoulders or slightly higher.

**6** Squeeze the dumbbells back while you contract the rear deltoid muscles as hard as you can. Hold this contraction for one second.

**7** From this point, slowly begin lowering the dumbbells, making sure that you make the rear deltoid muscles continue to work during the lowering portion of the exercise.

**8** As you reach the bottom (start) position, do not rest. Once again, slowly begin lifting the dumbbells out to each side of your body in a smooth, controlled and fluid motion, without using momentum.

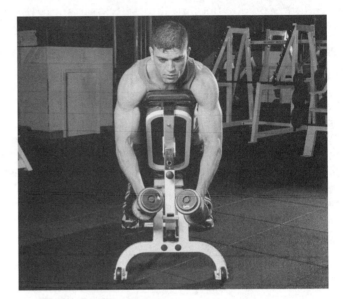

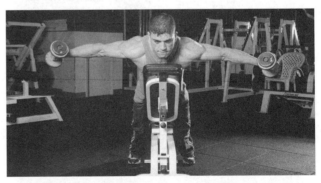

**FAQ:**

*I don't feel the stimulation in my rear deltoids as much as I feel it in my triceps and upper back muscles. Why is this?*

**ANSWER:**

If this is the case, try bringing your arms a little further in front of your body as you lift. This slight variation should redirect the stimulation to the rear deltoids. As far as the triceps are involved, you must work to maintain that slight bend in the elbows throughout the exercise. Otherwise, you will experience triceps involvement. The place where this customarily happens is at the top of the movement, where the elbow is extended.

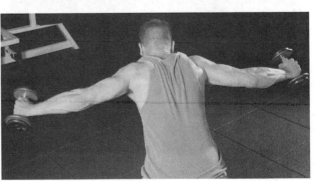

# Two-Arm Cable Lateral Raise

Using cables to perform laterals provides resistance during the positive and negative phases of your repetition. You may need to use lighter weights than usual for this exercise. If you feel any pain in your neck, this is an indication that the weight you are lifting may be too heavy. Make sure to keep your head in line with your spine throughout this exercise.

## PROPER ALIGNMENT

**1** Place the pins at the desired weights in the cable machine.

**2** Stand in the center of the cables, lean slightly forward from your hips while maintaining erect posture.

**3** Keep your knees bent and your abdominals engaged. Hold a handle in each hand.

**4** Pull the handles in until your arms cross under your chest.

## TECHNIQUE AND FORM

**1** Extend your arms in an upward arc-like movement, until they are parallel to the floor.

**2** At the top position, hold for a couple of seconds before returning to the crossed position.

**3** Repeat for the desired number of repetitions.

# Two-Arm Cable Lateral Raise

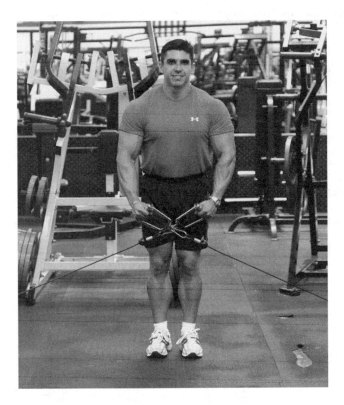 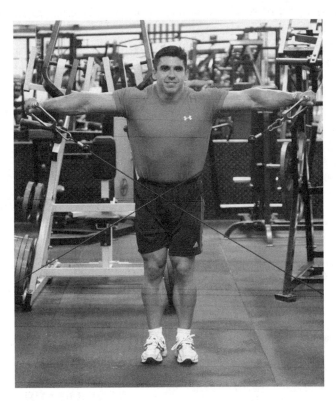

# Seated Rear-Delt Machine

The seated rear-delt machine is a great exercise to use for variety in your shoulder training arsenal. It will give you the ability to really focus on isolating the rear delts without the possibility of lower back injury and the burden of having to bend over at the hips. This is a perfect exercise for those who feel dizzy when bent over, or feel too much chest compression from having to lean on the incline bench, or who have lower back problems.

**VARIATION:** A variation you can try without a machine uses a bench and one dumbbell. Simply place one knee and one hand on a bench, bend over, keeping the lumbar curve in your lower back, and lift the dumbbell up, bending your elbow so your arm creates a 90-degree angle.

## PROPER ALIGNMENT

❶ Seat yourself on the machine and position your body so that you are sitting upright with your chest flush against the vertical pad. There should be a seat adjustment that will allow you to raise and lower the seat. Bring the seat to a height where your chin can rest neutrally on the edge of the pad in front of you. This is a good height to optimize the proper anatomical position for this shoulder exercise.

❷ Keep your feet flat on the floor and pointing straight ahead during the movement. Also, keep your knees pointing straight ahead at all times. On most rear-delt machines, you will find inner thigh pads for added stability. Keep your thighs snug against the pads to give you the added support needed to secure your core musculature.

❸ This machine is often used as a pec deck and gives you the option of adjusting the arm bars to your liking. For this particular exercise, you will want the arm bars brought to the back position so they are just about touching one another. You also might have the option of taking your handgrip in a palms facing position or an over-hand position. Take the overhand position, since this will take much stress off the wrists and allow better muscle control and isolation of the rear shoul-

ders, thus negating the triceps muscles as much as possible from the movement.

❹ Make sure that you keep a slight bend in the elbows at all times. This bend of the arms will help ensure that you keep the focus of resistance on the rear delts and off the triceps. You might reach a level of fatigue where you are forced to use the triceps muscles to move the weight. When you reach this point, either resist the temptation or simply lower the weight.

❺ Keep your chest cavity against the chest pad at all times during the exercise, with your torso totally upright.

## TECHNIQUE AND FORM

❶ Begin the exercise with your feet flat on the floor, thighs pinned snugly against the thigh pads, and body upright with chest against the pad and chin rested on the edge.

❷ With hands holding the grips in an overhand position, make sure that your elbows are pointed directly out to the sides. This is very important for isolation of the rear-delt muscles.

❸ Before you begin the movement, make sure you are consciously focused on the rear-delt muscles and begin to isometrically contract them before moving the weight. This might take some practice to perfect,

but you will soon multiply your muscle isolation abilities ten-fold.

❹ Begin bringing the bars away from each other and maintain your anatomical positioning at all times. Bring the bars as far back as possible without jerking or using momentum to do so.

❺ As you reach the top of the movement, with arms fully extended outwards, try to hold this position for one count while feeling the rear shoulder muscles taking the brunt of the resistance. At this point, really squeeze the rear delts.

❻ Slowly allow the arms to return to the start position, resisting the bars on the negative portion of the exercise.

❼ Once you have reached the position where the bars are just about touching each other, do not allow the weight stack to touch the bottom. You want to keep constant tension on the muscles and must stop right before the weights touch bottom. From here immediately begin to bring the bars apart once again with great form.

# Seated Rear-Delt Machine

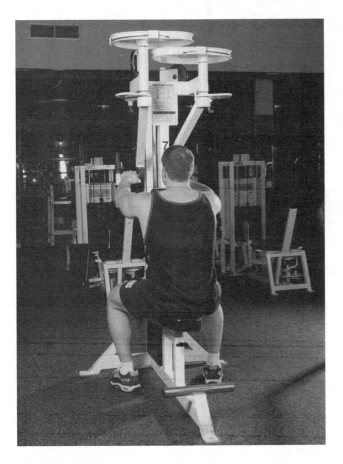

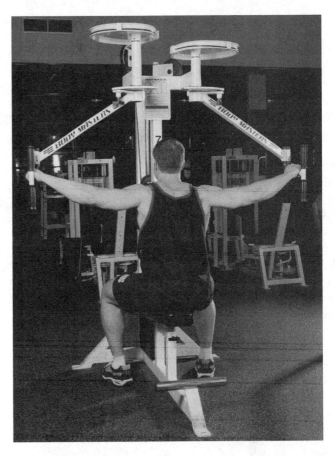

## VARIATION

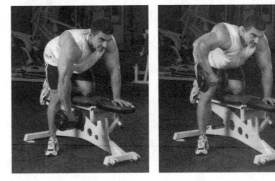

**FAQ:**

*The overhand grip hurts my wrists. Can I use another grip?*

**ANSWER:**

Yes. There are several other grips available on this machine. Try a couple to see which one feels comfortable and helps to elicit the best recruitment of the rear-deltoid muscles.

235

# Rotator Cuff

The four small muscles of the rotator cuff need strengthening, as they are prone to injury. You will need to use a noticeably lighter weight for this exercise than for other arm exercises. To make sure that you get the maximum benefit from this, make sure you maintain the 90-degree angle in the arms throughout the range of motion.

## PROPER ALIGNMENT

❶ Stand in a neutral position. Your feet should be just under shoulder-width apart, your knees slightly bent, your shoulders back, and your chest out.

❷ You should be holding a light weight in each hand, your palms facing behind you.

❸ Bend your arms so that the upper and lower arms are at a 90-degree angle, your arms parallel to the floor and extended before you.

## TECHNIQUE AND FORM

❶ Exhale and rotate your shoulders so that your hands rise above your elbows and your palms face front.

❷ Slowly return to the start position. At no time should your arms not be in a 90-degree angle, as this could cause stress or injury on your rotator cuff.

❸ Repeat for the desired number of repetitions.

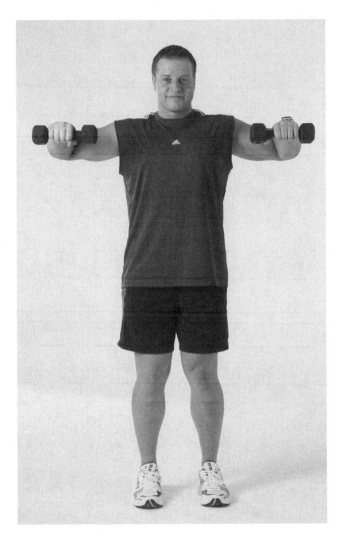
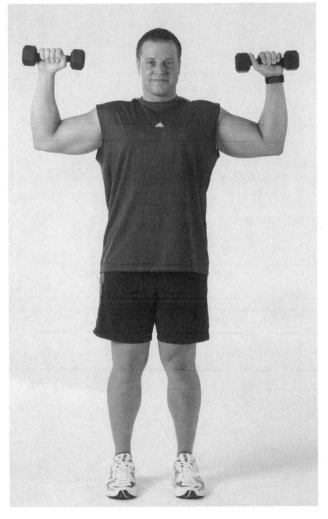

# Chapter 10
## Triceps

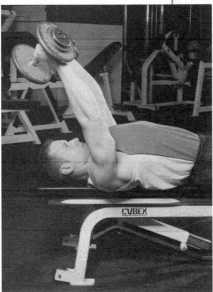

The triceps muscle, located on the back of the upper arm, is a three-headed muscle with a horseshoe appearance that requires different angles of training for full development. A lot of people don't realize that just one exercise for most body parts simply won't cut it, unless you want a simple looking body with simple looking muscles. Specific exercises will stimulate specific muscles to work primarily and incorporate other muscles to work as the secondary muscles.

While most guys who want big arms usually focus on the biceps, 2/3 of the arm size is provided by the triceps! Therefore, if you want big arms, you cannot afford to neglect the triceps. The following exercises incorporate all angles of training, providing total triceps muscle development.

For immediate Body Sculpting Bible support & coaching directly from James & Hugo, please visit www.BodySculptingBible.com

**10**

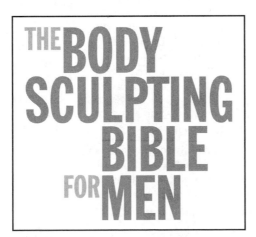

# Overhead Dumbbell Extension

## (Using one dumbbell supported by two hands)

The overhead dumbbell extension focuses on the middle and inner heads of the triceps muscles. You can do this exercise either while seated or while standing. We recommend you do it seated as you will be less likely to use momentum. One very important thing to remember with this exercise is to keep the elbows pointed to the ceiling above you at all times during the movement. This will help create a full range of motion for the triceps. You also need to hold the upper arms close to your head as you extend the weight overhead. Finally, one of the most important things to remember and perfect with this exercise is your handgrip on the dumbbell. It is not easy to get a perfectly even grip for both hands with this exercise. If you fail to grip the dumbbell evenly, you may end up directing the force of the dumbbell resistance to one arm more than the other. This will create muscle imbalance between the two arms. To fix this, you must learn to either grip the top, inner portion of the dumbbell with a separate, even grip for both hands or with an overlapping grip, having one hand overlap the other. We recommend that you choose, if available, a dumbbell that adequately allows two separate and even handgrips. Unfortunately, most dumbbells will not allow a great deal of space to securely grip in this fashion. In this case, you must learn to perfect your overlapping grip for better balance and muscle symmetry.

## PROPER ALIGNMENT

**❶** Choose a weight that you believe to be light enough to practice perfect form. Place the dumbbell on top of your thigh. You can also have someone hand the dumbbell to you from behind. This is especially useful when using very heavy weight and to avoid injuring the shoulder joints.

**❷** Sit on a bench with a 90-degree angled back pad.

**❸** Sit all the way back into the seat, making sure that your back is flat against the pad at all times during the movement.

**❹** Before lifting the weight into position overhead, make sure that your feet are placed flat on the floor and pointed straight ahead. Make sure that your knees are also pointing straight ahead. Keep the head level and facing straight ahead at all times during the movement.

**❺** Position the dumbbell overhead or have someone hand it to you from behind. Grasp the dumbbell with your grip of choice.

**❻** Point your elbows straight to the ceiling above you while holding your arms and elbows close to your head for triceps isolation.

## TECHNIQUE AND FORM

**❶** With the dumbbell overhead and in position, begin lowering the dumbbell while keeping the elbows pointed directly to the ceiling. It is important to do this because it will help isolate the triceps muscle and provide a full range of productive motion. It will also help you avoid hitting the dumbbell on the back of your head while extending and lowering the dumbbell.

**❷** As you lower the dumbbell, focus on the triceps muscles and feel the stretch. Always take this negative portion slow and stay in control.

**❸** Lower the dumbbell to a point where your forearms are slightly below parallel to the ground. You should feel a big stretch in the triceps.

**❹** Without any rest and avoiding the use of momentum, begin pressing the weight back up to the top position. Make sure that you are using perfect form, while maintaining the correct postural alignment.

**❺** All of your attention must be on the triceps muscles, focusing on the isolation of the muscles.

**❻** As you approach the top of the movement, contract the triceps muscles as hard as you possibly can while avoiding intensely locking out the elbow joints.

**❼** Hold this contraction for 1-2 seconds and begin your descent, lowering the dumbbell in a slow, controlled, and fluid manner.

# Overhead Dumbbell Extension

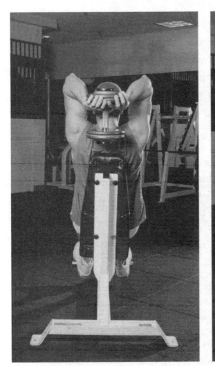
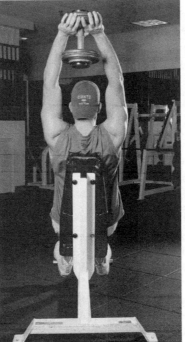

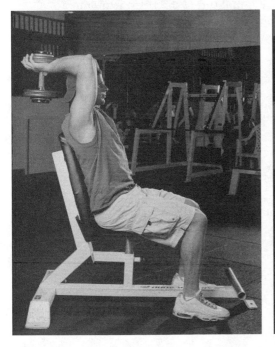
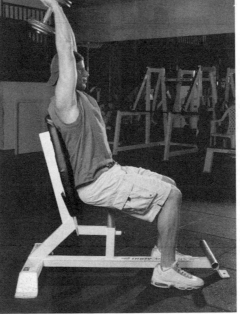

# Lying Dumbbell Extension

**(Using two dumbbells simultaneously)**

This exercise is a one of our favorites (second only to triceps dips). The lying position provides greater stability to lift more safely, preventing a chance of injury to your lower back. It also allows greater leverage to occur, much like the flat dumbbell press, allowing better strength output with a smoother exercise movement. Always make sure to move the dumbbells slowly from start to finish and squeeze the triceps muscles at the top of the movement to really feel the triceps working.

## PROPER ALIGNMENT

❶ Pick up two dumbbells, making sure that they are light enough for you to practice perfect form or for simply warming up your triceps muscles.

❷ Sit at the end of a flat bench with the weights positioned upright on top of your thighs.

❸ It is very important to grip both dumbbell handles all the way at the end closest to your thighs. Make sure to slide your hands all the way to the bottom of the handle so that the pinky side of your hand is up against the weight plate. Doing this will help you control the weight better while also allowing you to contract the triceps muscles harder at the top of the movement.

❹ Thrust each dumbbell up just as you would when doing a dumbbell bench press.

❺ Lay back on the bench and place your feet flat onto the floor.

❻ As you are lying down, keeping the long side of the dumbbells and the palms of your hands facing each other at all times, press the weights up using your chest muscles (chest press). You will begin the exercise in this position to avoid stressing the elbow joint. If you start at the bottom position of this exercise, you can easily create too much pressure on the elbow joint capsule, risking long-term injury. Remember, throughout the movement, the palms of your hands and your inner elbows must always face each other. You want to make sure that your whole arm is directly in line with your front shoulder (anterior deltoid).

❼ You must also make sure that your elbows are pointing directly at the ceiling at all times during the exercise.

❽ Begin the exercise with the arms fully extended overhead, holding the dumbbells high to the ceiling.

## TECHNIQUE AND FORM

❶ Once you are in the proper body alignment with the dumbbells overhead, slowly lower the dumbbells toward your shoulders. While doing this, your elbows will remain pointing directly at the ceiling, and your entire arm from the elbows to the shoulders will be frozen at all times. These steps are necessary for proper triceps stimulation during this exercise. Remember to consciously focus all of your attention on proper form and stimulation of the triceps muscles.

❷ As you lower the dumbbells, stop just before the dumbbells reach your shoulders and begin to slowly and smoothly extend your arms from the elbows to the hands back up to the starting position of the exercise. Remember to keep your upper arms frozen in place.

❸ As you reach the top of the exercise, contract the triceps muscles as hard as you possibly can for complete muscle stimulation. Make sure that you avoid excessively locking the elbow joint. Once you reach the position of full elbow extension, do not thrust the elbow joint into a locked position. Instead, contract the triceps muscles as hard as you possibly can. Practice using light weights with this technique as practice will make for perfect execution of the exercise and better results. Also, make sure that there is a smooth transition when switching directions from lowering the dumbbells to raising the dumbbells. Do not rest between lowering and raising the dumbbell.

# Lying Dumbbell Extension

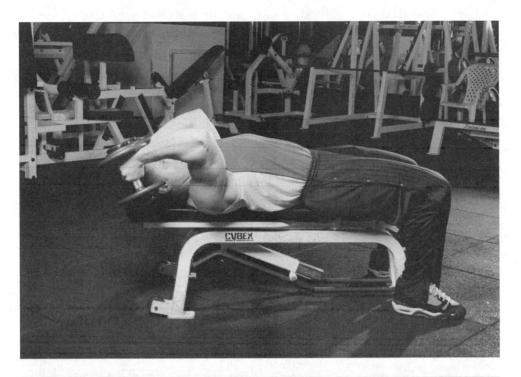

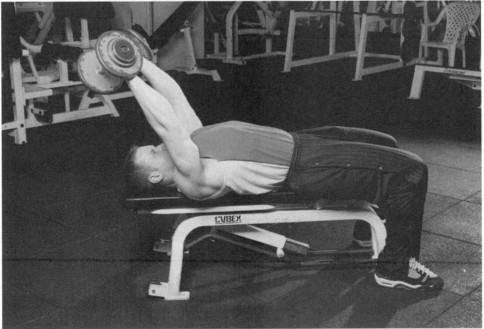

# Lying E-Z Bar Extension

This triceps exercise is one that will fully stimulate all three muscles of the triceps. It is performed with an E-Z curl bar, a curved bar usually found in the free weight section of your gym or health club. If you don't have access to this type of bar, just stick with the lying dumbbell triceps extension, as they are both very similar to one another. You can also use this exercise to build your strength and coordination in preparation for the lying dumbbell triceps extension.

## PROPER ALIGNMENT

❶ Set up a cambered bar (E-Z curl bar) with some light weight on each side or get one that is already pre-weighted. You can rest the curl bar on your thighs and lay back, set it in place so that it is at the base of your head while you lie down, or simply have someone hand it to you when you are already lying down.

❷ Before lifting the bar or having it handed to you, lay back on the bench and place your feet flat onto the floor, pointing straight ahead.

❸ As you are lying down, lift the bar into place by pressing it up using your chest muscles (like the chest press). Hold it up above your head and stay there. You will begin the exercise in this position to avoid stressing the elbow joint. If you start at the bottom position of this exercise, you can easily create too much pressure on the elbow joint capsule, risking long-term injury. Once you begin the movement from the top, the pressure in the elbow joints will be reduced as you reach the bottom position.

❹ Remember, the palms of your hands and inner elbows must always face each other during the exercise.

❺ Make sure that your whole arm is directly in line with your front shoulder (anterior deltoid).

❻ This exercise will slightly differ from the lying two-dumbbell extension. Take a grip on the bar and position your hands about 8 to 10 inches apart. Bring the E-Z bar overhead and position your elbows so that they are pointing directly to the ceiling above you, but now you will point your elbows slightly behind you and toward the ceiling on an angle. Doing this with the E-Z curl bar in your hands will automatically distribute the resistance from resting on the elbow joints to the triceps muscles. We don't recommend that you do this with the lying dumbbell extension because the two movements will stimulate different areas of the triceps muscles.

Begin the exercise just as we described it to you and maintain that technique, form, and postural alignment throughout the exercise.

## TECHNIQUE AND FORM

❶ Once you are in the proper body alignment with the E-Z curl bar overhead, slowly begin to lower the bar down toward your forehead. While doing this, your elbows will remain pointing slightly behind you at an angle toward the ceiling.

❷ Make sure that your entire arm from the elbows to your shoulders is frozen in place at all times during the exercise. These steps are necessary for proper triceps stimulation during this exercise.

❸ Remember to consciously focus all of your attention on proper form and stimulation of the triceps muscles.

---

**FAQ:**

*I feel the same pain and pressure as I did with the overhead dumbbell extension.*

**ANSWER:**

Your elbows are under the same pressure here. However, you can take a bit of the shearing force off of the elbow joints by making sure to keep your arms angled back throughout the exercise. If you still feel discomfort, switch this exercise with another.

# Lying E-Z Bar Extension

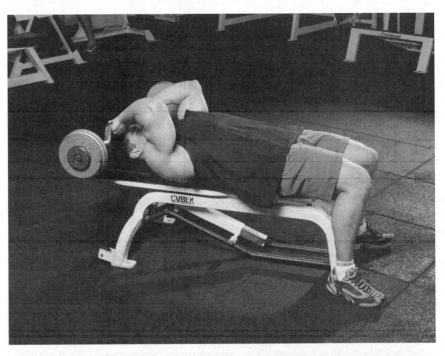

**❹** As you lower the bar, stop just before it reaches your forehead and begin to slowly and smoothly extend your arms back up to the starting position of the exercise.

**❺** As you reach the top of the exercise, make sure you are consciously contracting the triceps muscles as hard as you possibly can for complete muscle stimulation.

**❻** Hold this contraction for one second.

**❼** Make sure there is a smooth transition when switching directions. There should be no rest at all when switching from the bottom position to the upward extension of the bar.

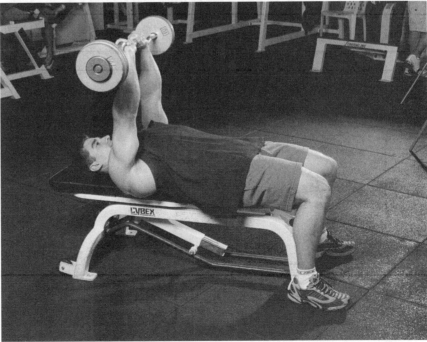

# Triceps Dip

The triceps dip is a great muscle-enhancing exercise focusing on the lower triceps, which are closer to the elbow. There is a major difference between the triceps dip and the chest dip. When we discussed the chest dips, we told you to bend at the knees, lock your feet, and bend forward as you lower yourself. You must stay bent over to keep the focus of resistance in the chest muscles. But with the triceps dip we are trying to isolate the triceps muscles and instead avoid stimulation of the chest muscles. To do this you will need a dip station or machine. If you are working out in your home, you can purchase an inexpensive dip unit from one of the sports-related retail chains or a wholesale fitness supply store.

## PROPER ALIGNMENT

**1** First, place your hands on the parallel bars as you position yourself for postural alignment. The best way to do this is to raise yourself up onto the dip bars by locking out your arms. Align your body starting with your head and moving down to your feet. We have found a fantastic way of doing triceps dips that makes it very easy to isolate the triceps muscles. To make it as easily understood as possible, your entire body from head to toes should be as straight as possible throughout the exercise.

**2** As you lower yourself from the lockout position, keep your head in a neutral or level position.

**3** Your chest and shoulders must be completely upright and as straight as possible.

**4** Your arms and elbows will ride close to your body as you lower yourself and when pushing to triceps lockout.

**5** Your abdominal muscles should be contracted slightly to hold you in position.

**6** Your legs must be completely straight, and your feet flat as if you were standing. Now, don't think that because the set-up is easy, the exercise will be easily executed. Yes, the set-up for the exercise is easier than most; but this easy set-up makes the triceps isolation and stimulation incredibly powerful.

## TECHNIQUE AND FORM

**1** As you lower yourself, lean back to help hold your body in the upright position.

**2** Lower yourself slowly while resisting your bodyweight all the way to the bottom position.

**3** Keep the elbows close to your body, helping to better isolate the triceps muscles.

**4** Keeping your legs straight and feet flat to the floor, lower yourself to the floor. You can do two things here: You can either stop lowering your body right before your feet touch, or you can lower yourself to the point where you tap your feet flat on the ground and immediately begin your return upward. We prefer the latter since we know that when we tap bottom, we have completed the full range of motion for complete muscle stimulation and should explode into the upward press. Some people will not be tall enough to touch their feet at the bottom of the training apparatus being used. Also, you would never want to lower yourself to a point where you could injure yourself just to touch your feet flat on the floor. There is such a point! In any of these cases, just lower your body until your upper arms (from your elbows to your shoulders) are parallel to the floor. Then, immediately begin your return upward.

**5** No matter what technique you use at the bottom position, after you've reached that point, slowly and with a smooth transition begin to press your body upward, maintaining your upright posture.

**6** As you begin pressing upward, make sure that all of your focus is directed to your triceps muscles. This alone will help stimulate the triceps by increased muscle control and as a reminder to maintain proper alignment.

# Triceps Dip

❼ As you near the top of the motion, your goal is not to lock the joint but instead to contract and squeeze the triceps muscles as hard as you possibly can for 1-2 seconds. It is important to let the triceps muscles hold you in this position rather than lock the elbow joints. Otherwise, you can injure the joint, plus you take all of the resistance off the triceps muscles and put it onto the joints, and bones. Remember that there should be no rest at the top of the exercise after the contraction period. From that lockout position, once again slowly lower yourself back to the bottom position as you resist the weight of your body. If you get to a point where your body weight is too light for the exercise, you may use a dip belt to hook some additional weight to your body, thus increasing the resistance. Please make sure that if you add weight, you do so in incremental stages.

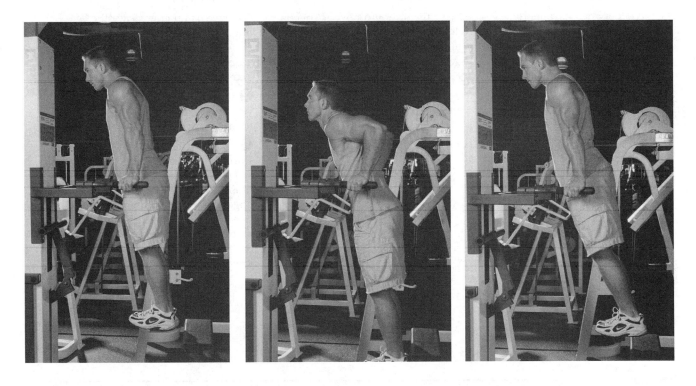

**FAQ:**

*When I do triceps dips, I feel a lot of pressure and pain in my shoulders. Why?*

**ANSWER:**

The triceps dip can be a very powerful and productive exercise. You do, however, need to make sure that you protect yourself from injury. Keep a few things in mind when doing the triceps dip. Don't go too heavy, unless you know your muscles, joints, and connective tissue can handle it. Although you may be very strong and feel that your flexibility it great, you still may not be as strong as necessary to do this exercise at its full capacity.

# Bench Dip

Triceps dips can also be performed between benches if you are unable to perform them on the parallel-bars, for whatever reason. Just like parallel bar triceps dips, this exercise will primarily focus on all three heads of the triceps. We guarantee you that this exercise will help you achieve those big and ripped horseshoe triceps that you are looking for, thus adding inches to your arm girth. Remember, triceps make up 2/3 of the arm size, so neglecting them is not a good idea. This is a great exercise for developing the strength necessary to do the triceps dip exercise on the parallel-dip bar unit.

## PROPER ALIGNMENT

❶ Place two benches parallel to each other (side by side) with sufficient space in between them to allow for your palms to be on one bench and the back of your feet on top of the other.

❷ Sit between the two benches with your palms on the bench behind you and with your legs on top of the other bench. If you are aligned correctly, your body should resemble an L.

## TECHNIQUE AND FORM

❶ Use the strength of your triceps to lower your body towards the ground in a gradual and controlled movement.

❷ Continue to lower yourself until the upper arms and the forearms create a 90-degree angle.

❸ Use your triceps to push yourself back up to the starting position.

## Important Notes

❶ Once again guys, leave the ego outside of the gym. Do not move up and down in a jerky or uncontrolled manner, as this exercise can place extreme stress on the shoulder girdle.

❷ If unable to perform this exercise, you may use a partner's assistance to support part of your weight.

❸ As you get stronger, you may want to have a partner put plates on top of your quadriceps muscles as illustrated in the picture on the next page. However, ensure that the partner is always there providing weight stability and also ensure that the weight is never placed on top of the knee joint.

---

*FAQ:*

*I saw someone perform this with five 45-pound plates on his lap. Is this safe?*

*ANSWER:*

It may be safe for him, but if you're not used to this exercise, you should start with your bodyweight first. This can be a very effective triceps exercise, but you'll want to perfect your form before progressing too quickly. Just be careful not to strain your shoulders with this exercise. Just like the chest and triceps dips, going too low can seriously damage your shoulders.

# Bench Dip

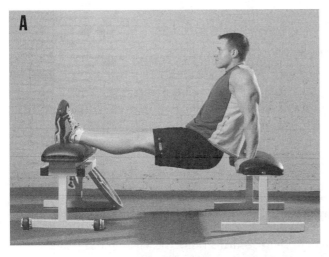

**A**

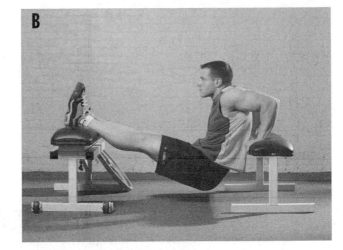

**B**

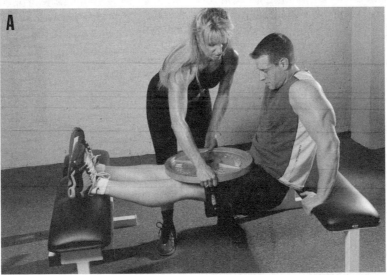

**A**

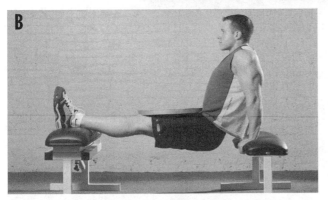

**B**

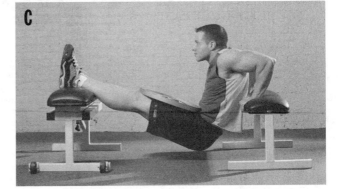

**C**

# E-Z Curl Bar Close-Grip Press

This exercise can be done one of two ways: alone as a triceps and inner chest exercise, or as a secondary superset exercise with the E-Z bar triceps extension exercise. We will explain this exercise in detail, and how you incorporate it will depend on the phase of training you have reached. The conventional way to do the close-grip bench press is with a barbell. It also calls for the arms to widen at the bottom, putting more emphasis on the inner chest muscles than the triceps. Our version of this exercise will obviously be done with the E-Z curl bar and with a different arm position than the conventional version. This puts emphasis on the triceps, with a secondary workload to the inner chest muscles.

## PROPER ALIGNMENT

This exercise will incorporate many of the same alignment positions as the lying E-Z bar triceps extension exercise.

❶ Set up the E-Z bar with some weight or get one that is pre-weighted. You can rest the bar on your thighs and bring it back overhead, setting it in place so that it is at the base of your head while you lie down, or you can simply have someone hand it to you when you are already lying down.

❷ Before lifting the bar or having it handed to you, lay back on the bench and place your feet flat on the floor, pointing straight ahead.

❸ As you are lying down lift the bar into place by pressing it up using your chest muscles (just like the chest press). Hold it above your head and stay there. You will begin the exercise in this position to avoid stressing the elbow joint.

❹ Remember to make sure that your whole arm is in direct line with your front shoulder (anterior deltoid). Your arms must stay close to your body and follow in a straight line from shoulder, to elbow, to arm. This is what will create primary isolation of the triceps muscles and allow better control of the bar.

❺ Take a position on the bar so that your hands are in the outer curved position. The inner curved position will create too much wrist strain. The proper width will be about 8-10 inches apart.

## TECHNIQUE AND FORM

❶ Once you are in proper alignment with the E-Z curl bar overhead, slowly begin to lower the bar as if you were lowering the bar during a bench press movement. But remember, your arms will now stay close to your body with your front shoulders and arms in a straight line.

❷ As you lower the bar, keep your arms riding closely to the sides of your body. This technique is essential for proper triceps stimulation.

❸ Remember to consciously focus all of your attention on proper form and intense stimulation of the triceps during the movement.

❹ As you continue to lower the bar, do so in a controlled manner and bring the bar down to around midchest. Without resting, and without momentum, use your triceps muscles to push the bar off your chest and back to the start position. Remember to maintain proper form, with the arms riding close to the sides of your body.

❺ As you reach the top of the movement, squeeze the triceps muscles as hard as you can without locking out your elbow joints.

*FAQ:*

*I thought that it was necessary and much more effective to keep the hands close together in order to work the triceps.*

**ANSWER:**

Not at all. Keeping your hands too close together can seriously damage your wrists and shoulders. You will get more than enough triceps stimulation by keeping your hands 8 to 10 inches apart.

# E-Z Curl Bar Close-Grip Press

**6** Hold this contraction for 1 second.

**7** Make sure that there is a smooth transition when switching directions from the top position going into the lowering of the bar, and also from the bottom position going into the extension or raising of the bar. There should be no rest at all when switching from the bottom position into the upward extension of the bar.

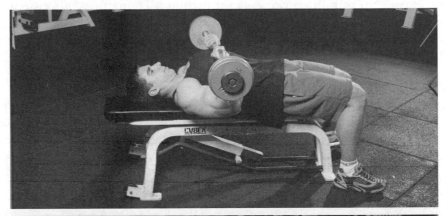

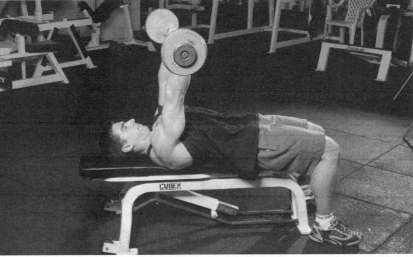

## VARIATION

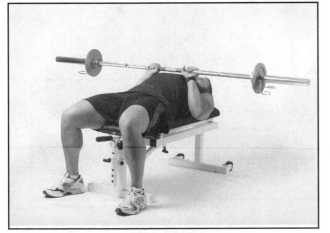

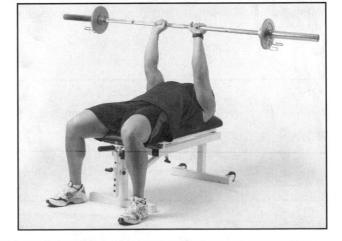

# Close-Grip Dumbbell Press

The close-grip dumbbell press is an excellent compound movement that not only targets the triceps muscle hard but also, as a bonus, targets the middle of your chest. The alignment used for this exercise is the same as the alignment used for chest exercises with the exception that you will need to retract the scapula in order to bring the chest above the shoulders.

## TECHNIQUE AND FORM

**1** With the dumbbells on your thighs, thrust one leg up, leveraging one dumbbell up to around chest level.

**2** Immediately thrust the second dumbbell upward while simultaneously allowing momentum and the dumbbells to guide you back into the lying position. Use your abdominal muscles to help safely ease you into position.

**3** Lay back and align your body using the alignment instructions presented for chest exercises, but retracting the scapula to bring the chest above the shoulders.

**4** Once you are in position, instead of bringing the dumbbells to the outside of the chest, hold them close to your chest. The handles of the dumbbells and palms of your hands must face each other with the elbows riding close to your body during movement. Your forearms must be perpendicular to the ceiling during the entire exercise. This close-grip movement will stimulate the inner chest muscles while a primary emphasis will be delivered to the triceps muscles as well.

**5** Because your shoulder muscles are more likely to move the weight than your chest muscles, you must retract the shoulder blades back or together against the flat bench. This slight variation will take the shoulders out of the chest movement, allowing the chest and triceps muscles to be the primary muscles working during the exercise.

**6** With the chest in its elevated position, the elbows out and wide, and the forearms perpendicular to the floor, press the dumbbells up toward the ceiling.

**7** As you press the weight up, put your mind into the chest and triceps muscles by concentrating on and feeling the muscles contract as you push upward.

**8** As you reach the top of the exercise, you must continue to consciously focus on the targeted muscles while physically contracting these muscles as hard as you possibly can. Your goal is to get the most intense contraction possible in the top position!

**9** In this position, squeeze and hold for a count of 1-2 seconds.

**10** Slowly begin lowering the weight while holding proper postural alignment throughout the exercise.

**11** As the dumbbells are lowered to the start position, they should touch your chest. This allows for a full stretch of the chest and triceps muscles.

**12** Without rest, slowly begin to press the dumbbells up again in a controlled, smooth, fluid motion, without using any momentum.

---

*FAQ:*

*When I do this exercise, I feel all the stimulation in my chest muscles instead of my triceps.*

*ANSWER:*

Because this exercise uses dumbbells, your range of motion is more open to improper form than that of an E-Z bar. Focus on keeping your arms pulled in close to your sides and it will put the emphasis of the resistance on your triceps.

# Close-Grip Dumbbell Press

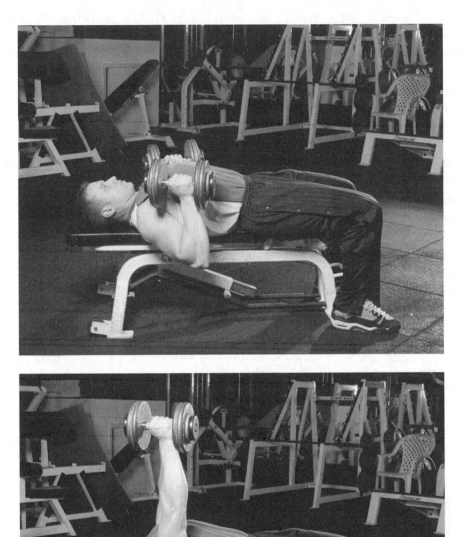

# Triceps Pushdown

This exercise often is performed incorrectly. Some common mistakes include the following:

1. Too much bending at the hips, which incorporates chest muscle activity. Proper form for this exercise means staying as straight as possible with a very slight bend to prevent lower back injury.

2. Bending over with the cable set on one side of the head. This causes the crucial balance of the resistance to be thrown off because force is greater at one side of the body than the other. Many professional trainers and athletes do this all the time. For proper form, keep the cable right at the center of your body.

3. Allowing the arms to come up during the negative portion of the exercise. Proper form calls for the upper arms (from the elbows to the shoulders) to stay locked at the sides of the body and remain there until the end of the exercise, when you have to return to the start position. Only the forearms should move.

This is a great exercise if done correctly. Follow the proper form and techniques and you will soon have the fat-free, firm triceps you desire.

## PROPER ALIGNMENT

You have the option of using a v-bar, a short cambered bar attachment, a rope, or a straight bar attachment for this exercise. Choose the bar that gives you the most comfortable grip. You can also change bars over time in order to add variety to your program.

❶ Stand in front of the cable and take hold of the bar. Bring the bar down by bringing your arms (from the elbow to the shoulder) to the sides of your body and lock them there.

❷ Position your feet shoulder-width apart with your feet pointing straight ahead.

❸ Slightly bend your knees and keep your torso upright throughout the movement.

❹ Keep your head pointing straight ahead and avoid looking down; otherwise you will tend to bend over.

## TECHNIQUE AND FORM

❶ Holding the bar with your arms positioned in place at your sides, begin by isometrically contracting the triceps muscles before moving the bar down.

❷ Begin pushing the bar down while keeping your elbows pinned to your sides.

❸ Push down until you have reached full extension. Avoid locking the elbow joint out hard. Make sure you squeeze the triceps muscles as hard as you possibly can at lockout. You are to focus on squeezing the triceps muscles hard, not the elbow joint. There is a major difference that practice will perfect.

❹ When you've reached the bottom position, squeeze the triceps muscles and hold for a count of 1 second.

❺ Begin to allow the bar to rise while maintaining your posture and arms at the sides.

❻ Let the bar come up to the point where your forearms are slightly higher than parallel to the floor. At this point, without resting, begin once again pushing down to the bottom position.

❼ Follow this form throughout this exercise and your triceps will burn with delight. If you continue with this proper alignment, technique and form, your triceps will very soon develop into arms of beauty!

# Triceps Pushdown

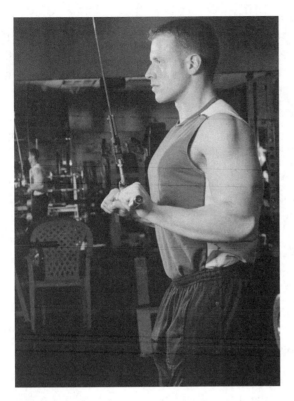 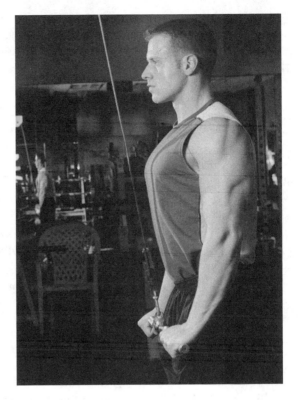

## VARIATION

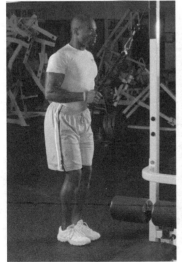 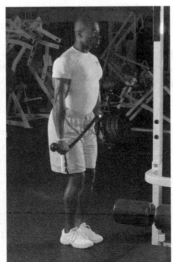

**FAQ:**

*I always see people doing this exercise with their bodies in line with the cable, but with their heads to one side.*

**ANSWER:**

Pulling your head to one side of the cable will create an imbalance in the distribution of weight. One side will be working much more than the other, and there are risks to your spine, as it is enduring the lateral pull to your core.

To avoid this, keep your head directly in the middle of the cable, stand up straight to avoid the chest muscles' involvement, keep your elbows pointed to the ground, and lock those shoulders in place. Don't let them flex upward.

# Triceps Kickback

This is a great isolation exercise if you settle for using lighter weights and just concentrate on using good form. Sloppy or incorrect technique will not allow you to get any benefit out of this exercise. This exercise will provide you with a killer contraction at the top of the movement. Try to hold that contraction for a second or two in order to really fry those triceps!

### PROPER ALIGNMENT

**1** With this exercise, you will be training one arm at a time. Starting with the right triceps, lean down on a flat bench and place your left knee and your left hand on the bench for support. Your right leg will remain in a semi-straight position, with the foot flat on the floor. Maintain a flat back throughout the exercise.

**2** Pick up a dumbbell with the right hand using an overhand grip, making sure that the weight is light enough to maintain proper form throughout the exercise.

**3** In the bent-over position, place the upper arm (right humerus) flush against the right side of your body. Make sure to allow your lower arm to remain loose.

**4** Take note that when you are ready to begin this exercise the upper and lower arm of the triceps should form a 90-degree angle.

**5** Reverse the same protocol when training the left triceps.

### TECHNIQUE AND FORM

**1** Once again, make sure that the lower and upper arm are at a 90-degree angle, and the dumbbell is held with an overhand grip.

**2** Begin the exercise by extending the lower arm back until it is at full extension.

**3** Make sure that you keep the upper arm pressed against the right side of the body during the exercise.

**4** Once the elbow reaches the point of full extension, contract the triceps as hard as possible. Make sure to avoid hyperextension of the elbow.

**5** Slowly lower the dumbbell back to the 90-degree angle.

---

*FAQ:*

*I'm not sure if I'm getting the dumbbell up high enough for a full range of motion.*

*ANSWER:*

There's nothing wrong with looking in the mirror every so often to check if your form and technique are good. If you see that you aren't bringing the dumbbell up high enough, maybe you need to go lighter with the weights. Make sure to avoid momentum.

# Triceps Kickback

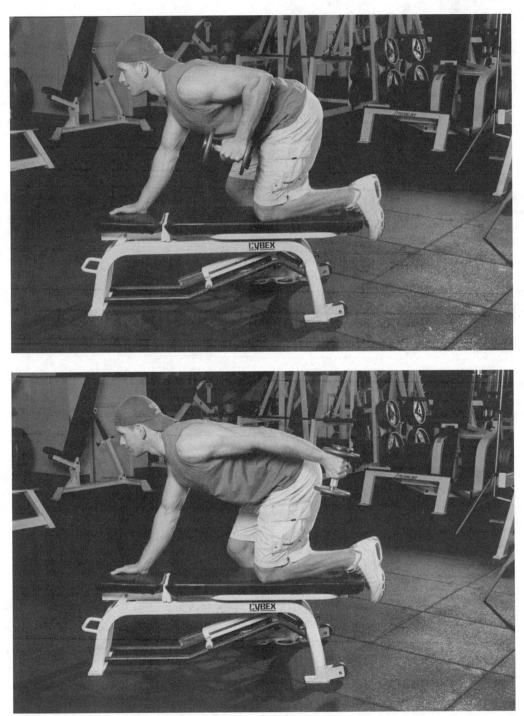

# Fixed-Bar Bodyweight Triceps Extension

This is a very advanced exercise that should only be performed by people with strength and gym experience.

### PROPER ALIGNMENT

❶ Fix a horizontal bar in front of you at waist height.  Do this by using the bar of a Smith machine or a regular Olympic bar placed at the end of a squat rack with adjustable pins.

❷ Grasp the bar at shoulder width with an overhand (pronated) grip. Your arms should extend forward at an angle of about 50 degrees from the head to the arms.

❸ Keep the rest of the torso straight but slanted forward so your arms are holding your weight and your legs are behind you like a modified push-up position.

❹ Keep your arms stationary and your elbows in.

### TECHNIQUE AND FORM

❶ Inhale, bend at the elbows, and lower your body until your forehead lightly touches the bar.

❷ Use your triceps to press against the bar, and then exhale while bringing your torso back to the starting position.

# Fixed-Bar Bodyweight Triceps Extension

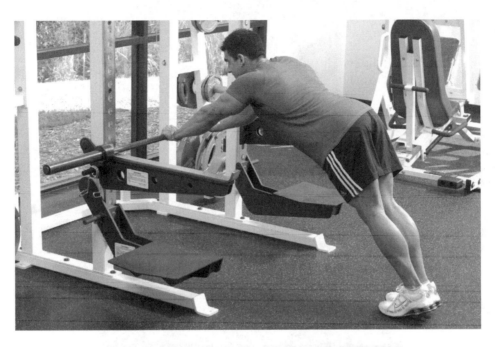

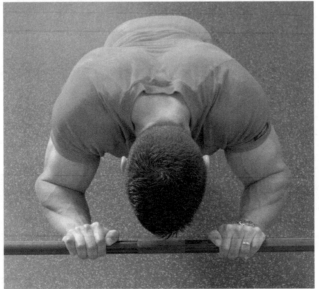

# Chapter 11
# Biceps

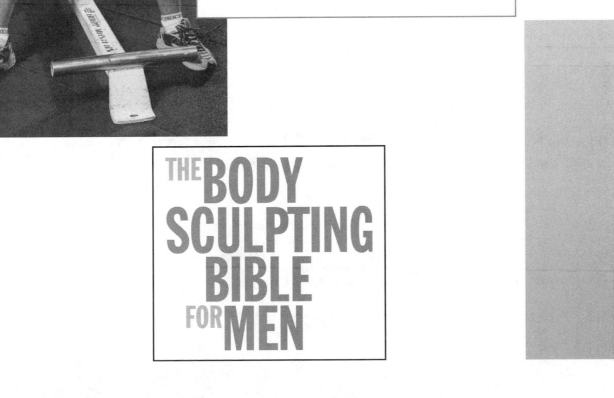

The biceps muscles are located on the front of the upper arms and are a two-headed muscle that serves to lift the forearms upwards. Biceps are probably one of the simplest muscles to train. However, just like chest muscles, you can go to any gym in the country and probably see that 90 percent of the people training them are using incorrect form.

For immediate Body Sculpting Bible support & coaching directly from James & Hugo, please visit www.BodySculptingBible.com

**11**

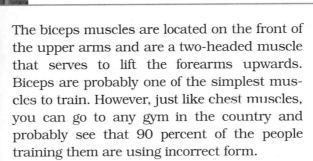

# Dumbbell Curl

**(Using two dumbbells simultaneously, while standing)**
The dumbbell biceps curl is a great exercise for building the biceps muscles. We suggest that you do this exercise standing up and supporting yourself against a wall for good body mechanics and strict form.

## PROPER ALIGNMENT

❶ Choose two light dumbbells so that you can practice perfect form.

❷ With the dumbbells in hand, begin the alignment of your body by placing your feet about shoulder-width apart with the toes pointing straight ahead.

❸ Slightly bend at the knees.

❹ Allow the dumbbells to hang down at your sides with your palms and dumbbells facing forward, as shown in the picture.

❺ Make sure that your elbows stay pointed to the ground at all times during the biceps curl exercise. Do not allow them to move from that position.

❻ Keep your upper body straight by sticking out your chest and keeping your shoulder blades squared off.

❼ Keep your head level, and your eyes pointing straight ahead of you.

## TECHNIQUE AND FORM

❶ Once you are in proper postural alignment and against the wall, make sure to focus all of your attention on the biceps muscles and the exercise you are about to do. It is very easy to get distracted during exercise, but the rewards of staying focused throughout your training sessions will be well worth your efforts.

❷ With the dumbbells at your sides, begin curling them up, making sure to keep your elbows pointed toward the ground.

❸ Once you've reached the top position of the exercise, contract the biceps muscles as hard as you possibly can and hold that contraction for a count of 2 seconds.

❹ From the top position, slowly and smoothly begin to lower the dumbbells back to the starting position.

❺ As you reach the bottom of the exercise, immediately begin curling the weights up toward your shoulders again. Make sure that there is a smooth transition when switching directions from both the top position and also from the bottom position. Both scenarios must be done with no rest in between either of the direction changes, unless you are so fatigued by the end of the set that you need a few seconds of rest in order to get a couple more repetitions.

## VARIATION: SUPINATION

For added stimulation of the biceps muscles, you can try a technique called supination. Instead of beginning the exercise with your palms facing forward, begin with your palms facing in toward the sides of the body. As you lift the weights, rotate your wrists until the dumbbells and palms of your hands are facing back toward you by the time you reach the top of the movement. Supination or rotation of your wrists should last the entire distance from the sides of your body up to your shoulders. In other words, don't just rotate your hands completely at the bottom position; allow them to gradually rotate during the entire distance. When you reach the top position of the exercise, your pinkies should be above your thumbs. Make sure your elbows remain pointed to the ground. Then, as you lower the weight, reverse the supination by rotating the wrists in the opposite direction, again making sure you prolong the rotation throughout the entire distance. When you finish, the palms of your hands and dumbbells should once again face the sides of your body.

# Dumbbell Curl

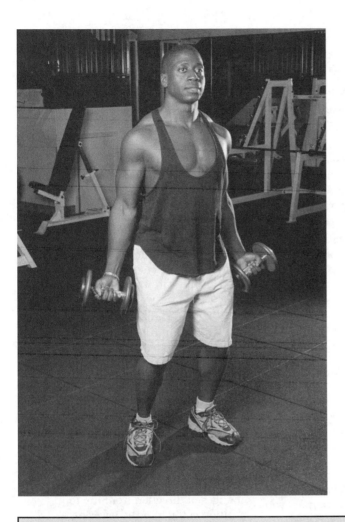 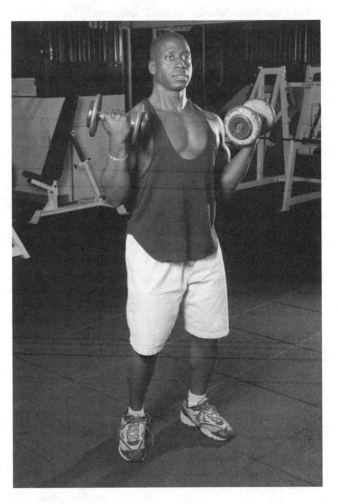

**FAQ:**

*Why don't my biceps get larger?*

**ANSWER:**

Your biceps are really not a very big muscle. Beginners might see some dramatic difference, but the more advanced you are the less likely you will see larger biceps. If you want to get the most out of your biceps training, make sure that you avoid momentum, keep those elbows pointed to the ground, and stop allowing those shoulders to flex upward. Remember to squeeze and contract fully at the top of each repetition!

# Incline Dumbbell Curl

**(Using two dumbbells simultaneously)**

The incline dumbbell curl is a great exercise for developing great looking biceps muscles. It was one of Arnold Schwarzenegger's favorite exercises because of the stretch that it provides at the bottom of the movement. Because the exercise requires strict form and isolation, you should start doing the exercise with a weight lighter than what you'd usually use for a regular dumbbell curl. Remember, form is everything. Make sure to avoid momentum and keep the form strict. Do not sacrifice good form for heavy weight and ego!

## PROPER ALIGNMENT

**1** Go to an incline bench and set the bench incline to a 45-degree angle. Due to the full stretch and range of motion of this exercise, it is designed to work the full length of the biceps with added emphasis on the outer head of the biceps muscle.

**2** Pick two dumbbells with a weight that you can handle using perfect form. This exercise must be done very strictly in order to receive the desired effects.

**3** Decide if you'd rather start the exercise holding the dumbbells at the sides of your body or with them resting on top of your thighs, which we prefer. Starting with the dumbbells on your thighs will give you some quality time to visualize and focus on the exercise you are about to do. This preparation can set up the proper mindset for even greater lifting performance.

**4** Lean all the way back into the bench so that your entire back is lying flat against the back pad. Stay that way for the entire exercise and do not take your back off the bench until the exercise is complete. Once you are properly positioned and ready to begin, take a firm grip on the dumbbells and allow them to hang at your sides.

**5** Make sure that the palms of your hands are facing the wall in front of you for the entire exercise. Refrain from supination or hand twisting with this exercise.

**6** Make sure to keep your elbows pointed directly at the floor during the entire exercise. When people usually do any type of biceps curl, they allow their elbows to drift up with the curling movement, allowing the shoulders to flex forward. When this happens, you can forget about fully stimulating the biceps muscles since the anterior shoulders become the prime movers of the weight being curled. There is only one instance when you may lift the shoulders while doing a biceps curl. That is when you have come to a point in your training where you add additional repetitions (forced reps) with the help of a spotter. Before you reach this point in your training, you must follow the earlier described form of keeping the elbows to the ground for full and proper stimulation of the biceps muscles.

## TECHNIQUE AND FORM

**1** Once you are in position, focus all of your attention on the exercise you are about to do and on the biceps muscle itself.

**2** Begin curling the dumbbells at the same time, making sure that the elbows stay positioned towards the ground without moving upward as you curl.

**3** Curl the weights up until you can no longer curl while simultaneously contracting the biceps muscles as hard as you can. Hold that position for a second or two.

**4** Slowly and smoothly begin to lower the dumbbells until your arms are fully elongated and back at your sides.

**5** Without rest and without using any momentum, slowly and steadily begin curling the dumbbells back up toward your shoulders. If you jerk or in any way use momentum to begin curling the dumbbells, you risk serious injury to the biceps muscles. Once again, make sure that the changes of direction from the top position going into the lowering phase, and from the bottom position going into the curling phase, are always smooth and controlled.

# Incline Dumbbell Curl

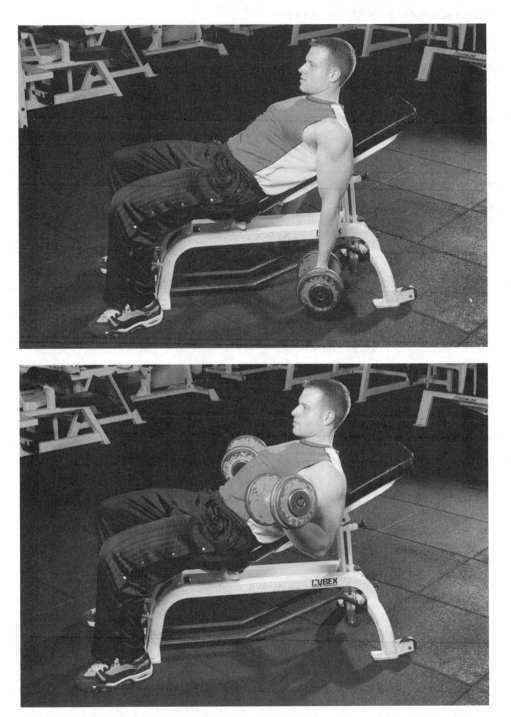

# One-Arm Preacher Curl

**(Using a preacher machine or inclined bench)**

Larry Scott, the first Mr. Olympia, attributed his 21-inch guns to this exercise. Preacher curls develop the lower portion of the biceps muscle, helping to build balance in the biceps. For this exercise, you may use two dumbbells together or one at a time, which will help to create concentration and balance for this particular exercise. This exercise will also cause a greater contraction at the top of the movement because of the independent range of motion involved. It can be done on a preacher bench or simply on the back support of an incline bench. Because the exercise is very strict, it is important that you choose a dumbbell weight you can handle while practicing perfect form.

## PROPER ALIGNMENT

❶ If using a preacher machine, sit on the machine's seat and bring your chest against the pad in front of you. If using an incline bench, stand at the end of the bench so the incline portion is touching your stomach.

❷ Position your feet flat on the floor and keep them there for the entire exercise.

❸ Allow one arm to hang over the angled support of the preacher bench or incline bench. Support yourself with your other arm. Make sure that the back of your arm is positioned flat against the angled support and lying in a straight line. In order to comfortably keep the arm in this position, you may have to angle your body to one side, making sure you are not using leveraging techniques to assist you in the curl.

❹ It is important to focus all of your attention on the biceps muscles while doing the exercise instead of calling upon the assistance of other muscles to help curl the weight.

Also, as you curl the weight up, make sure that you lean into the front chest support rather than lean back for cheating leverage. Make sure that the majority of the resistance is being focused on the biceps muscles throughout the exercise. When you reach the top position of the exercise, you must contract the biceps muscle as hard as you possibly can. Because you are on an angled support, the upper position of this exercise makes it very easy for you to rest the weight of the dumbbell on the bones rather than the biceps muscle. You must overcome this bone support with a very hard contraction of the biceps muscle.

## TECHNIQUE AND FORM

❶ Once you are in position with one arm lying flat against the angled support, hold the body steady and begin curling the weight up toward your shoulder.

❷ Focus all of your attention on the arm you are exercising, making sure to squeeze hard on the curling phase

and resisting the weight as you come back down.

❸ As you begin curling, relax the shoulder on the arm you are training as it can assist in the lift.

❹ As you reach the top of this exercise, again contract the biceps muscles as hard as you can for a count of two seconds.

❺ Slowly return to the starting position of the exercise.

❻ As you reach the bottom position, immediately once again begin curling the weight up toward your shoulder. Once you are done with the desired amount of repetitions with that arm, switch arms and do the same amount of repetitions.

# One-Arm Preacher Curl

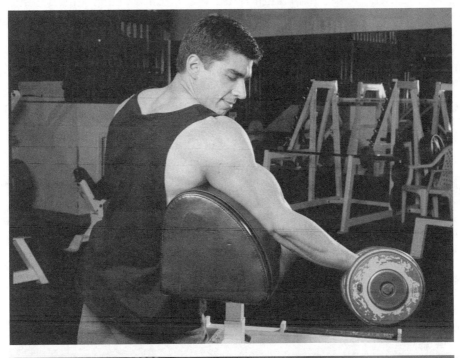

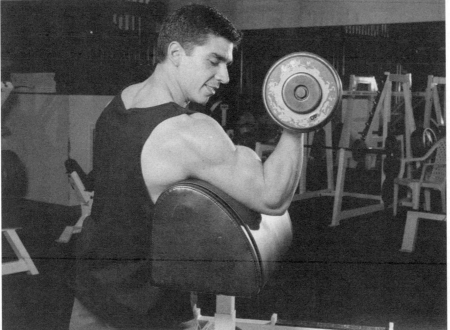

# E-Z Reverse Preacher Curl

This exercise targets the brachialis, also known as the outer biceps, and forearm muscles. Remember to keep your head level, looking straight ahead, and to engage your abdominals to avoid using your lower back.

There are a couple variations, including the regular preacher curl, which requires grasping the E-Z bar with your palms facing you. You can also use a low pulley with an E-Z bar attachment instead of an E-Z bar. You will need to position the bench in front of the pulley, and may also use a closer grip. You can use a straight bar as well—just remember that straight bars place more stress on the wrist joint.

## PROPER ALIGNMENT

**1** This exercise requires a preacher bench and an E-Z bar. Have your spotter hand you the bar or use the front bar rest. Grasp the E-Z curl bar at the wide outer handle with the palms of you hands facing downward due to the shape of the bar, arms fully extended. Your thumb should be higher than your little finger.

**2** Position your chest and upper arms against the preacher bench pad and hold the E-Z curl bar at shoulder length.

**3** Keep your head and eyes facing straight ahead throughout the movement.

## TECHNIQUE AND FORM

**1** As you inhale, slowly lower the bar until your upper arm is extended and the biceps are fully stretched.

**2** Exhale and use the biceps to curl the weight up until your biceps are fully contracted and the bar is at shoulder height.

# E-Z Reverse Preacher Curl

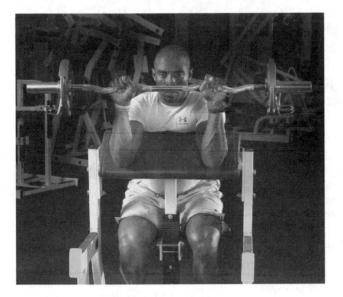

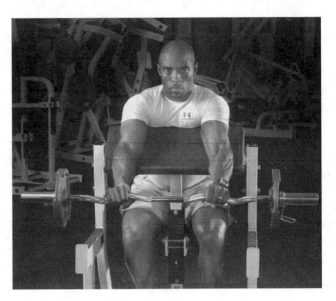

**VARIATION**

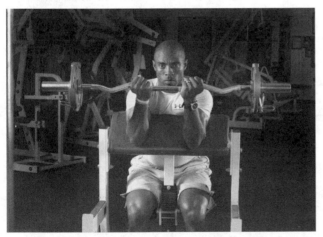

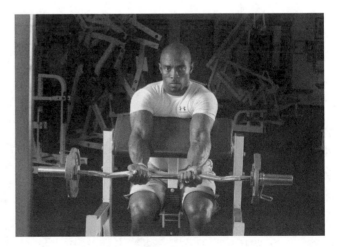

# Concentration Curl

**(One arm at a time)**

The name concentration curl should not just be applied to this version of the biceps curl. It should be applied to every exercise we've discussed or will discuss in the book. Putting your mind into the muscle and focusing every bit of your attention on the exercise you are about to do is the surest way of reaching your fitness goals in the quickest amount of time possible. In the picture of our model demonstrating the concentration curl, look at his eyes and how they are focused on the exercise movement. His results and the results you will soon achieve are a direct result of the focus and intensity you put into every set and rep of an exercise.

## PROPER ALIGNMENT

❶ You can do the concentration curl either in a sitting position or while standing.

❷ Whatever position you choose, bend over at the hips and take a dumbbell in one hand. The dumbbell weight should at first be light so that you can practice perfect form.

❸ Sit at the edge of a bench and support your arm by resting your elbow on your thigh.

## TECHNIQUE AND FORM

❶ Do not curl the weight straight up to your chest. You must curl the weight with your arm angled in toward your body. This will help make certain that the exercise motion is correct, following the direction towards your shoulders rather than your chest. To start, bend over at the hips and fully extend the arm that you will be exercising while the other arm is resting on your thigh.

❷ Begin curling the weight while you also begin rotating your wrist.

❸ Curl the weight towards your shoulder and contract the biceps muscle as hard as you possibly can, while keeping your arm pointing at the ground.

❹ Once you reach the top of the movement, hold for a 2-second count.

❺ Slowly lower the dumbbell back to the starting position, resisting the weight the entire way down.

❻ Without rest or momentum, once again start curling the weight towards the shoulder with great focus and concentration. Once you have completed the desired amount of repetitions, switch arms and do the same amount of repetitions.

**FAQ:**

*Why do I feel this exercise more than any other biceps exercise?*

**ANSWER:**

You can bet that it's because you're focused on truly squeezing and contracting the biceps at the top of the movement. Most people just go through the motions of exercises and pay little attention to making sure that they are consciously squeezing and contracting. This additional bit of mental focus really works your muscles. This applies to all exercises!

# Concentration Curl

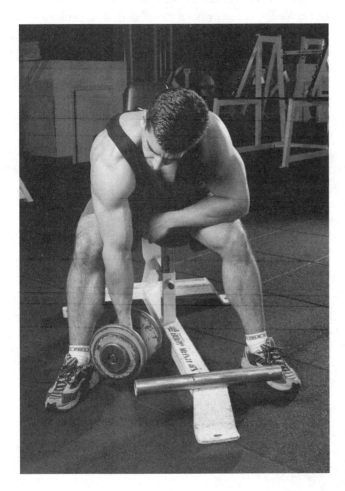
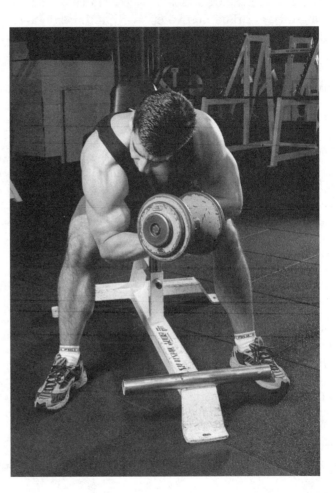

# Standing E-Z Bar Curl

Do not underestimate this exercise because of its name. The E-Z bar curl is a versatile exercise that allows you to use heavy weight while being much easier on the wrists than straight bar curls. If you have a pending strain such as tennis elbow or tendonitis, we would recommend this exercise over straight bar curls. The two-curved hand positions on the bar allow you to do both close-grip and wide-grip curls. The inner grip will enable you to develop the outer biceps, and the outer grip will enable you to develop the inner biceps.

## PROPER ALIGNMENT

❶ First, decide which hand position you will take on the bar. Remember what we discussed earlier about assessing your body and focusing on the unbalanced or weak body parts to create muscle balance and symmetry. Look at your biceps muscles and assess the inner and outer muscle heads. Decide if one head needs more work then the other. If you find a weakness or imbalance in one of the two muscle heads, then address that problem by simply using the hand position that will bring the smaller portion of the biceps muscle up to par with the others.

❷ Hold the bar across your thighs with your palms facing away from your body.

❸ Position your feet shoulder-width apart and point them straight ahead. Next, bend your knees slightly.

❹ Slightly contract the abdominal muscles.

❺ Stand straight up and stay that way throughout the movement.

❻ Stick your chest out and keep the shoulders back, which will help you maintain a straight back.

❼ Keep your head level and do not move it from that position for the rest of the exercise.

## TECHNIQUE AND FORM

❶ With the bar across your thighs, lock your elbows to the sides of your body and begin curling the bar up towards your shoulders in an arc-like motion.

❷ Keep the elbows pointing directly to the ground as you curl upward to avoid using the shoulders in the curling motion.

❸ As you curl upward to the shoulders with an arc-like movement, concentrate and focus all of your attention on the biceps muscles. Feel the muscles contracting as you curl the bar upward.

❹ As you reach the top of the movement with the bar close to your shoulders, contract the biceps muscles as hard as you possibly can.

❺ Hold this position for a count of 1-2 seconds.

❻ Slowly begin lowering the bar while making sure that the biceps endure the negative resistance on the way down to the bottom position.

❼ As you reach the start position with the arms fully straightened, do not rest. Begin curling the bar once again in a smooth controlled and fluid motion without using momentum.

**FAQ:**

*Why do my wrists and forearms hurt when I do this exercise?*

**ANSWER:**

This exercise can definitely stress those areas. If you feel discomfort, we recommend warming up a bit more or simply switching the exercise to something more effective.

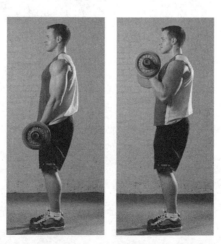

# Standing E-Z Bar Curl

**WIDE GRIP**

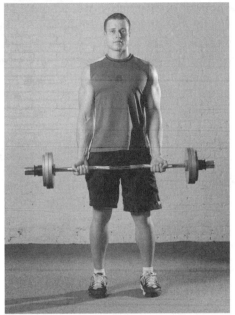 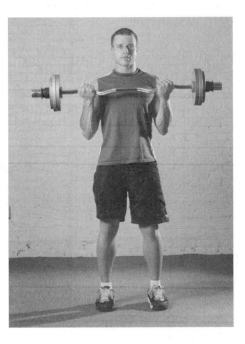

**NARROW GRIP**

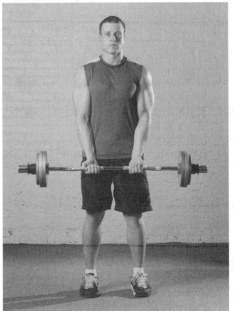 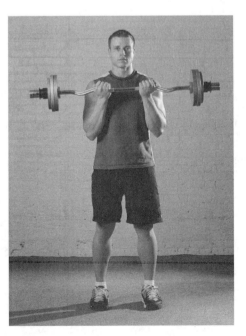

# Hammer Curl

**(Outer biceps and forearms)**

The dumbbell hammer curl is a great exercise for building the outer head of the biceps, or brachialis muscles. It also builds the extensor muscles of the forearms. This exercise is done in the same way as standing dumbbell curls, except that you hold the dumbbells with the palms facing each other throughout the entire exercise. You can do this exercise either sitting, which will make it much stricter, or standing which will allow you to go a bit heavier. We suggest that you include both versions in your training routine.

**VARIATION:** To get an additional burn in your forearms, try this same movement on an incline bench.

## PROPER ALIGNMENT

**1** Choose two light dumbbells so that you can practice perfect form.

**2** With the dumbbells in hand, begin the alignment of your body by placing your feet about shoulder-width apart with your feet pointing straight ahead of you.

**3** Slightly bend your knees.

**4** Allow the dumbbells to hang down at your sides with your palms and dumbbells facing the sides of your body.

**5** Make sure that your elbows stay pointed at the ground at all times during the biceps curl exercise.

**6** Keep your upper body straight by contracting your abdominal muscles slightly, sticking out your chest and keeping your shoulder blades squared off.

**7** Keep your head level, and your eyes pointing straight ahead of you.

## TECHNIQUE AND FORM

**1** Once you are in proper postural alignment stand against a wall. Make sure to focus all of your attention on the biceps and forearm muscles. It is very easy to get distracted during exercise, but the rewards of staying focused throughout your training sessions will be well worth your efforts.

**2** Begin curling your dumbbells up with palms and dumbbells facing each other.

**3** Focus on driving your thumbs to your front shoulders, concentrating on feeling the biceps and forearm muscles working.

**4** Once you've reached the top position of the exercise, contract the biceps and forearm muscles as hard as you possibly can and hold that contraction for a count of 1-2 seconds.

**5** From the top position, slowly and smoothly begin to lower the dumbbells back to the starting position.

**6** As you reach the bottom of the exercise, the palms of your hands and dumbbells should remain facing each other and pressed to the sides of your body.

**7** Make sure that there is a smooth transition when switching directions from both the top position going into the lowering of the dumbbells, and also from the bottom position going into the curling or raising of the dumbbells. Both scenarios must be done with no rest in between either of the direction changes, unless you are so fatigued by the end of the set that you need a few seconds rest in order to do a couple more repetitions.

# Hammer Curl

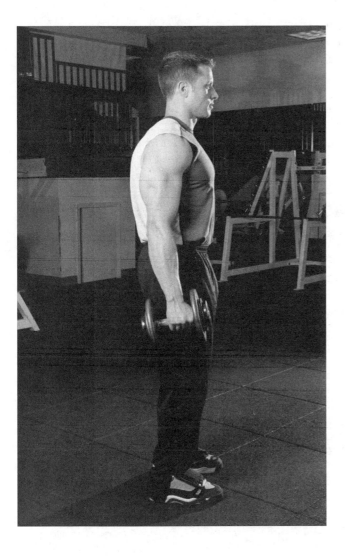

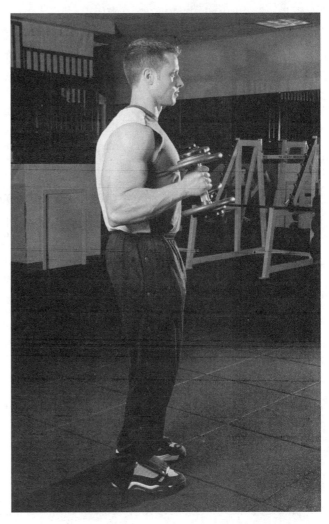

**FAQ:**

*I don't feel this in my biceps.*

**ANSWER:**

That's fine. You should instead feel it in your forearm extensor muscles (the backs of your forearms). The secondary muscles here are the brachiallis muscles of the upper arm (the outer biceps).

## VARIATION

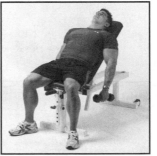
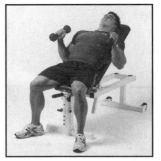

# Reverse Curl

This exercise is best performed with an E-Z bar and it targets both the brachialis and the upper forearms muscles. The exercise alignment and execution is the same as that of the E-Z curls except that the hands are holding the bar with the palms facing the thighs on the outer handles of the bar for direct forearm stimulation.

## PROPER ALIGNMENT

To prepare for the exercise, you will align your body similar to the way you did with the standing dumbbell biceps curl.

**1** First, take your hand position by placing your hands with an overhand grip on the outer handles of the bar.

Hold the bar across your thighs with your palms facing towards your body.

**2** Position your feet shoulder width apart and point them straight ahead. Next, bend your knees slightly.

**3** Slightly contract the abdominal muscles.

**4** Stand straight up and stay that way throughout the movement.

**5** Stick your chest out and keep your shoulders back, which will help you maintain a straight back.

**6** Keep your head level and do not move it from that position for the rest of the exercise.

## TECHNIQUE AND FORM

**1** Now in position with the bar across your thighs, lock your elbows to the sides of your body and begin curling the bar up towards your shoulders in an arc-like motion.

**2** Keep the elbows pointing directly to the ground as you curl upward to avoid using the shoulders in the curling motion.

**3** As you curl upward to the shoulders with an arc-like movement, concentrate and focus all of your attention on forearms and biceps muscles. Feel the muscles contracting as you curl the bar upward.

**4** As you reach the top of the movement with the bar close to your shoulders, contract the biceps muscles as hard as you possibly can.

**5** Hold this position for a count of 1-2 seconds.

**6** Slowly begin lowering the bar while making sure that the forearms and biceps endure the negative resistance on the way back down to the bottom position.

**7** As you reach the start position with the arms fully straightened, do not rest. Begin curling the bar once again in a smooth and controlled, fluid motion without using momentum.

---

**FAQ:**

*I feel like I tend to rest at the top of the exercise when the bar is just under my chin.*

**ANSWER:**

If this is happening to you, try using an E-Z bar cable attachment, and stand in front of that cable machine. Because of the line of pull, it keeps tension on the muscles, even at the top of the movement.

# Reverse Curl

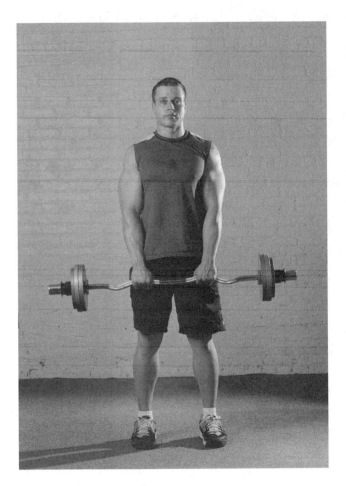
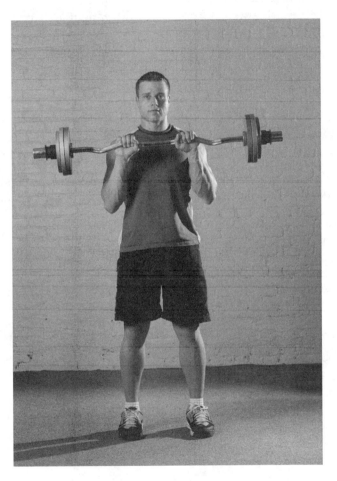

# Neutral-Grip Chin-Up

If you are new to this exercise and do not have the strength to perform it, use a pull-up assist machine if available. These machines use weight to help you push your body weight. Otherwise a spotter holding your legs can help. If neither of these two options is available, then substitute a pull-down using a v-bar attachment.

More advanced lifters can add weight to the exercise by using a weight belt that allows the addition of weighted plates.

**VARIATION:** Try a variation of this exercise, the close grip chin-up, by grasping the pull-up bar with your palms facing your torso in a reverse grip closer than shoulder width.

## PROPER ALIGNMENT

**1** You will need access to a v-bar (the triangular bar with two handles used for the low pulley rows) and a pull-up bar. Start by placing the middle of the v-bar in the middle of the pull-up bar. The v-bar handles will be facing down so that you can hang from the pull-up bar through the use of the handles.

**2** After securely placing the v-bar, take hold of the bar from each side and hang from it. Stick your chest out while keeping your torso as straight as possible in order to limit the engagement of the lats and maximize biceps stimulation.

## TECHNIQUE AND FORM

**1** Using your biceps, pull your torso up while leaning your head back slightly so you do not hit yourself with the chin-up bar.

**2** Exhale and continue until your head nearly touches the v-bar and your biceps are contracted (there should be an angle less than 90 degrees between the upper arm and the lower arm).

**3** After holding for 1 second in the contracted position, slowly lower your body back to the starting position as you breathe in.

**4** Repeat for the desired number of repetitions.

# Neutral-Grip Chin-Up

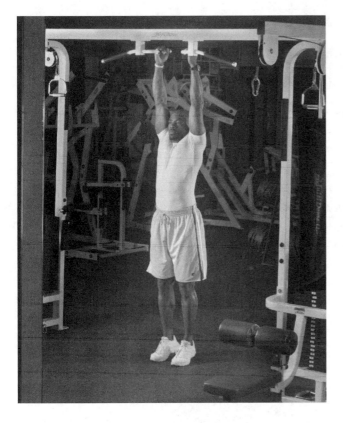

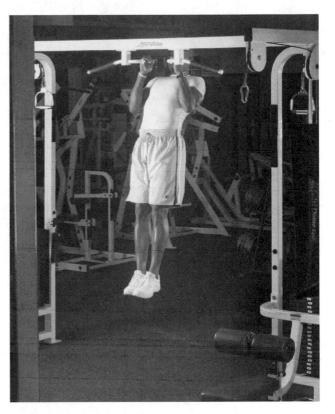

## VARIATION

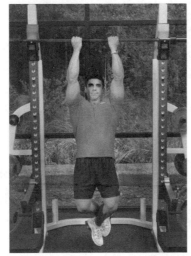

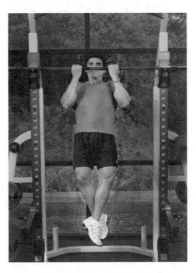

# High Cable Curl

This movement targets the biceps brachii with a secondary emphasis on the brachialis.

You may slant your torso a bit backward to maintain good balance when you grab the bar before starting the exercise, but remember that your upper arms must remain stationary, moving them will take off stimulation from the biceps.

## PROPER ALIGNMENT

**1** Stand in front of a pull-down machine with a bar attached to the pulley.

**2** Grab the bar using a shoulder-width grip and position your upper arms so that they are parallel to the floor with your palms facing up.

## TECHNIQUE AND FORM

**1** Exhale and curl the bar toward you until it is close to your forehead while flexing your biceps. The upper arms should remain still-only the forearms should move. Hold for 1 second in the contracted position.

**2** Slowly bring your arms back to the starting position as you inhale.

**3** Repeat for the recommended number of repetitions.

# High Cable Curl

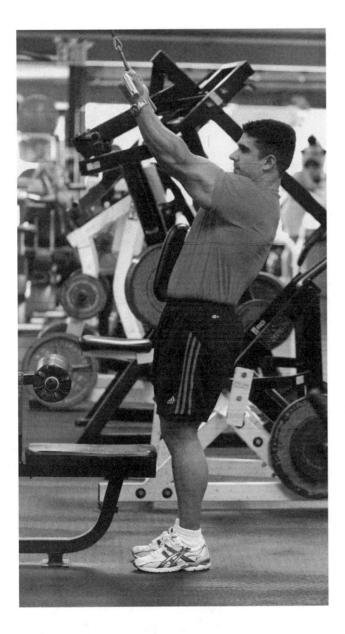
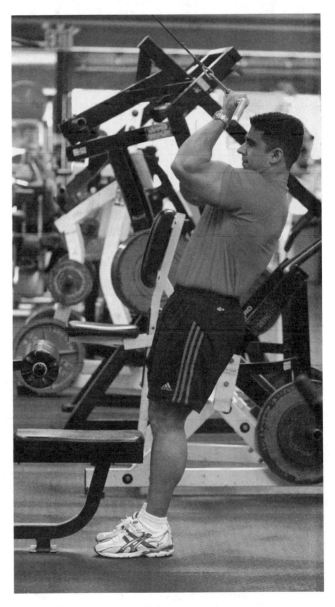

# Chapter 12
## Abdominals

In this section we will talk about how to exercise the most visually stunning and most sought after muscles: the abdominals. Let us recall that these exercises only firm up and build these muscles. In order to increase the visibility of the abdominal muscles, both diet and aerobic training have to be in order as these two are the components that burn body fat.

For immediate Body Sculpting Bible support & coaching directly from James & Hugo, please visit www.BodySculptingBible.com

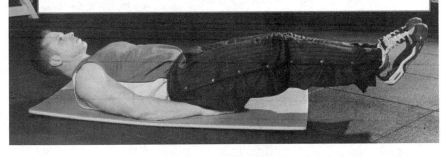

**12**

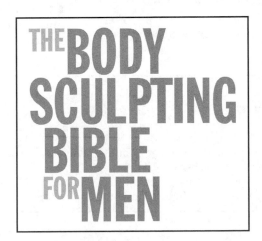

THE **BODY**
**SCULPTING**
**BIBLE**
FOR **MEN**

# Crunch

Crunches are a great exercise for the abdominal muscles. They are easier to do than the traditional sit-up (which should never be done by anyone with lower back problems), but just because they're easy doesn't mean they don't produce great results. By far, crunches are one of the best abdominal exercises for creating great looking abs, as they mimic the exact function of the abdominal muscles.

**VARIATION:** A variation of this exercise is a crunch on the ball. For this, you use a fitness ball which allows for greater range of motion and increased recruitment of core stabilizers. Simply sit on a fitness ball, then slide down until your lower back is on the ball. Elevate your shoulders and upper back, keep your feet flat on the floor, focus your eyes on the ceiling, and crunch slightly to your feet. Lift one foot off of the ground for an even more advanced technique. You'll be keeping your head in line with your spine.

## PROPER ALIGNMENT

Crunches are by far one of the premier abdominal exercises for ultimate looking abs.

**1** Lay down with your back flat on a carpet or mat.

**2** Bend your knees and lay your feet flat on the floor.

**3** Cross your hands at the chest and put a thumb on each side of your chin. This will help keep your head in a neutral position throughout the movement.

## TECHNIQUE AND FORM

**1** To really optimize this exercise you'll want to focus on the motion of bringing your chest plate to your pelvic area. Our focus is to squish the stomach area between the chest and pelvis. The abdominal muscles are what will actually move your chest towards your pelvic region, so what better than to crunch them in-between the two? The reason we say this is because many trainers simply teach their clients to "crunch." Many times, instead of flexing their spines with their abdominal muscles these clients often end up using their hip flexors as the primary muscles to "crunch."

**2** Begin by isometrically contracting the abdominal muscles before moving.

**3** As you begin the crunch, focus on moving your chest (not your head) toward your pelvis.

**4** Exhale as you move up toward your knees. This will allow you to get a more forceful contraction of the abs.

**5** Remember that the distance from start position to end position is not very far at all. It is not like a sit-up. Once again, your focus is not just to move but also to crunch your abs in between your chest and pelvis. Makes sense now doesn't it?

**6** As you reach the top (end) position, make sure that you are contracting the abdominal muscles as hard as you possibly can. This is the most important position of the exercise.

**7** Hold the contraction for 1-2 seconds.

**8** Return to the bottom position and, without rest or momentum, return to the upward movement.

---

*FAQ:*

*My neck hurts when I keep my thumbs under my chin.*

*ANSWER:*

You can put your hands behind your head, but make sure not to pull on your head to assist in the exercise. You can also stretch your hands out to the sides of your body. Imagine trying to touch an object a bit far in front of you. This will both help to take your mind off the ab muscle burn, while making sure that you are really squeezing and contracting those ab muscles. This also applies to the trunk curl and crunch.

# Crunch

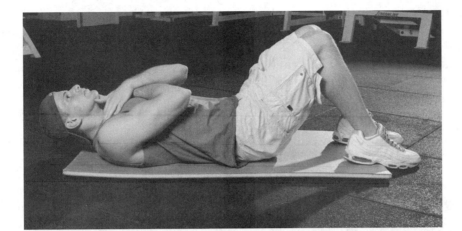

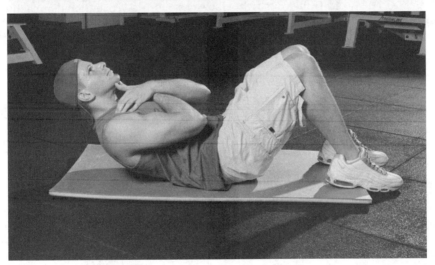

## VARIATION

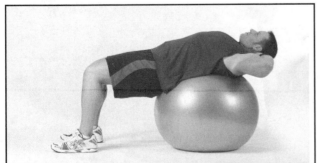

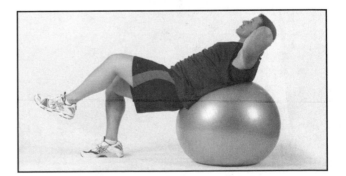

# Bicycle Crunch

This exercise, commonly known as the bicycle, is very effective when done properly. In a study conducted by the American Council on Exercise, it was found to be one of the most effective exercises you can do to stimulate the muscle fibers in the abdominal area. You cannot add resistance to this exercise but you can concentrate on perfect execution and slow speed.

## PROPER ALIGNMENT

**1** Lay on your back, flat on the floor, keeping your hands behind your head and your knees bent. Press your lower back to the ground. Be careful not to strain your neck as you perform this exercise. Try to keep your back pressed against the floor; avoid having it arch up.

**2** Lift your shoulders into the crunch position.

**3** Bring your knees up until they are perpendicular to the floor, with your lower legs parallel to the floor.

## TECHNIQUE AND FORM

**1** Now simultaneously go through a pedal motion, kicking forward with the right leg and bringing in the knee of the left leg. The extended leg should be a few inches off the floor; if you place it too close to the floor you can strain your back.

**2** Bring your right elbow close to your left knee by crunching to the side as you breathe out. When you twist toward your knee actively think about twisting with your waist, rather than with your elbow. If you feel that you are pulling against your neck, you may be using your arms rather than your waist to twist.

**3** Go back to the starting position as you breathe in.

**4** Immediately crunch to the opposite side as you cycle your legs and bring your left elbow closer to your right knee and exhale.

**5** Continue alternating in this manner until all of the recommended repetitions for each side have been completed.

# Bicycle Crunch

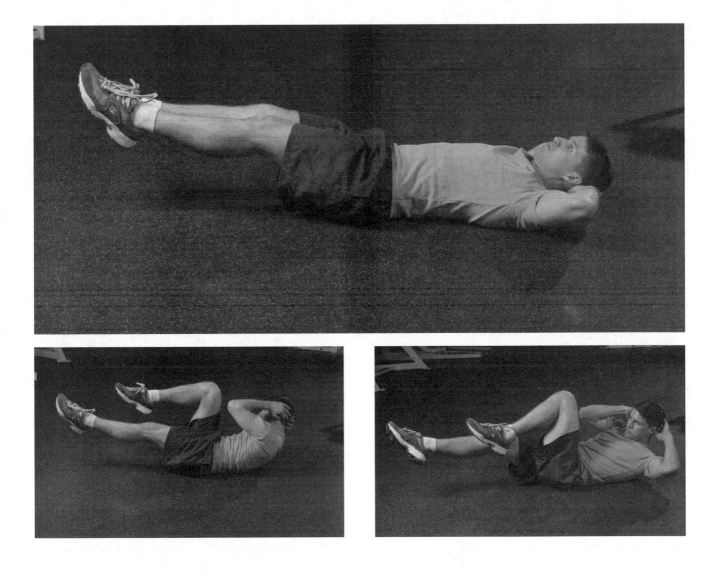

# Trunk Curl and Crunch

This is yet another incorporation exercise, simultaneously working the upper and lower abs. You should find this easier than the v-up but just as effective. The object is to bring the knees to the chest and chest to the knees at the same time.

### PROPER ALIGNMENT

❶ Lay flat on your back with knees bent, but lower legs and feet suspended (The correct thigh and lower leg position should look like the number 7).

❷ As you did with the crunch curl, cross your hands across your chest with your thumbs touching each side of your chin.

❸ Once again, the object will be to simultaneously crunch your chest to your knees and your knees to your chest. The elbows will meet with the knees as an indicator of one full rep.

### TECHNIQUE AND FORM

❶ Cross your hands over your chest and bring the thighs and feet away from your body in front of you. This will provide a full range of motion for this exercise.

❷ Isometrically contract the abdominal muscles before moving.

❸ At the same time, crunch your chest to your knees and bring your knees to your chest. Your back should come off the ground while your buttocks should also slightly lift off the ground.

❹ By touching your elbows to the knees and vice-versa you will know you have done one full rep. It is at this point that you should squeeze the abdominal muscles as hard as you possibly can. Do not cheat by failing to bring your thighs away from your body in front of you. With each rep, reach out with your feet and allow the lower abs to bring them back in for the knee-elbow touch. At the same time, do not fail to effectively crunch your upper body from the bottom of the floor up to the elbow-knee touch.

# Trunk Curl and Crunch

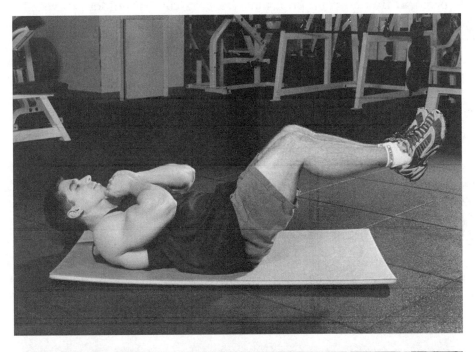

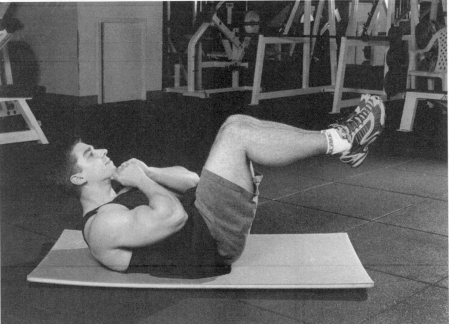

# Twist on the Ball

This exercise maximizes recruitment of the obliques while working the entire core. If you do not have a fitness ball, perform this exercise on a mat, keeping your shoulders elevated throughout the exercise as you twist from side to side. Make sure you are leading with your shoulder and not pulling on your neck.

To increase the challenge of this exercise, lift your opposite leg off the ball as you perform the twist.

## PROPER ALIGNMENT

❶ Position yourself on the ball so your lower back is supported.

❷ Your arms should be bent at the elbows and your head should be relaxed into the palms of your hands.

❸ Your chest should be open.

❹ Keep your feet flat on the floor and facing forward for balance.

## TECHNIQUE AND FORM

❶ Exhale, lift your chest, and twist over to your left knee, leading with your right shoulder.

❷ Hold for one second and return to the starting position.

❸ Lift and twist, leading with your left shoulder, to your right knee.

❹ Return to the start position.

❺ Repeat for the desired number of repetitions, alternating the leading shoulder on each repetition.

# Twist on the Ball

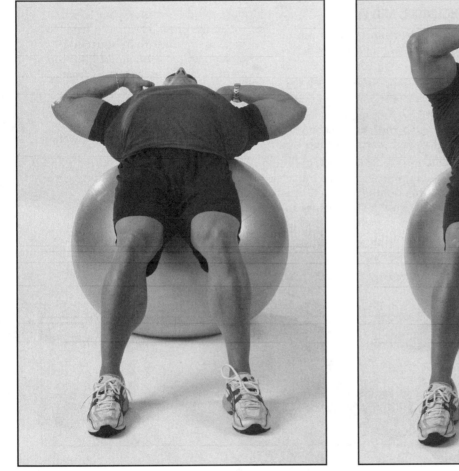
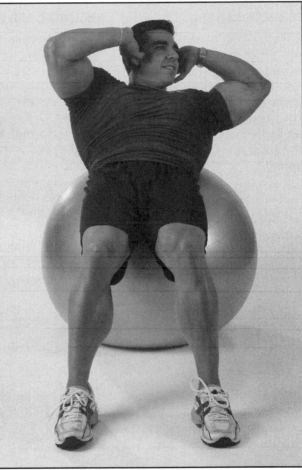

# V-Up

This is a very good incorporation exercise for the upper and lower abdominal muscles. It is a variation of the crunch, but much more intense. You will simultaneously exercise the upper and lower abs. Start out easy, but try! You will soon breeze through these like a person who has an amazingly strong mid-section, because that's exactly what you'll have!

## PROPER ALIGNMENT

❶ Sit on the floor, making sure you are on a carpet or mat.

❷ Put your arms by your side for support, slightly behind your torso. Your torso should be at an incline of 45 degrees between your lower back and the floor.

❸ Keep the legs straight and flat on the ground.

❹ Focus on keeping the head and neck in line with your chest.

❺ The object is to simultaneously lift your legs and torso, thus crunching your mid-section.

## TECHNIQUE AND FORM

❶ Begin by isometrically contracting the abdominal muscles before moving.

❷ At the same time, crunch forward by moving your torso toward your feet (as if trying to make your chest touch your legs), while you lift your legs and reverse crunch.

❸ You must truly focus on the contraction of your abdominal muscles here. If you do, the contraction will be very intense; a sure sign of amazing abs soon to come!

❹ Hold the crunched position for a count of 1 second.

❺ Slowly return to the start position, but do not allow your legs to touch the ground. This is a true measure of time under muscular tension and is very important if you want to obtain great results from your efforts.

❻ Without rest or momentum slowly begin once again to lift your chest and legs to the middle meeting point.

**FAQ:**

*I don't feel this one very much in my lower abs.*

**ANSWER:**

You may be sitting too far upright. This can engage the hip flexors to a higher degree. Try leaning back a bit more and concentrate on those lower abdominals. This also applies to the knee-in.

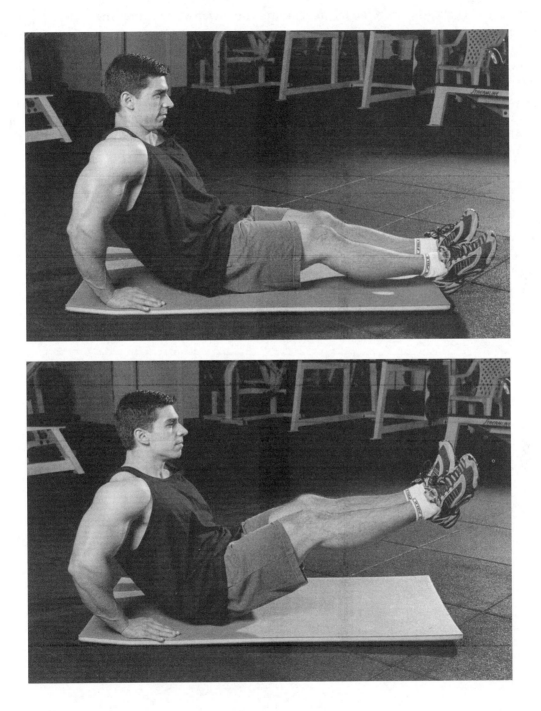

# Knee-In

This is another great variation exercise for developing the lower abdominal muscles.

It is more convenient than some of the other lower abdominal exercises and just as effective. This exercise also gives you the ability to really squeeze the lower abs when the knees are brought in towards your chest. For a change of pace, vary your speed from one workout to the next. The next time you do this or any of the exercises we recommend, move slowly while exercising. Deliberately squeeze the abdominal muscles at the peak contraction position. Then the next time you train your abdominal muscles again, go a little quicker. Varying the speed of your movements will help to keep your body from hitting a plateau, while keeping you motivated by changing the pace of your movements.

### PROPER ALIGNMENT

❶ Sit on the floor (or on the edge of a chair or exercise bench) with your legs extended in front of you.

❷ Your hands should be holding on to the sides of the bench or to the floor for support.

### TECHNIQUE AND FORM

❶ Keeping your knees together, pull them in towards your chest until you can go no farther.

❷ Keeping the tension on your lower abdominal muscles, return to the start position.

❸ Repeat the movement until you have completed your set.

# Knee-In

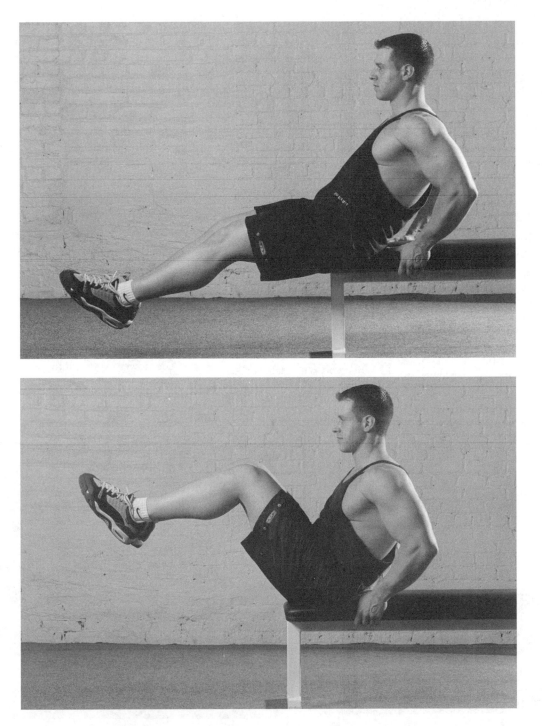

# Lying Leg Raise

Leg raises are a great lower abdominal exercise. It is not enough though to simply lift the legs off the floor. Doing so can hurt the lower back and will do nothing to improve your lower abdominal muscles. You must focus and feel the abdominal muscles actually working while you raise your legs. When you are ready for the next step, WATCH OUT! The advanced version of the leg raise will not only blow your mind, but will blast your abdominal results into the stratosphere!

**VARIATION:** There are a few variations for this exercise. Try lying leg raise on the ball, where you lie on a ball, holding onto a rack with your arms extended behind you, and raise your legs up and down. There is also the hanging leg raise, which requires an overhead bar. You will be hanging with your arms fully extended, using either wide or medium grip, and then raising and lowering your legs.

### PROPER ALIGNMENT

❶ Lay flat on the floor with your legs straight and flat on the floor as well.

❷ Put your hands face down underneath your buttocks, with fingertips facing each other. Your ring finger and pinky finger will most likely sit between the insertion point of your buttocks and hamstrings. This is a preventative measure against lower back injury.

❸ You will also bend your knees very slightly for the same reason.

### TECHNIQUE AND FORM

❶ Begin by lifting your legs about 5 inches off the ground and holding. This is for preparation.

❷ Lift your legs straight up until they are perpendicular to the ground.

❸ Make sure you are focused on the abdominal muscles working while you move the legs up.

❹ When you reach the vertical point, squeeze the abs as hard as you can and hold momentarily.

❺ Slowly return the legs to the bottom position but remember to stop 5 inches from the floor. From here you will once again lift the legs up.

### ADVANCED VERSION

This time, when your legs reach the point the perpendicular position, holding the vertical position, lift your buttocks off of your hands and reach your feet into the air as if you are trying to put footprints on the ceiling. This little movement will greatly enhance the stimulation of the lower abdominal section. It is like doing an instant super-set and is sure to be one of your favorites.

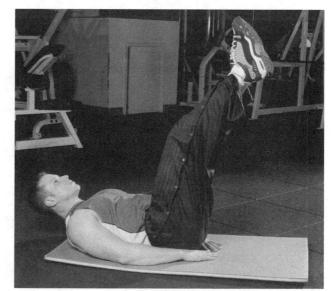

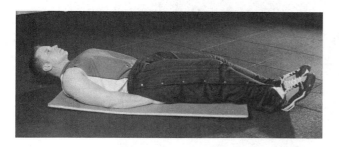

# Lying Leg Raise

## VARIATION

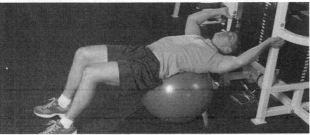

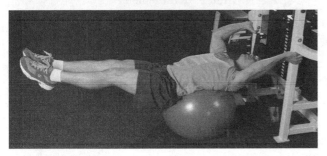

## VARIATION

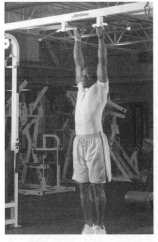 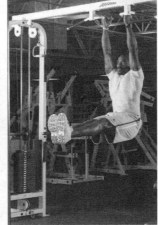

## ADVANCED

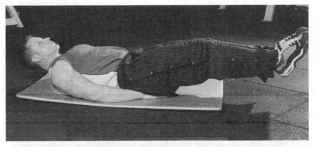

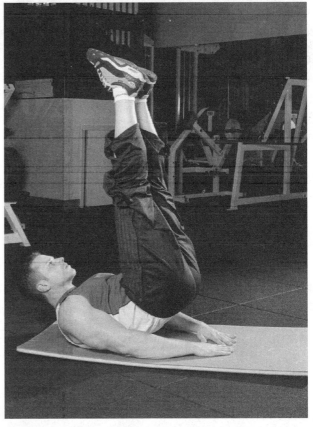

---

**FAQ:**

*I don't feel this one very much in my lower abs.*

**ANSWER:**

You may be lying too far upright. This can engage the hip flexors to a higher degree. Try leaning back a bit more and concentrate on those lower abdominals. This also applies to the knee-in.

# Crunch/Pelvic Lift Combination

This exercise targets both the inner and outer abdominals. Try not to bring your shoulders down to the floor for the entire set. By keeping them slightly elevated, you maintain tension and work the muscles throughout the range of motion. A great variation is the reverse crunch with ball. In this exercise, you lay on a mat, your arms extended to your sides, and hold a ball between your legs, lifting and raising for a predetermined number of repetitions.

## PROPER ALIGNMENT

**1** Lie on your back with your legs extended so that the soles of your feet face the ceiling. Your legs should make a 90-degree angle with your body.

**2** Bend your arms behind your head.

**3** Make sure you keep your head back and that your neck is relaxed.

## TECHNIQUE AND FORM

**1** Exhale and slowly lift your torso, keeping your head in line with your spine.

**2** At the same time, press your heels up to the ceiling by pressing your abs deep down through your spine. For the pelvic lift segment of the exercise is it important that you mentally focus on the lower part of your abdominals. Try to minimize action in the hips. The movement is very small—your buttocks should rise just an inch or two from the floor.

**3** Hold at the top position for a second or two before returning to a point where your shoulders do not quite touch the floor.

**4** Repeat for the desired number of repetitions.

# Crunch/Pelvic Lift Combination

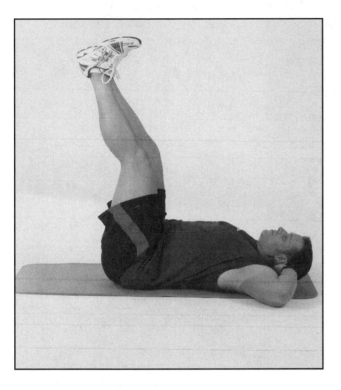
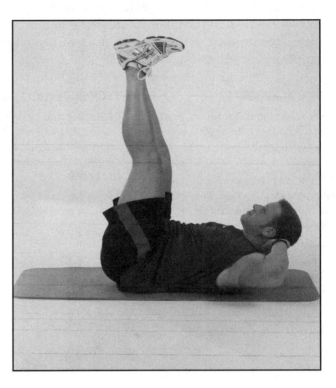

**VARIATION**

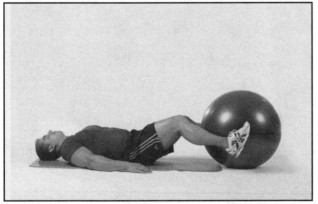
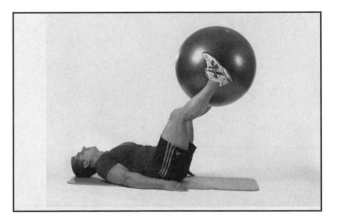

# Incline Board Partial Sit-Up

This exercise can be hard on the lower back, so avoid it if you have an unhealthy back. Avoid performing this exercise by swinging your torso as this leads to injury. Varying the angle of this exercise by choosing smaller or steeper inclines can increase or decrease the difficulty. Beginners should always start with no angle. As you become more advanced, weight can be added by holding a plate to your chest.

## PROPER ALIGNMENT

❶ Set the abdominal board to an incline. The more advanced you are, the steeper the incline you should choose.

❷ Hook your feet under the foot brace provided and lie on it with your hands crossed on top of your chest or kept alongside your body.

❸ Keep your head straight and your eyes looking ahead.

## TECHNIQUE AND FORM

❶ Exhale and raise your torso from the bench by bending at the waist and hips until you achieve a 30-degree angle between the torso and the bench.

❷ Slowly return to the starting position as you inhale.

# Incline Board Partial Sit-Up

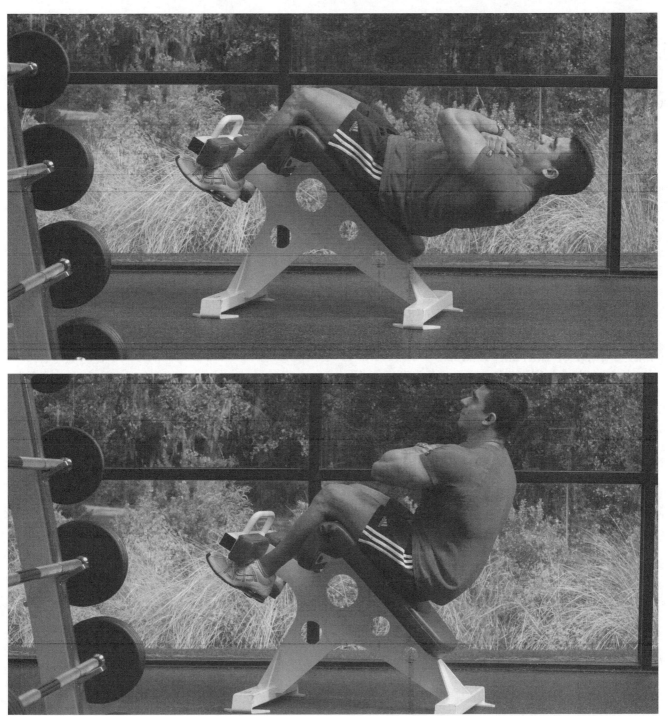

# Ab Bench Crunch

For this exercise you will need a bench created by Ironman called the ab bench. It has a rounded back that allows for a full stretch of the abdominals. As always, be very careful when adding weight to this exercise—if you add too much too quickly you could injure yourself.

## PROPER ALIGNMENT

**1** Sit on the ab bench with your back on the rounded pad and hold onto the handlebars.

**2** Your feet should be firm on the ground and your torso should be tilted back to stretch the abdominals.

**3** Keep your head steady and your eyes looking straight ahead for the duration of the exercise.

## TECHNIQUE AND FORM

**1** Exhale and pull your torso forward and maintain full contact with the back pad. Hold this contraction for a second.

**2** Inhale and slowly return to the starting position.

## FINAL POINTERS ON EXERCISE FORM

Remember that without knowing how to perform an exercise correctly, no matter how good your routine is you will not get the fast results that you want and deserve.

Also keep in mind that before starting any exercise, you should think about or visualize yourself doing the movement. This helps prepare you better for the exercise. When you begin the exercise, mentally focus on the muscle you are trying to stimulate. Use the Zone-Tone technique.

Remember how powerful the mind is and what it can do! By focusing your attention and "putting your mind in the muscle" you will double the intensity of muscle stimulation and therefore double your results. This is opposed to simply allowing any available muscle in the body to move the weight merely by going through the motions. You must learn to be connected as one with the muscle, observant of the connection every moment during the movement. Picture your muscle as toned and as lean as you want it to be. It's really much easier than you would expect to master the mind-to-muscle connection and you'll soon see remarkable results from your newfound knowledge and dedication.

# Ab Bench Crunch

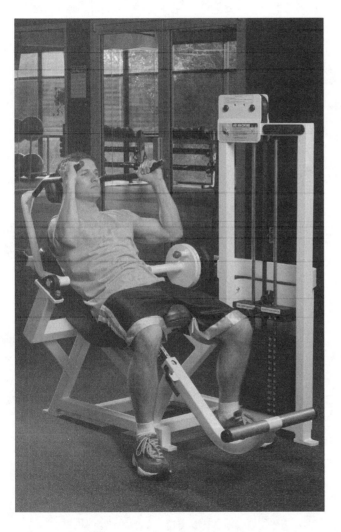 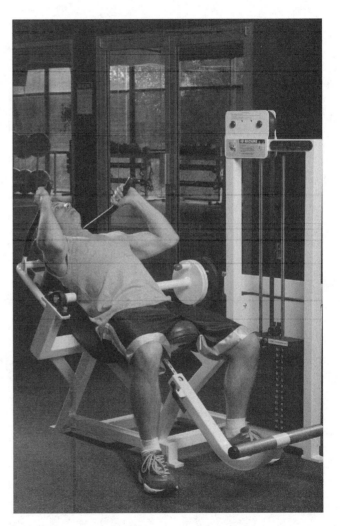

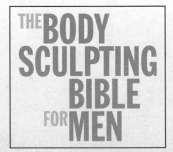

THE **BODY**
**SCULPTING**
**BIBLE**
FOR **MEN**

# Part 4
# Workout Charts

# Chapter 13
## Workout Charts

For immediate Body Sculpting Bible support & coaching directly from James & Hugo, please visit www.BodySculptingBible.com

13

## THE BREAK-IN PROGRAM

In this program, you will train with weights four days a week and perform aerobic activity two days a week. In this book, we use Sundays as your off days. You may do Day 1 on Mondays and Thursdays, Day 2 on Tuesdays and Fridays and Day 3 on Wednesdays and Saturdays.

This program is designed to be performed in the comfort of your home with minimum equipment, namely a pair of dumbbells or a pair of dumbbells with an adjustable bench. As you get stronger you may wish to purchase a pair of secure adjustable dumbbells such as Powerblocks.

You will notice that we present two Break-In Routines. The first routine is designed on the assumption that the only equipment available is a pair of dumbbells. The second routine is based on the assumption that you also have access to an adjustable exercise bench with a leg curl/leg extension attachment. Choose the routine that you can do with the equipment you have available.

## HOW TO PROGRESS WITH BREAK-IN ROUTINES 1 & 2

For the first six weeks, follow the routine exactly as it is laid out. The reason for this is that if you have never worked out before, it will take your body approximately six weeks to adjust and get used to the movements, while making it most efficient for recruiting muscle fibers. It will also give your cardiovascular system a chance to start getting back into shape. By the end of the six weeks, you should have lost a significant amount of weight and you should start seeing more muscle tone and definition in your body. You should also be able to reach your target heart rate by the end of this period.

After week six, add one more set to all of the exercises. You will now be performing three sets instead of two. Increase the weights and perform fewer repetitions (13-15; except for abs and calves where the repetition range stays the same). Also, increase your aerobic activity to 20 minutes. Follow this workout for the next four weeks.

After week 10, you are ready to go up to four sets per exercise and 30 minutes of cardio. Increase the weights and perform fewer repetitions (10-12; except for abs and calves where the repetition range stays the same). Follow this workout for three more weeks and then you should not only look dramatically different, but you are also in perfect shape to start the 14-Day Body Sculpting Workout.

## THE 14-DAY BODY SCULPTING WORKOUT

In this program, you will train with weights four days a week and perform aerobic activity two days a week. Sundays are your off days. You may do Day 1 on Mondays and Thursdays, Day 2 on Tuesdays and Fridays and Day 3 on Wednesdays and Saturdays.

This program is designed to be performed in the comfort of your home with minimum equipment, namely a pair of dumbbells or a pair of dumbbells with an adjustable bench. As you get stronger you may wish to purchase a pair of secure adjustable dumbbells such as Powerblocks.

You will notice that we present three 14-Day Body Sculpting Workouts. The first routine is designed on the assumption that the only equipment available is a pair of dumbbells. The second routine is based on the assumption that you also have access to an adjustable exercise bench with a leg curl/leg extension attachment. Choose the routine that you can do with the equipment that you have available.

## THE 14-DAY RAPID BODY SCULPTING WORKOUT

This program was created especially for men who do not have a lot of time to work out. The program is very fast paced and will get you the most effective and efficient workout possible in 30 minutes or less!

Use this program either as a means to introduce variety into your workouts after you have gone through the 14-Day Body Sculpting Workouts #1 and #2 or use the 14-Day Rapid Body Sculpting Workout right after the Break-In Routines if 30 minutes is all the time that you can devote to exercise.

The 14-Day Rapid Body Sculpting Workout comes in two workouts. Workout #1 only requires a pair of dumbbells, while workout #2 also requires a weight bench.

## THE ADVANCED 14-DAY BODY SCULPTING PROGRAM

In this program, you will train with weights six days a week and perform aerobic activity six days a week. Sundays are your off days. You may do Day 1 on Mondays and Thursdays, Day 2 on Tuesdays and Fridays and Day 3 on Wednesdays and Saturdays.

This program is designed to be performed at either a commercial gym or a very well equipped home gym. The reason for this is that we will be using a variety of exercises and training different angles and areas of the muscles in order to stimulate all muscle fibers.

Note that these routines provide alternate exercises. Alternate exercises are to be performed the next time that you perform the workout for that specific body part in order to provide varied stimulation. For example, if on Tuesday of week one you perform reverse curls as your first biceps exercise, on Friday you will perform preacher curls instead. This variation will help to avoid a plateau, keeping your muscle building capabilities in paramount shape.

Cardio and abs are to be performed on a daily basis preferably first thing in the morning on an empty stomach. The weight training workouts are to be performed in the afternoon or at any other convenient time. If your schedule does not allow for two separate sessions, then you may merge both sessions by performing the abs first, and then the weight training followed by the cardiovascular exercise.

## THE 14-DAY BODY SCULPTING MASS WORKOUT

This program was created for those people with faster metabolisms—and consequently, low body fat—who are interested only in gaining muscle. We created the program with the assumption that you will be working out at a well-equipped gym. If you are working out at home, just substitute exercises that you can do with your equipment for those designed for the gym. However, be aware that to add serious muscle you will have to lift some heavy weights, which means that you need sturdy, high-quality equipment. At this point, you should have already completed the Break-In Routines described earlier. If you are a complete beginner, start with the Break-In Routines. Once you have completed them, you can graduate to this level.

You will notice that every two weeks the exercises change along with the set, rep and rest schemes to provide a fresh shock to the body. If you work out at a gym, once you have completed this routine, feel free to add other exercises, such leg press hack squats for the leg routines. As long as the exercises are basic (using mostly free weights), there is no problem with substituting them for other exercises.

# THE 14-DAY BODYWEIGHT BODY SCULPTING WORKOUT

This program was created for people who, for one reason or another, do not have access to any weight-bearing equipment. This is also a great workout to do if you are traveling. All you need is a portable pull-up bar, which you can find at any sporting goods store. This is also a great functional program for soldiers who may be overseas and have limited access to weights.

While you won't be able to manipulate the amount of repetitions in the same manner that you would with the other Body Sculpting Workouts, you can certainly manipulate the number of sets and rest time in between sets in order to get the results you want. You will notice that there is no direct shoulder work, but due to the compound nature of the exercises used, you will be giving your shoulders plenty of stimulation.

You will be training with bodyweight exercises four days a week while you perform aerobic activity twice a week. This is how your schedule will look:

**Monday/Thursday (Day 1):**
Chest/Back/Biceps/Triceps

**Tuesday/Friday (Day 2):**
Thighs/Hamstrings/Calves/Abs

**Wednesday/Saturday (Day 3):** Cardio

# Break-In Routine #1

<table>
<tr><td colspan="2">SPECIAL INSTRUCTIONS FOR WEEKS 1 & 2</td></tr>
</table>

**SPECIAL INSTRUCTIONS FOR WEEKS 1 & 2**

Use modified compound supersets. Perform modified compound supersets by performing the first exercise, resting for the prescribed rest period, performing the second exercise, resting the prescribed rest period, and going back to the first exercise. Continue in this manner until you have performed all of the prescribed number of sets. Then continue with the next modified compound superset. You will repeat Day 1 on Monday and Thursday, Day 2 on Tuesday and Friday, and Day 3 on Wednesday and Saturday.

## DAY 1 — MONDAY/THURSDAY

| EXERCISE | PAGE NO. | REPS | SETS | REST |
|---|---|---|---|---|
| **MODIFIED COMPOUND SUPERSET # 1** | | | | |
| Back—Dumbbell One-Arm Row | 170 | 15-20 | 2 | 90 seconds |
| Chest—Push-Up | 210 | 15-20 | 2 | 90 seconds |
| (against the wall if unable to perform on the floor) | | | | |
| **MODIFIED COMPOUND SUPERSET # 2** | | | | |
| Back—Two-Arm Rows | 172 | 15-20 | 2 | 90 seconds |
| Chest —Flat Dumbbell Fly | 200 | 15-20 | 2 | 90 seconds |
| (performed on the floor if you don't | | | | |
| have access to an exercise bench) | | | | |
| **MODIFIED COMPOUND SUPERSET # 3** | | | | |
| Biceps—Dumbbell Curl | 262 | 15-20 | 2 | 90 seconds |
| Triceps—Lying Dumbbell Extension | 242 | 15-20 | 2 | 90 seconds |
| **MODIFIED COMPOUND SUPERSET # 4** | | | | |
| Biceps—Hammer Curl | 274 | 15-20 | 2 | 90 seconds |
| Triceps—Overhead Dumbbell Extension | 240 | 15-20 | 2 | 90 seconds |

**PUSH-UP**

Depending on your bodyweight, you may find this exercise difficult to do in the traditional manner. If this is the case, then start by performing them standing against the wall (stand 1.5 to 2 feet in front of the wall, extend your arms and perform the exercise) as in this manner you will not be lifting your full bodyweight. As you become stronger, you may perform them on the floor in the "halfway" position. This is when you will kneel down and perform the push-up the same way you would regularly with the exception of not keeping your legs straight  Once you master that position, you will be able to perform the traditional push-up.

## DAY 2                            TUESDAY/FRIDAY

| EXERCISE | PAGE NO. | REPS | SETS | REST |
|---|---|---|---|---|
| **MODIFIED COMPOUND SUPERSET # 1** | | | | |
| Thighs—Dumbbell Squat | 122 | 15-20 | 2 | 90 seconds |
| Hamstrings—Dumbbell Lunge | 132 | 15-20 | 2 | 90 seconds |
| **MODIFIED COMPOUND SUPERSET # 2** | | | | |
| Thighs—Ballet Squat | 124 | 15-20 | 2 | 90 seconds |
| Hamstrings—Stiff-Legged Deadlift | 144 | 15-20 | 2 | 90 seconds |
| **MODIFIED COMPOUND SUPERSET # 3** | | | | |
| Calves—Standing Calf Raise (one leg) | 152 | 15-25 | 2 | 90 seconds |
| Shoulders—Dumbbell Shoulder Press | 216 | 15-20 | 2 | 90 seconds |
| **MODIFIED COMPOUND SUPERSET # 4** | | | | |
| Calves—Standing Calf Raise (two legs using dumbbells) | 152 | 15-25 | 2 | 90 seconds |
| Shoulders—Bent-Over Lateral Raise | 220 | 15-20 | 2 | 90 seconds |

## DAY 3                           WEDNESDAY/SATURDAY

| EXERCISE | PAGE NO. | REPS | SETS | REST |
|---|---|---|---|---|
| **MODIFIED COMPOUND SUPERSET # 1** | | | | |
| Lower Abs—Lying Leg Raise | 296 | 15-25 | 2 | 90 seconds |
| Upper Abs—Crunch | 284 | 15-25 | 2 | 90 seconds |

**ABS**

If you cannot perform the desired amount of repetitions for abdominal exercises, just do as many as you can and as your strength allows, increase the number of reps.

**AEROBIC ACTIVITY**

10 minutes of fast walking, stationary bike, or any other type of aerobic activity that you like. Don't be concerned at this stage with reaching the target heart rate. Just concentrate on performing the activity at a comfortable but steady pace.

**REPETITIONS**

You will note that the repetition ranges are higher than what we normally recommend, which means using lighter weights, for the following reasons:

•To start getting the joints and muscles accustomed to weight training exercise while preventing injuries.

•To start creating neural pathways (links) between the brain and the muscles so that you start gaining better control and feel of the muscles in your body.

Please refer to www.BodySculptingBible.com for updated workouts and additional cardio routines.

# Break-In Routine #2

---

### SPECIAL INSTRUCTIONS FOR WEEKS 1 & 2

Use modified compound supersets. Perform modified compound supersets by performing the first exercise, resting for the prescribed rest period, performing the second exercise, resting the prescribed rest period, and going back to the first exercise. Continue in this manner until you have performed all of the prescribed number of sets. Then continue with the next modified compound superset. You will repeat Day 1 on Monday and Thursday, Day 2 on Tuesday and Friday, and Day 3 on Wednesday and Saturday.

---

| DAY 1 | | | | MONDAY/THURSDAY |
|---|---|---|---|---|
| **EXERCISE** | **PAGE NO.** | **REPS** | **SETS** | **REST** |
| **MODIFIED COMPOUND SUPERSET # 1** | | | | |
| Back—Dumbbell One-Arm Row (one arm, alternate with two-arm rows on the next workout) | 170 | 15-20 | 2 | 90 seconds |
| Chest—Incline Dumbbell Press | 196 | 15-20 | 2 | 90 seconds |
| **MODIFIED COMPOUND SUPERSET # 2** | | | | |
| Back—Dumbbell Pullover | 186 | 15-20 | 2 | 90 seconds |
| Chest—Incline Dumbbell Fly (alternate with Push-Up on the next workout) | 202 | 15-20 | 2 | 90 seconds |
| **MODIFIED COMPOUND SUPERSET # 3** | | | | |
| Biceps—Dumbbell Curl | 262 | 15-20 | 2 | 90 seconds |
| Triceps—Lying Dumbbell Extension | 242 | 15-20 | 2 | 90 seconds |
| **MODIFIED COMPOUND SUPERSET # 4** | | | | |
| Biceps—Concentration Curl (alternate with Hammer Curl, 274) | 270 | 15-20 | 2 | 90 seconds |
| Triceps—Triceps Kickback (alternate with Overhead Dumbbell Extension, 240) | 256 | 15-20 | 2 | 90 seconds |

**PUSH-UP**

Depending on your bodyweight, you may find this exercise difficult to do in the traditional way. If this is the case, start by performing them standing against the wall (stand 1.5 to 2 ft in front of the wall, extend your arms and perform the exercise) as in this manner you will not be lifting your full bodyweight. As you become stronger, you may perform them on the floor in the "halfway" position. This is when you will kneel down and perform the push-up the same way you would regularly with the exception of not keeping your legs straight. Once you master that position, you will be able to perform the traditional push-up.

## DAY 2 — TUESDAY/FRIDAY

| EXERCISE | PAGE NO. | REPS | SETS | REST |
|---|---|---|---|---|
| **MODIFIED COMPOUND SUPERSET # 1** | | | | |
| Thighs—Dumbbell Squat (alternate with Ballet Squat, 124) | 122 | 15-20 | 2 | 90 seconds |
| Hamstrings—Lying Leg Curl (alternate with Dumbbell Lunge, 132) | 138 | 15-20 | 2 | 90 seconds |
| **MODIFIED COMPOUND SUPERSET # 2** | | | | |
| Thighs—Ballet Squat (alternate with Leg Extension, 136) | 124 | 15-20 | 2 | 90 seconds |
| Hamstrings—Stiff-Legged Deadlift (Alternate with Standing Leg Curl, 142) | 144 | 15-20 | 2 | 90 seconds |
| **MODIFIED COMPOUND SUPERSET # 3** | | | | |
| Calves—Standing Calf Raise (one leg) | 152 | 15-25 | 2 | 90 seconds |
| Shoulders—Dumbbell Shoulder Press (alternate with Dumbbell Upright Row, 226) | 216 | 15-20 | 2 | 90 seconds |
| **MODIFIED COMPOUND SUPERSET # 4** | | | | |
| Calves—Standing Calf Raise (two legs) | 152 | 15-25 | 2 | 90 seconds |
| Shoulders—Bent-Over Lateral Raise | 220 | 15-20 | 2 | 90 seconds |

## DAY 3 — WEDNESDAY/SATURDAY

| EXERCISE | PAGE NO. | REPS | SETS | REST |
|---|---|---|---|---|
| **MODIFIED COMPOUND SUPERSET # 1** | | | | |
| Lower Abs—Lying Leg Raise | 296 | 15-25 | 2 | 90 seconds |
| Upper Abs—Crunch | 284 | 15-25 | 2 | 90 seconds |

**ABS**

If you cannot perform the desired amount of repetitions for abdominal exercises, just do as many as you can. As your strength allows, increase the number of reps.

**AEROBIC ACTIVITY**

10 minutes of fast walking, stationary bike, or any other type of aerobic activity that you like. Don't be concerned at this stage with reaching the target heart rate. Just concentrate on performing the activity at a comfortable but steady pace.

**REPETITIONS**

You will note that the repetition ranges are higher than what we normally recommend, which means using lighter weights, for the following reasons in order to start getting the joints and muscles accustomed to weight training exercise while preventing injuries, and to start creating neural pathways between the brain and muscles so you start gaining better control and feel of the muscles in your body.

**ALTERNATE EXERCISES**

Alternate exercises are added as a means to introduce variety into the weight-training program. Variety is good as it prevents the body from getting used to the exercise routine, helping to avoid boredom. It also helps to intensify your workouts by providing additional angles of movement for diversified muscular stimulation.

These alternate exercises are to be performed in the second workout of the week. For instance, if you did a ballet squat on Tuesday, then do a leg extension instead on Friday.

Please refer to www.BodySculptingBible.com for updated workouts and additional cardio routines.

# 14-Day Body Sculpting Workout #1

**SPECIAL INSTRUCTIONS FOR WEEKS 1 & 2**

Use modified compound supersets. Perform modified compound supersets by performing the first exercise, resting for the prescribed rest period, performing the second exercise, resting the prescribed rest period, and going back to the first exercise. Continue in this manner until you have performed all of the prescribed number of sets. Then continue with the next modified compound superset. You will repeat Day 1 on Monday and Thursday, Day 2 on Tuesday and Friday, and Day 3 on Wednesday and Saturday.

## DAY 1 — MONDAY/THURSDAY

| EXERCISE | PAGE NO. | REPS | SETS | REST |
|---|---|---|---|---|
| **MODIFIED COMPOUND SUPERSET # 1** | | | | |
| Back—Dumbbell One-Arm Row | 170 | 12-15 | 2 | 90 seconds |
| Chest—Push-Up (against the wall if unable to perform on the floor) | 210 | 12-15 | 2 | 90 seconds |
| **MODIFIED COMPOUND SUPERSET # 2** | | | | |
| Back—Two-Arm Row | 172 | 12-15 | 2 | 90 seconds |
| Chest—Flat Dumbbell Fly (performed on the floor if you don't have access to an exercise bench) | 200 | 12-15 | 2 | 90 seconds |
| **MODIFIED COMPOUND SUPERSET # 3** | | | | |
| Biceps—Dumbbell Curl | 262 | 12-15 | 2 | 90 seconds |
| Triceps—Lying Dumbbell Extension | 242 | 12-15 | 2 | 90 seconds |
| **MODIFIED COMPOUND SUPERSET # 4** | | | | |
| Biceps—Hammer Curl | 274 | 12-15 | 2 | 90 seconds |
| Triceps—Overhead Dumbbell Extension | 240 | 12-15 | 2 | 90 seconds |

| DAY 2 | | | | TUESDAY/FRIDAY |
|---|---|---|---|---|
| **EXERCISE** | **PAGE NO.** | **REPS** | **SETS** | **REST** |
| **MODIFIED COMPOUND SUPERSET # 1** | | | | |
| Thighs—Dumbbell Squat (alternate with Ballet Squat, 124) | 122 | 12-15 | 2 | 90 seconds |
| Hamstrings—Dumbbell Lunge | 132 | 12-15 | 2 | 90 seconds |
| **MODIFIED COMPOUND SUPERSET # 2** | | | | |
| Thighs—Ballet Squat | 124 | 12-15 | 2 | 90 seconds |
| Hamstrings—Stiff-Legged Deadlift | 144 | 12-15 | 2 | 90 seconds |
| **MODIFIED COMPOUND SUPERSET # 3** | | | | |
| Calves—Standing Calf Raise (one leg) | 152 | 12-15 | 2 | 90 seconds |
| Shoulders—Dumbbell Shoulder Press | 216 | 12-15 | 2 | 90 seconds |
| **MODIFIED COMPOUND SUPERSET # 4** | | | | |
| Calves—Standing Calf Raise (two legs) | 152 | 12-15 | 2 | 90 seconds |
| Shoulders—Bent-Over Lateral Raise | 220 | 12-15 | 2 | 90 second |

| DAY 3 | | | | WEDNESDAY/SATURDAY |
|---|---|---|---|---|
| **EXERCISE** | **PAGE NO.** | **REPS** | **SETS** | **REST** |
| **MODIFIED COMPOUND SUPERSET # 1** | | | | |
| Lower Abs—Lying Leg Raise | 296 | 15-25 | 2 | 90 seconds |
| Upper Abs—Crunch | 284 | 15-25 | 2 | 90 seconds |

**AEROBIC ACTIVITY**

20 minutes of fast walking, stationary bike, or any other type of aerobic activity that you like at the target heart rate.

Please refer to www.BodySculptingBible.com for updated workouts and additional cardio routines.

# 14-Day Body Sculpting Workout #1

---

**SPECIAL INSTRUCTIONS FOR WEEKS 3 & 4**

Use supersets. Perform supersets by pairing exercises with no rest period in between. Only rest after the two exercises have been performed consecutively. Repeat for the prescribed number of sets and then move on to the next pair of exercises. You will repeat Day 1 on Monday and Thursday, Day 2 on Tuesday and Friday, and Day 3 on Wednesday and Saturday.

---

| DAY 1 | | | | MONDAY/THURSDAY |
|---|---|---|---|---|
| **EXERCISE** | **PAGE NO.** | **REPS** | **SETS** | **REST** |
| **SUPERSET # 1** | | | | |
| Back—Dumbbell One-Arm Row | 170 | 10-12 | 3 | No Rest |
| Chest—Push-Up (against the wall if unable to perform on the floor) | 210 | 10-12 | 3 | 60 seconds |
| **SUPERSET # 2** | | | | |
| Back—Two-Arm Row | 172 | 10-12 | 3 | No Rest |
| Chest—Flat Dumbbell Fly (performed on the floor if you don't have access to an exercise bench) | 200 | 10-12 | 3 | 60 seconds |
| **SUPERSET # 3** | | | | |
| Biceps—Dumbbell Curl | 262 | 10-12 | 3 | No Rest |
| Triceps—Lying Dumbbell Extension | 242 | 10-12 | 3 | 60 seconds |
| **SUPERSET # 4** | | | | |
| Biceps—Hammer Curl | 274 | 10-12 | 3 | No Rest |
| Triceps—Overhead Dumbbell Extension | 240 | 10-12 | 3 | 60 seconds |

# Weeks 3 & 4

| DAY 2 | | | | TUESDAY/FRIDAY |
|---|---|---|---|---|
| EXERCISE | PAGE NO. | REPS | SETS | REST |
| **SUPERSET # 1** | | | | |
| Thighs—Dumbbell Squat | 122 | 10-12 | 3 | No Rest |
| Hamstrings—Dumbbell Lunge | 132 | 10-12 | 3 | 60 seconds |
| **SUPERSET # 2** | | | | |
| Thighs—Ballet Squat | 124 | 10-12 | 3 | No Rest |
| Hamstrings—Stiff-Legged Deadlift | 144 | 10-12 | 3 | 60 seconds |
| **SUPERSET # 3** | | | | |
| Calves—Standing Calf Raise (one leg) | 152 | 12-15 | 3 | No Rest |
| Shoulders—Dumbbell Shoulder Press | 216 | 10-12 | 3 | 60 seconds |
| **SUPERSET # 4** | | | | |
| Calves—Standing Calf Raise (two legs) | 152 | 12-15 | 3 | No Rest |
| Shoulders—Bent-Over Lateral Raise | 220 | 10-12 | 3 | 60 seconds |

| DAY 3 | | | | WEDNESDAY/SATURDAY |
|---|---|---|---|---|
| EXERCISE | PAGE NO. | REPS | SETS | REST |
| **SUPERSET # 1** | | | | |
| Lower Abs—Lying Leg Raise | 296 | 15-25 | 3 | No Rest |
| Upper Abs—Crunch | 284 | 15-25 | 3 | 90 seconds |

**AEROBIC ACTIVITY**

30 minutes of fast walking, stationary bike, or any other type of aerobic activity that you like at your target heart rate.

Please refer to www.BodySculptingBible.com for updated workouts and additional cardio routines.

# 14-Day Body Sculpting Workout #1

**SPECIAL INSTRUCTIONS FOR WEEKS 5 & 6**

Use giant sets. Perform giant sets by performing four exercises with no rest period in between. Only rest after the four exercises have been performed consecutively. Repeat for the prescribed number of sets and then move on to the second group of exercises. You will repeat Day 1 on Monday and Thursday, Day 2 on Tuesday and Friday, and Day 3 on Wednesday and Saturday.

## DAY 1 — MONDAY/THURSDAY

| EXERCISE | PAGE NO. | REPS | SETS | REST |
|---|---|---|---|---|
| **GIANT SET # 1** | | | | |
| Back—Dumbbell One-Arm Row | 170 | 8-10 | 4 | No Rest |
| Chest—Push-Up (against the wall if unable to perform on the floor) | 210 | 8-10 | 4 | No Rest |
| Back—Two-Arm Row | 172 | 8-10 | 4 | No Rest |
| Chest—Flat Dumbbell Fly (performed on the floor if you don't have access to an exercise bench) | 200 | 8-10 | 4 | 60 seconds |
| **GIANT SET # 2** | | | | |
| Biceps—Dumbbell Curl | 262 | 8-10 | 4 | No Rest |
| Triceps—Lying Dumbbell Extension | 242 | 8-10 | 4 | No Rest |
| Biceps—Hammer Curl | 274 | 8-10 | 4 | No Rest |
| Triceps—Overhead Dumbbell Extension | 240 | 8-10 | 4 | 60 seconds |

| DAY 2 | | | | TUESDAY/FRIDAY |
|---|---|---|---|---|
| **EXERCISE** | **PAGE NO.** | **REPS** | **SETS** | **REST** |
| **GIANT SET # 1** | | | | |
| Thighs—Dumbbell Squat | 122 | 8-10 | 4 | No Rest |
| Hamstrings—Dumbbell Lunge | 132 | 8-10 | 4 | No Rest |
| Thighs—Ballet Squat | 124 | 8-10 | 4 | No Rest |
| Hamstrings—Stiff-Legged Deadlift | 144 | 8-10 | 4 | 60 seconds |
| **GIANT SET # 2** | | | | |
| Calves—Standing Calf Raise (one leg) | 152 | 15-25 | 4 | No Rest |
| Shoulders—Dumbbell Shoulder Press | 216 | 15-25 | 4 | No Rest |
| Calves—Standing Calf Raise (two legs) | 152 | 15-25 | 4 | No Rest |
| Shoulders—Bent-Over Lateral Raise | 220 | 15-25 | 4 | 60 seconds |

| DAY 3 | | | | WEDNESDAY/SATURDAY |
|---|---|---|---|---|
| **EXERCISE** | **PAGE NO.** | **REPS** | **SETS** | **REST** |
| **GIANT SET # 1** | | | | |
| Lower Abs—Lying Leg Raise | 296 | 15-25 | 4 | No Rest |
| Upper Abs—Crunch | 284 | 15-25 | 4 | No Rest |

**Note:** Continue until all four sets of each exercise have been done. Don't worry if you are not able to perform all of the recommended reps the first few times that you perform this abdominal workout. As you get used to this rigorous workout, your body will adapt and get stronger.

**AEROBIC ACTIVITY**

40 minutes of fast walking, stationary bike, or any other type of aerobic activity that you like at your target heart rate.

Please refer to www.BodySculptingBible.com for updated workouts and additional cardio routines.

# 14-Day Body Sculpting Workout #2

---

### SPECIAL INSTRUCTIONS FOR WEEKS 1 & 2

Use modified compound supersets. Perform modified compound supersets by performing the first exercise, resting for the prescribed rest period, performing the second exercise, resting the prescribed rest period and going back to the first exercise. Continue in this manner until you have performed all of the prescribed number of sets. Then continue with the next modified compound superset. You will repeat Day 1 on Monday and Thursday, Day 2 on Tuesday and Friday, and Day 3 on Wednesday and Saturday.

---

| DAY 1 | | | | MONDAY/THURSDAY |
|---|---|---|---|---|
| **EXERCISE** | **PAGE NO.** | **REPS** | **SETS** | **REST** |
| **MODIFIED COMPOUND SUPERSET # 1** | | | | |
| Back—Dumbbell One-Arm Row (Alternate with Two-Arm Row, 172) | 170 | 12-15 | 2 | 90 seconds |
| Chest—Incline Dumbbell Press | 196 | 12-15 | 2 | 90 seconds |
| **MODIFIED COMPOUND SUPERSET # 2** | | | | |
| Back—Dumbbell Pullover | 186 | 12-15 | 2 | 90 seconds |
| Chest—Incline Dumbbell Fly (alternate with Push-Up, 210) | 202 | 12-15 | 2 | 90 seconds |
| **MODIFIED COMPOUND SUPERSET # 3** | | | | |
| Biceps—Dumbbell Curl | 262 | 12-15 | 2 | 90 seconds |
| Triceps—Lying Dumbbell Extension | 242 | 12-15 | 2 | 90 seconds |
| **MODIFIED COMPOUND SUPERSET # 4** | | | | |
| Biceps—Concentration Curl (alternate with Hammer Curl, 274) | 270 | 12-15 | 2 | 90 seconds |
| Triceps—Triceps Kickback (alternate with Overhead Dumbbell Extensions, 240) | 256 | 12-15 | 2 | 90 seconds |

| DAY 2 | | | | TUESDAY/FRIDAY |
|---|---|---|---|---|
| **EXERCISE** | **PAGE NO.** | **REPS** | **SETS** | **REST** |
| **MODIFIED COMPOUND SUPERSET # 1** | | | | |
| Thighs—Dumbbell Squat (alternate with Ballet Squat, 124) | 122 | 12-15 | 2 | 90 seconds |
| Hamstrings—Lying Leg Curl (alternate with Dumbbell Lunge, 132) | 138 | 12-15 | 2 | 90 seconds |
| **MODIFIED COMPOUND SUPERSET # 2** | | | | |
| Thighs—Ballet Squat (alternate with Leg Extension, 136) | 124 | 12-15 | 2 | 90 seconds |
| Hamstrings—Stiff-Legged Deadlift (alternate with Standing Leg Curl, 142) | 144 | 12-15 | 2 | 90 seconds |
| **MODIFIED COMPOUND SUPERSET # 3** | | | | |
| Calves—Standing Calf Raise (one leg) | 152 | 12-15 | 2 | 90 seconds |
| Shoulders—Dumbbell Shoulder Press (alternate with Dumbbell Upright Row, 226) | 216 | 12-15 | 2 | 90 seconds |
| **MODIFIED COMPOUND SUPERSET # 4** | | | | |
| Calves—Standing Calf Raise (two legs) | 152 | 12-15 | 2 | 90 seconds |
| Shoulders—Bent-Over Lateral Raise | 220 | 12-15 | 2 | 90 seconds |

| DAY 3 | | | | WEDNESDAY/SATURDAY |
|---|---|---|---|---|
| **EXERCISE** | **PAGE NO.** | **REPS** | **SETS** | **REST** |
| **MODIFIED COMPOUND SUPERSET # 1** | | | | |
| Lower Abs—Lying Leg Raise | 296 | 15-25 | 2 | 90 seconds |
| Upper Abs—Crunch | 284 | 15-25 | 2 | 90 seconds |

**AEROBIC ACTIVITY**

20 minutes of fast walking, stationary bike, or any other type of aerobic activity that you like at your target heart rate.

Please refer to www.BodySculptingBible.com for updated workouts and additional cardio routines.

# 14-Day Body Sculpting Workout #2

**SPECIAL INSTRUCTIONS FOR WEEKS 3 & 4**

Use supersets. Perform supersets by pairing exercises with no rest period in between. Only rest after the two exercises have been performed consecutively. Repeat for the prescribed number of sets and then move on to the next pair of exercises. You will repeat Day 1 on Monday and Thursday, Day 2 on Tuesday and Friday, and Day 3 on Wednesday and Saturday.

| DAY 1 | | | | MONDAY/THURSDAY |
|---|---|---|---|---|
| **EXERCISE** | **PAGE NO.** | **REPS** | **SETS** | **REST** |
| **SUPERSET # 1** | | | | |
| Back—Dumbbell One-Arm Row (Alternate with Two-Arm Row, 172) | 170 | 10-12 | 3 | No Rest |
| Chest—Incline Dumbbell Press | 196 | 10-12 | 3 | 60 seconds |
| **SUPERSET # 2** | | | | |
| Back—Dumbbell Pullover | 186 | 10-12 | 3 | No Rest |
| Chest—Incline Dumbbell Fly (alternate with Push-Up, 210) | 202 | 10-12 | 3 | 60 seconds |
| **SUPERSET # 3** | | | | |
| Biceps—Dumbbell Curl | 262 | 10-12 | 3 | No Rest |
| Triceps—Lying Dumbbell Extension | 242 | 10-12 | 3 | 60 seconds |
| **SUPERSET # 4** | | | | |
| Biceps—Concentration Curl (alternate with Hammer Curl, 274) | 270 | 10-12 | 3 | No Rest |
| Triceps—Triceps Kickback (alternate with Overhead Dumbbell Extension, 240) | 256 | 10-12 | 3 | 60 seconds |

# Weeks 3 & 4

| DAY 2 | | | | TUESDAY/FRIDAY |
|---|---|---|---|---|
| EXERCISE | PAGE NO. | REPS | SETS | REST |
| **SUPERSET # 1** | | | | |
| Thighs—Dumbbell Squat (alternate with Ballet Squat, 124) | 122 | 10-12 | 3 | No Rest |
| Hamstrings—Lying Leg Curl (alternate with Dumbbell Lunge, 132) | 138 | 10-12 | 3 | 60 seconds |
| **SUPERSET # 2** | | | | |
| Thighs—Ballet Squat (alternate with Leg Extension, 136) | 124 | 10-12 | 3 | No Rest |
| Hamstrings—Stiff-Legged Deadlift (alternate with Standing Leg Curl, 142) | 144 | 10-12 | 3 | 60 seconds |
| **SUPERSET # 3** | | | | |
| Calves—Standing Calf Raise (one leg) | 152 | 12-15 | 3 | No Rest |
| Shoulders—Dumbbell Shoulder Press (alternate with Dumbbell Upright Row, 226) | 216 | 10-12 | 3 | 60 seconds |
| **SUPERSET # 4** | | | | |
| Calves—Standing Calf Raise (two legs) | 152 | 12-15 | 3 | No Rest |
| Shoulders—Bent-Over Lateral Raise | 220 | 10-12 | 3 | 60 seconds |

| DAY 3 | | | | WEDNESDAY/SATURDAY |
|---|---|---|---|---|
| EXERCISE | PAGE NO. | REPS | SETS | REST |
| **SUPERSET # 1** | | | | |
| Lower Abs—Lying Leg Raise | 296 | 15-25 | 3 | No Rest |
| Upper Abs—Crunch | 284 | 15-25 | 3 | 90 seconds |

**AEROBIC ACTIVITY**

30 minutes of fast walking, stationary bike, or any other type of aerobic activity that you like at your target heart rate.

Please refer to www.BodySculptingBible.com for updated workouts and additional cardio routines.

# 14-Day Body Sculpting Workout #2

---

**SPECIAL INSTRUCTIONS FOR WEEKS 5 & 6**

Use giant sets. Perform giant sets by performing four exercises with no rest period in between. Only rest after the four exercises have been performed consecutively. Repeat for the prescribed number of sets and then move on to the second group of exercises. You will repeat Day 1 on Monday and Thursday, Day 2 on Tuesday and Friday, and Day 3 on Wednesday and Saturday.

---

## DAY 1                                                                 MONDAY/THURSDAY

| EXERCISE | PAGE NO. | REPS | SETS | REST |
|---|---|---|---|---|
| **GIANT SET # 1** | | | | |
| Back—Dumbbell One-Arm Row (Alternate with Two-Arm Row, 172) | 170 | 8-10 | 4 | No Rest |
| Chest—Incline Dumbbell Press (alternate with Push-Up, 210) | 196 | 8-10 | 4 | No Rest |
| Back—Dumbbell Pullover | 186 | 8-10 | 4 | No Rest |
| Chest—Incline Dumbbell Fly (alternate with Push-Up, 210) | 202 | 8-10 | 4 | 60 seconds |
| **GIANT SET # 2** | | | | |
| Biceps—Dumbbell Curl | 262 | 8-10 | 4 | No Rest |
| Triceps—Lying Dumbbell Extension | 242 | 8-10 | 4 | No Rest |
| Biceps—Concentration Curl (alternate with Hammer Curl, 274) | 270 | 8-10 | 4 | No Rest |
| Triceps—Triceps Kickback (alternate with Overhead Dumbbell Extension, 240) | 256 | 8-10 | 4 | 60 seconds |

| DAY 2 | | | | TUESDAY/FRIDAY |
|---|---|---|---|---|
| **EXERCISE** | **PAGE NO.** | **REPS** | **SETS** | **REST** |
| **GIANT SET # 1** | | | | |
| Thighs—Dumbbell Squat (alternate with Ballet Squat, 124) | 122 | 8-10 | 4 | No Rest |
| Hamstrings—Lying Leg Curl (alternate with Dumbbell Lunge, 132) | 138 | 8-10 | 4 | No Rest |
| Thighs—Ballet Squat (alternate with Leg Extension, 136) | 124 | 8-10 | 4 | No Rest |
| Hamstrings—Stiff-legged Deadlift (alternate with Standing Leg Curl, 142) | 144 | 8-10 | 4 | 60 seconds |
| **GIANT SET # 2** | | | | |
| Calves—Standing Calf Raise (one leg) | 152 | 15-25 | 4 | No Rest |
| Shoulders—Dumbbell Shoulder Press (alternate with Dumbbell Upright Row, 226) | 216 | 15-25 | 4 | No Rest |
| Calves—Standing Calf Raise (two legs) | 152 | 15-25 | 4 | No Rest |
| Shoulders—Bent-Over Lateral Raise | 220 | 15-25 | 4 | 60 seconds |

| DAY 3 | | | | WEDNESDAY/SATURDAY |
|---|---|---|---|---|
| **EXERCISE** | **PAGE NO.** | **REPS** | **SETS** | **REST** |
| **GIANT SET # 1** | | | | |
| Lower Abs—Lying Leg Raise | 296 | 15-25 | 4 | No Rest |
| Upper Abs—Crunch | 284 | 15-25 | 4 | No Rest |

**Note:** Continue until all four sets of each exercise have been done. Don't worry if you are not able to perform all of the recommended reps the first few times you perform this abdominal workout. As you get used to this rigorous workout, your body will adapt and get stronger.

**AEROBIC ACTIVITY**

40 minutes of fast walking, stationary bike, or anyother type of aerobic activity that you like at your target heart rate.

Please refer to www.BodySculptingBible.com for updated workouts and additional cardio routines.

# 14-Day Body Sculpting Workout #3

**SPECIAL INSTRUCTIONS FOR WEEKS 1 & 2**

Use modified compound supersets. Perform modified compound supersets by performing the first exercise, resting for the prescribed rest period, performing the second exercise, resting the prescribed rest period, and going back to the first exercise. Continue in this manner until you have performed all of the prescribed number of sets. Then continue with the next modified compound superset. You will repeat Day 1 on Monday and Thursday, Day 2 on Tuesday and Friday, and Day 3 on Wednesday and Saturday.

| DAY 1 | | | | MONDAY/THURSDAY |
|---|---|---|---|---|
| **EXERCISE** | **PAGE NO.** | **REPS** | **SETS** | **REST** |
| **MODIFIED COMPOUND SUPERSET # 1** | | | | |
| Back—Wide-Grip Pull-Up (or Pull-Down to Front, 180) | 174 | 12-15 | 3 | 90 seconds |
| Chest—Incline Dumbbell Bench Press | 196 | 12-15 | 3 | 90 seconds |
| **MODIFIED COMPOUND SUPERSET # 2** | | | | |
| Back—Neutral Grip Pull-Up (or Straight-Arm Pull-Down, 188) | 178 | 12-15 | 2 | 90 seconds |
| Chest—Chest Dip | 204 | 12-15 | 2 | 90 seconds |
| **MODIFIED COMPOUND SUPERSET # 3** | | | | |
| Biceps—Incline Dumbbell Curl | 264 | 12-15 | 3 | 90 seconds |
| Triceps—Triceps Push-Down | 254 | 12-15 | 3 | 90 seconds |
| **MODIFIED COMPOUND SUPERSET # 4** | | | | |
| Biceps—Hammer Curl | 274 | 12-15 | 2 | 90 seconds |
| Triceps—Overhead Dumbbell Extension | 240 | 12-15 | 2 | 90 seconds |

# Weeks 1 & 2

| DAY 2 | | | | TUESDAY/FRIDAY |
|---|---|---|---|---|
| **EXERCISE** | **PAGE NO.** | **REPS** | **SETS** | **REST** |
| **MODIFIED COMPOUND SUPERSET # 1** | | | | |
| Thighs—Leg Press | 134 | 12-15 | 3 | 90 seconds |
| Hamstrings—Lying Leg Curl | 138 | 12-15 | 3 | 90 seconds |
| **MODIFIED COMPOUND SUPERSET # 2** | | | | |
| Thighs—Ballet Squat | 124 | 12-15 | 2 | 90 seconds |
| Hamstrings—Stiff Legged Deadlift | 144 | 12-15 | 2 | 90 seconds |
| **MODIFIED COMPOUND SUPERSET # 3** | | | | |
| Calves—Seated Machine Calf Raise | 154 | 12-15 | 3 | 90 seconds |
| Shoulders—Bent-Over Lateral Raise on Incline Bench | 230 | 12-15 | 3 | 90 seconds |
| **MODIFIED COMPOUND SUPERSET # 4** | | | | |
| Calves—Calf Press | 158 | 12-15 | 2 | 90 seconds |
| Shoulders—Standing Bent-Over Lateral Raises | 220 | 12-15 | 2 | 90 seconds |

| DAY 3 | | | | WEDNESDAY/SATURDAY |
|---|---|---|---|---|
| **EXERCISE** | **PAGE NO.** | **REPS** | **SETS** | **REST** |
| **MODIFIED COMPOUND SUPERSET # 1** | | | | |
| Lower Abs—Lying Leg Raise | 296 | 12-15 | 3 | 90 seconds |
| Upper Abs—Crunch On The Ball | 284 | 12-15 | 2 | 90 seconds |

**AEROBIC ACTIVITY**

20 minutes of fast walking, stationary bike, or any other type of aerobic activity that you like at the target heart rate.

Please refer to www.BodySculptingBible.com for updated workouts and additional cardio routines.

# 14-Day Body Sculpting Workout #3

<table>
<tr><td colspan="2">SPECIAL INSTRUCTIONS FOR WEEKS 3 & 4</td></tr>
</table>

**SPECIAL INSTRUCTIONS FOR WEEKS 3 & 4**

Use supersets. Perform supersets by pairing exercises with no rest period in between. Only rest after the two exercises have been performed consecutively. Repeat for the prescribed number of sets and then move on to the next pair of exercises. You will repeat Day 1 on Monday and Thursday, Day 2 on Tuesday and Friday, and Day 3 on Wednesday and Saturday.

| DAY 1 | | | | MONDAY/THURSDAY |
|---|---|---|---|---|
| **EXERCISE** | **PAGE NO.** | **REPS** | **SETS** | **REST** |
| **SUPERSET # 1** | | | | |
| Back—Close Grip Pull-Up | 176 | 10-12 | 4 | No Rest |
| Chest—Incline Dumbbell Press | 196 | 10-12 | 4 | 60 seconds |
| **SUPERSET # 2** | | | | |
| Back—Dumbbell One-Arm Row | 170 | 10-12 | 3 | No Rest |
| Chest—Flat Dumbbell Press | 198 | 10-12 | 3 | 60 seconds |
| **SUPERSET # 3** | | | | |
| Biceps—Incline Hammer Curl | 274 | 10-12 | 4 | No Rest |
| Triceps—Close-Grip Dumbbell Press | 252 | 10-12 | 4 | 60 seconds |
| **SUPERSET # 4** | | | | |
| Biceps—Reverse Curl | 276 | 10-12 | 3 | No Rest |
| Triceps—Triceps Dip | 246 | 10-12 | 3 | 60 seconds |

## DAY 2 — TUESDAY/FRIDAY

| EXERCISE | PAGE NO. | REPS | SETS | REST |
|---|---|---|---|---|
| **SUPERSET # 1** | | | | |
| Thighs—Barbell Squat | 120 | 10-12 | 4 | No Rest |
| Hamstrings—Lying Leg Curl | 138 | 10-12 | 4 | 60 seconds |
| **SUPERSET # 2** | | | | |
| Thighs—Hack Squat | 128 | 10-12 | 3 | No Rest |
| Hamstrings—Leg Press (feet high on platform, pressing with heels) | 134 | 10-12 | 3 | 60 seconds |
| **SUPERSET # 3** | | | | |
| Calves—Standing Calf Raise | 152 | 12-15 | 4 | No Rest |
| Shoulders—Dumbbell Upright Row | 226 | 10-12 | 4 | 60 seconds |
| **SUPERSET # 4** | | | | |
| Calves—Standing Calf Raise (One-Legged with Dumbbell) | 152 | 12-15 | 3 | No Rest |
| Shoulders—Bent-Over Lateral Raise on Incline Bench | 230 | 10-12 | 3 | 60 seconds |

## DAY 3 — WEDNESDAY/SATURDAY

| EXERCISE | PAGE NO. | REPS | SETS | REST |
|---|---|---|---|---|
| **SUPERSET #1** | | | | |
| Lower Abs-Crunch/Pelvic Lift Combination | 298 | 12-15 | 4 | No Rest |
| Upper Abs-Bicycle Crunch | 286 | 12-15 | 3 | 60 seconds |

**AEROBIC ACTIVITY**

30 minutes of fast walking, stationary bike, or any other type of aerobic activity that you like at your target heart rate.

Please refer to www.BodySculptingBible.com for updated workouts and additional cardio routines.

# 14-Day Body Sculpting Workout #3

<table>
<tr><td colspan="5">**SPECIAL INSTRUCTIONS FOR WEEKS 5 & 6**<br>Use giant sets. Perform giant sets by performing four exercises with no rest period in between. Only rest after the four exercises have been performed consecutively. Repeat for the prescribed number of sets and then move on to the second group of exercises. You will repeat Day 1 on Monday and Thursday, Day 2 on Tuesday and Friday, and Day 3 on Wednesday and Saturday.</td></tr>
</table>

## DAY 1 — MONDAY/THURSDAY

| EXERCISE | PAGE NO. | REPS | SETS | REST |
|---|---|---|---|---|
| **GIANT SET # 1** | | | | |
| Back—Wide Grip Pull-Up to Front | 174 | 8-10 | 4 | No Rest |
| Chest—Incline Dumbbell Press | 196 | 8-10 | 4 | No Rest |
| Back—Bent-Over Barbell Row | 166 | 8-10 | 4 | No Rest |
| Chest—Flat Dumbbell Press | 198 | 8-10 | 4 | 60 seconds |
| **GIANT SET # 2** | | | | |
| Biceps—Reverse Curl | 276 | 8-10 | 4 | No Rest |
| Triceps—Triceps Dip | 246 | 8-10 | 4 | No Rest |
| Biceps—E-Z Preacher Curl | 268 | 8-10 | 4 | No Rest |
| Triceps—Close-Grip Dumbbell Press | 252 | 8-10 | 4 | 60 seconds |

## DAY 2 — TUESDAY/FRIDAY

| EXERCISE | PAGE NO. | REPS | SETS | REST |
|---|---|---|---|---|
| **GIANT SET # 1** | | | | |
| Thighs—Ballet Squat | 124 | 8-10 | 4 | No Rest |
| Hamstrings—Barbell Lunge | 132 | 8-10 | 4 | No Rest |
| Thighs—Barbell Squat | 120 | 8-10 | 4 | No Rest |
| Hamstrings—Barbell Stiff-Legged Deadlift | 144 | 8-10 | 4 | 60 seconds |
| **GIANT SET # 2** | | | | |
| Calves—Calf Press | 158 | 12-15 | 4 | No Rest |
| Shoulders—Military Press | 222 | 8-10 | 4 | No Rest |
| Calves—Standing Calf Raise | 152 | 12-15 | 4 | No Rest |
| Shoulders—Bent-Arm Bent-Over Row | 228 | 8-10 | 4 | 60 seconds |

| DAY 3 | | | | WEDNESDAY/SATURDAY |
|---|---|---|---|---|
| EXERCISE | PAGE NO. | REPS | SETS | REST |
| **GIANT SET # 1** <br> Lower Abs—Trunk Curl and Crunch with Legs Extended | 288 | 12-15 | 4 | No Rest |
| Upper Abs—Incline Board Partial Sit-Up | 300 | 12-15 | 4 | No Rest |

**Note**: Continue until all four sets of each exercise have been done. Don't worry if you are not able to perform all of the recommended reps the first few times that you perform this abdominal workout. As you get used to this rigorous workout, your body will adapt and get stronger.

**AEROBIC ACTIVITY**

40 minutes of fast walking, stationary bike, or any other type of aerobic activity that you like at your target heart rate.

Please refer to www.BodySculptingBible.com for updated workouts and additional cardio routines.

## WHAT TO DO AFTER WEEK 6?

By going through all three Body Sculpting Bible Workouts you have learned many useful exercises that target your muscles in a very efficient manner. After week six, you can retain the main structure of the workout but exchange the recommended exercises with similar ones. Don't be afraid to experiment!

Another alternative, if you want to take your body to the next level, is to try out the Advanced Routine. Or, if you want to gain more muscle mass, you may want to try the mass gaining program.

# 14-Day Rapid Body Sculpting Workout #1

---

**SPECIAL INSTRUCTIONS FOR WEEKS 1 & 2**

Use modified compound supersets. Perform modified compound supersets by performing the first exercise, resting for the prescribed rest period, performing the second exercise, resting the prescribed rest period, and going back to the first exercise. Continue in this manner until you have performed all of the prescribed number of sets. Then continue with the next modified compound superset. You will repeat Day 1 on Monday and Thursday, Day 2 on Tuesday and Friday, and Day 3 on Wednesday and Saturday.

---

| DAY 1 | | | | MONDAY/THURSDAY |
|---|---|---|---|---|
| **EXERCISE** | **PAGE NO.** | **REPS** | **SETS** | **REST** |
| **MODIFIED COMPOUND SUPERSET # 1** | | | | |
| Back – Dumbbell One-Arm Row | 170 | 12-15 | 2 | 30 seconds |
| Chest – Push-Up (against the wall if unable to perform on the floor) | 210 | 12-15 | 2 | 30 seconds |
| **MODIFIED COMPOUND SUPERSET # 2** | | | | |
| Back – Two-Arm Row | 172 | 12-15 | 2 | 30 seconds |
| Chest - Flat Dumbbell Fly (performed on the floor if you don't have access to an exercise bench) | 200 | 12-15 | 2 | 30 seconds |
| **MODIFIED COMPOUND SUPERSET # 3** | | | | |
| Biceps-Dumbbell Curl | 262 | 12-15 | 2 | 30 seconds |
| Triceps-Lying Dumbbell Extension | 242 | 12-15 | 2 | 30 seconds |
| **MODIFIED COMPOUND SUPERSET # 4** | | | | |
| Biceps-Hammer Curl | 274 | 12-15 | 2 | 30 seconds |
| Triceps-Overhead Dumbbell Extension | 240 | 12-15 | 2 | 30 seconds |

| DAY 2 | | | | TUESDAY/FRIDAY |
|---|---|---|---|---|
| **EXERCISE** | **PAGE NO.** | **REPS** | **SETS** | **REST** |
| **MODIFIED COMPOUND SUPERSET #1** | | | | |
| Thighs-Dumbbell Squat (alternate with Ballet Squat, 124) | 122 | 12-15 | 2 | 30 seconds |
| Hamstrings- Dumbbell Lunge | 132 | 12-15 | 2 | 30 seconds |
| **MODIFIED COMPOUND SUPERSET # 2** | | | | |
| Thighs-Ballet Squat | 124 | 12-15 | 2 | 30 seconds |
| Hamstrings-Stiff-Legged Deadlift | 144 | 12-15 | 2 | 30 seconds |
| **MODIFIED COMPOUND SUPERSET # 3** | | | | |
| Calves-Standing Calf Raise (one leg) | 152 | 12-15 | 2 | 30 seconds |
| Shoulders-Dumbbell Shoulder Press | 216 | 12-15 | 2 | 30 seconds |
| **MODIFIED COMPOUND SUPERSET # 4** | | | | |
| Calves-Standing Calf Raise (two legs) | 152 | 12-15 | 2 | 30 seconds |
| Shoulders-Bent-Over Lateral Raise | 220 | 12-15 | 2 | 30 seconds |

| DAY 3 | | | | WEDNESDAY/SATURDAY |
|---|---|---|---|---|
| **EXERCISE** | **PAGE NO.** | **REPS** | **SETS** | **REST** |
| **MODIFIED COMPOUND SUPERSET # 1** | | | | |
| Lower Abs-Lying Leg Raise | 296 | 15-25 | 2 | 30 seconds |
| Upper Abs-Crunch | 284 | 15-25 | 2 | 30 seconds |

**AEROBIC ACTIVITY**

15 minutes of fast walking, stationary bike, or any other type of aerobic activity that you like at the target heart rate.

Please refer to www.BodySculptingBible.com for updated workouts and additional cardio routines.

# 14-Day Rapid Body Sculpting Workout #1

<table>
<tr><td colspan="2">SPECIAL INSTRUCTIONS FOR WEEKS 3 & 4</td></tr>
<tr><td colspan="2">Use supersets. Perform supersets by pairing exercises with no rest period in between. Only rest after the two exercises have been performed consecutively. Repeat for the prescribed number of sets and then move on to the next pair of exercises. You will want to repeat Day 1 on Monday and Thursday, Day 2 on Tuesday and Friday, and Day 3 on Wednesday and Saturday.</td></tr>
</table>

| DAY 1 | | | | MONDAY/THURSDAY |
|---|---|---|---|---|
| **EXERCISE** | **PAGE NO.** | **REPS** | **SETS** | **REST** |
| **SUPERSET # 1** | | | | |
| Back – Dumbbell One-Arm Row | 170 | 10-12 | 3 | No Rest |
| Chest – Push-Up 1 | 210 | 10-12 | 3 | 30 seconds |
| (against the wall if unable to perform on the floor) | | | | |
| **SUPERSET # 2** | | | | |
| Back –Two-Arm Row | 172 | 10-12 | 2 | No Rest |
| Chest – Flat Dumbbell Fly (performed on the floor | | | | |
| if you don't have access to an exercise bench) | 200 | 10-12 | 2 | 30 seconds |
| **SUPERSET # 3** | | | | |
| Biceps-Dumbbell Curl | 262 | 10-12 | 3 | No Rest |
| Triceps-Lying Dumbbell Extension | 242 | 10-12 | 3 | 30 seconds |
| **SUPERSET # 4** | | | | |
| Biceps-Hammer Curl | 274 | 10-12 | 2 | No Rest |
| Triceps-Overhead Dumbbell Extension | 240 | 10-12 | 2 | 30 seconds |

# Weeks 3 & 4

| DAY 2 | | | | TUESDAY/FRIDAY |
|---|---|---|---|---|
| **EXERCISE** | **PAGE NO.** | **REPS** | **SETS** | **REST** |
| **SUPERSET # 1** | | | | |
| Thighs-Dumbbell Squat | 122 | 10-12 | 3 | No Rest |
| Hamstrings- Dumbbell Lunge | 132 | 10-12 | 3 | 30 seconds |
| **SUPERSET # 2** | | | | |
| Thighs-Ballet Squat | 124 | 10-12 | 2 | No Rest |
| Hamstrings-Stiff-Legged Deadlift | 144 | 10-12 | 2 | 30 seconds |
| **SUPERSET # 3** | | | | |
| Calves-Standing Calf Raise (one leg) | 152 | 12-15 | 3 | No Rest |
| Shoulders-Dumbbell Shoulder Press | 216 | 10-12 | 3 | 30 seconds |
| **SUPERSET # 4** | | | | |
| Calves-Standing Calf Raise (two legs) | 152 | 12-15 | 2 | No Rest |
| Shoulders-Bent-Over Lateral Raise | 220 | 10-12 | 2 | 30 seconds |

| DAY 3 | | | | WEDNESDAY/SATURDAY |
|---|---|---|---|---|
| **EXERCISE** | **PAGE NO.** | **REPS** | **SETS** | **REST** |
| **SUPERSET # 1** | | | | |
| Lower Abs-Lying Leg Raise | 296 | 15-25 | 3 | No Rest |
| Upper Abs-Crunch | 284 | 15-25 | 3 | 30 seconds |

**AEROBIC ACTIVITY**

20 minutes of fast walking, stationary bike, or any other type of aerobic activity that you like at your target heart rate.

Please refer to www.BodySculptingBible.com for updated workouts and additional cardio routines.

# 14-Day Rapid Body Sculpting Workout #1

## SPECIAL INSTRUCTIONS FOR WEEKS 5 & 6

Use giant sets. Perform giant sets by performing four exercises with no rest period in between. Only rest after the four exercises have been performed consecutively. Repeat for the prescribed number of sets and then move on to the second group of exercises. You will repeat Day 1 on Monday and Thursday, Day 2 on Tuesday and Friday, and Day 3 on Wednesday and Saturday.

### DAY 1 — MONDAY/THURSDAY

| EXERCISE | PAGE NO. | REPS | SETS | REST |
|---|---|---|---|---|
| **GIANT SET # 1** | | | | |
| Back – Dumbbell One-Arm Row | 170 | 8-10 | 3 | No Rest |
| Chest- Push-Up (against the wall if unable to perform on the floor) | 210 | 8-10 | 3 | No Rest |
| Back - Two-Arm Row | 172 | 8-10 | 3 | No Rest |
| Chest- Flat Dumbbell Fly (performed on the floor if you don't have access to an exercise bench) | 200 | 8-10 | 3 | 45 seconds |
| **GIANT SET #2** | | | | |
| Biceps-Dumbbell Curl | 262 | 8-10 | 3 | No Rest |
| Triceps-Lying Dumbbell Extension | 242 | 8-10 | 3 | No Rest |
| Biceps-Hammer Curl | 274 | 8-10 | 3 | No Rest |
| Triceps-Overhead Dumbbell Extension | 240 | 8-10 | 3 | 45 seconds |

### DAY 2 — TUESDAY/FRIDAY

| EXERCISE | PAGE NO. | REPS | SETS | REST |
|---|---|---|---|---|
| **GIANT SET # 1** | | | | |
| Thighs-Dumbbell Squat | 122 | 8-10 | 3 | No Rest |
| Hamstrings-Dumbbell Lunge | 132 | 8-10 | 3 | No Rest |
| Thighs-Ballet Squat | 124 | 8-10 | 3 | No Rest |
| Hamstrings-Stiff-Legged Deadlift | 144 | 8-10 | 3 | 45 seconds |
| **GIANT SET # 2** | | | | |
| Calves-Standing Calf Raise (one leg) | 152 | 15-25 | 3 | No Rest |
| Shoulders- Dumbbell Shoulder Press | 216 | 8-10 | 3 | No Rest |
| Calves-Standing Calf Raise (two legs) | 152 | 15-25 | 3 | No Rest |
| Shoulders –Bent-Over Lateral Raise | 220 | 8-10 | 3 | 45 seconds |

# Weeks 5 & 6

| DAY 3 | | | | WEDNESDAY/SATURDAY |
|---|---|---|---|---|
| EXERCISE | PAGE NO. | REPS | SETS | REST |
| GIANT SET # 1 | | | | |
| Lower Abs-Lying Leg Raise | 296 | 15-25 | 4 | No Rest |
| Upper Abs-Crunch | 284 | 15-25 | 4 | No Rest |

**Note**: Continue until all four sets of each exercise have been done. Don't worry if you are not able to perform all of the recommended reps the first few times that you perform this abdominal workout. As you get used to this rigorous workout, your body will adapt and get stronger.

### AEROBIC ACTIVITY

25 minutes of fast walking, stationary bike, or any other type of aerobic activity that you like at your target heart rate.

Please refer to www.BodySculptingBible.com for updated workouts and additional cardio routines.

# 14-Day Rapid Body Sculpting Workout #2

| DAY 1 | | | | MONDAY/THURSDAY |
|---|---|---|---|---|
| **EXERCISE** | **PAGE NO.** | **REPS** | **SETS** | **REST** |
| **MODIFIED COMPOUND SUPERSET # 1** | | | | |
| Back – Dumbbell One-Arm Row (alternate with Two-Arm Row, 172) | 170 | 12-15 | 2 | 30 seconds |
| Chest – Incline Dumbbell Press | 196 | 12-15 | 2 | 30 seconds |
| **MODIFIED COMPOUND SUPERSET # 2** | | | | |
| Back –Dumbbell Pullover | 186 | 12-15 | 2 | 30 seconds |
| Chest – Incline Dumbbell Fly (alternate with Push-Up, 210) | 202 | 12-15 | 2 | 30 seconds |
| **MODIFIED COMPOUND SUPERSET # 3** | | | | |
| Biceps-Dumbbell Curl | 262 | 12-15 | 2 | 30 seconds |
| Triceps-Lying Dumbbell Extension | 242 | 12-15 | 2 | 30 seconds |
| **MODIFIED COMPOUND SUPERSET # 4** | | | | |
| Biceps-Concentration Curl (alternate with Hammer Curl, 274) | 270 | 12-15 | 2 | 30 seconds |
| Triceps—Triceps Kickback (alternate with Overhead Dumbbell Extension, 240) | 256 | 12-15 | 2 | 30 seconds |

| DAY 2 | | | | **TUESDAY/FRIDAY** |
|---|---|---|---|---|
| **EXERCISE** | **PAGE NO.** | **REPS** | **SETS** | **REST** |
| **MODIFIED COMPOUND SUPERSET # 1** | | | | |
| Thighs-Dumbbell Squat (alternate with Ballet Squat, 124) | 122 | 10-12 | 2 | 30 seconds |
| Hamstrings-Lying Leg Curl (alternate with Dumbbell Lunge, 132) | 138 | 12-15 | 2 | 30 seconds |
| **MODIFIED COMPOUND SUPERSET # 2** | | | | |
| Thighs-Ballet Squat (alternate with Leg Extension, 136) | 124 | 12-15 | 2 | 30 seconds |
| Hamstrings-Stiff-Legged Deadlift (alternate with Standing Leg Curl, 142) | 144 | 12-15 | 2 | 30 seconds |
| **MODIFIED COMPOUND SUPERSET # 3** | | | | |
| Calves-Standing Calf Raise (one leg) | 152 | 12-15 | 2 | 30 seconds |
| Shoulders-Dumbbell Shoulder Press (alternate with Dumbbell Upright Row, 226) | 216 | 10-12 | 2 | 30 seconds |
| **MODIFIED COMPOUND SUPERSET # 4** | | | | |
| Calves-Dumbbell Calf Raise (two legs) | 152 | 12-15 | 2 | 30 seconds |
| Shoulders-Bent-Over Lateral Raise | 220 | 12-15 | 2 | 30 seconds |

| DAY 3 | | | | **WEDNESDAY/SATURDAY** |
|---|---|---|---|---|
| **EXERCISE** | **PAGE NO.** | **REPS** | **SETS** | **REST** |
| **MODIFIED COMPOUND SUPERSET # 1** | | | | |
| Lower Abs-Lying Leg Raise | 296 | 15-25 | 2 | 30 seconds |
| Upper Abs-Crunch | 284 | 15-25 | 2 | 30 seconds |

**AEROBIC ACTIVITY**

15 minutes of fast walking, stationary bike, or any other type of aerobic activity that you like at the target heart rate.

Please refer to www.BodySculptingBible.com for updated workouts and additional cardio routines.

# 14-Day Rapid Body Sculpting Workout #2

<table>
<tr><td colspan="5">SPECIAL INSTRUCTIONS FOR WEEKS 3 & 4<br>Use supersets. Perform supersets by pairing exercises with no rest period in between. Only rest after the two exercises have been performed consecutively. Repeat for the prescribed number of sets and then move on to the next pair of exercises. You will repeat Day 1 on Monday and Thursday, Day 2 on Tuesday and Friday, and Day 3 on Wednesday and Saturday.</td></tr>
</table>

| DAY 1 | | | | MONDAY/THURSDAY |
|---|---|---|---|---|
| **EXERCISE** | **PAGE NO.** | **REPS** | **SETS** | **REST** |
| **SUPERSET #1** | | | | |
| Back – Dumbbell One-Arm Row | 170 | 10-12 | 3 | No Rest |
| Chest – Incline Dumbbell Press | 196 | 10-12 | 3 | 30 seconds |
| **SUPERSET #2** | | | | |
| Back –Dumbbell Pullover | 186 | 10-12 | 2 | No Rest |
| Incline Dumbbell Fly (alternate with Push-Up, 210) | 202 | 10-12 | 2 | 30 seconds |
| **SUPERSET #3** | | | | |
| Biceps-Dumbbell Curl | 262 | 10-12 | 3 | No Rest |
| Triceps-Lying Dumbbell Extension | 242 | 10-12 | 3 | 30 seconds |
| **SUPERSET #4** | | | | |
| Biceps-Concentration Curl (alternate with Hammer Curl, 274) | 270 | 10-12 | 2 | No Rest |
| Triceps—Triceps Kickback (alternate with Overhead Dumbbell Extension, 240) | 256 | 10-12 | 2 | 30 seconds |

# Weeks 3 & 4

| DAY 2 | | | | TUESDAY/FRIDAY |
|---|---|---|---|---|
| **EXERCISE** | **PAGE NO.** | **REPS** | **SETS** | **REST** |
| **SUPERSET # 1** | | | | |
| Thighs-Dumbbell Squat (alternate with Ballet Squat, 124) | 122 | 10-12 | 3 | No Rest |
| Hamstrings- Lying Leg Curl (alternate with Dumbbell Lunge, 132) | 138 | 10-12 | 3 | 30 seconds |
| **SUPERSET # 2** | | | | |
| Thighs-Ballet Squat (alternate with Leg Extension, 136) | 124 | 10-12 | 2 | No Rest |
| Hamstrings-Stiff-Legged Deadlift (alternate with Standing Leg Curl, 142) | 144 | 10-12 | 2 | 30 seconds |
| **SUPERSET # 3** | | | | |
| Calves-Standing Calf Raise (one leg) | 152 | 12-15 | 3 | No Rest |
| Shoulders-Dumbbell Shoulder Press (alternate with Dumbbell Upright Row, 226) | 216 | 10-12 | 3 | 30 seconds |
| **SUPERSET # 4** | | | | |
| Calves-Standing Calf Raise (two legs) | 152 | 12-15 | 2 | No Rest |
| Shoulders-Bent-Over Lateral Raise | 220 | 10-12 | 2 | 30 seconds |

| DAY 3 | | | | WEDNESDAY/SATURDAY |
|---|---|---|---|---|
| **EXERCISE** | **PAGE NO.** | **REPS** | **SETS** | **REST** |
| **SUPERSET # 1** | | | | |
| Lower Abs-Lying Leg Raise | 296 | 15-25 | 3 | No Rest |
| Upper Abs-Crunch | 284 | 15-25 | 3 | 30 seconds |

**AEROBIC ACTIVITY**

20 minutes of fast walking, stationary bike, or any other type of aerobic activity that you like at your target heart rate.

Please refer to www.BodySculptingBible.com for updated workouts and additional cardio routines.

# 14-Day Rapid Body Sculpting Workout #2

**SPECIAL INSTRUCTIONS FOR WEEKS 5 & 6**

Use giant sets. Perform giant sets by performing four exercises with no rest period in between. Only rest after the four exercises have been performed consecutively. Repeat for the prescribed number of sets and then move on to the second group of exercises. You will repeat Day 1 on Monday and Thursday, Day 2 on Tuesday and Friday, and Day 3 on Wednesday and Saturday.

## DAY 1 — MONDAY/THURSDAY

| EXERCISE | PAGE NO. | REPS | SETS | REST |
|---|---|---|---|---|
| **GIANT SET # 1** | | | | |
| Back – Dumbbell One-Arm Row (alternate with Two-Arm Row, 172) | 170 | 8-10 | 3 | No Rest |
| Chest- Incline Dumbbell Press (alternate with Push-Up, 210) | 196 | 8-10 | 3 | No Rest |
| Back - Dumbbell Pullover | 186 | 8-10 | 3 | No Rest |
| Chest- Incline Dumbbell Fly (alternate with Push-Up, 210) | 202 | 8-10 | 3 | 45 seconds |
| **GIANT SET # 2** | | | | |
| Biceps-Dumbbell Curl | 262 | 8-10 | 3 | No Rest |
| Triceps-Lying Dumbbell Extension | 242 | 8-10 | 3 | No Rest |
| Biceps-Concentration Curl (alternate with Hammer Curl, 274) | 270 | 8-10 | 3 | No Rest |
| Triceps-Triceps Kickback (alternate with Overhead Dumbbell Extension, 240) | 256 | 8-10 | 3 | 45 seconds |

## DAY 2 — TUESDAY/FRIDAY

| EXERCISE | PAGE NO. | REPS | SETS | REST |
|---|---|---|---|---|
| **GIANT SET # 1** | | | | |
| Thighs-Dumbbell Squat (alternate with Ballet Squat, 124) | 122 | 8-10 | 3 | No Rest |
| Hamstrings-Lying Leg Curl (alternate with Dumbbell Lunge, 132) | 138 | 8-10 | 3 | No Rest |
| Thighs-Ballet Squat (alternate with Leg Extension, 136) | 124 | 8-10 | 3 | No Rest |
| Hamstrings-Stiff-Legged Deadlift (alternate with Standing Leg Curl, 142) | 144 | 8-10 | 3 | 45 seconds |
| **GIANT SET # 2** | | | | |
| Calves-Standing Calf Raise (one leg) | 152 | 15-25 | 3 | No Rest |
| Shoulders- Dumbbell Shoulder Press (alternate with Dumbbell Upright Row, 226) | 216 | 8-10 | 3 | No Rest |
| Calves-Standing Calf Raise (two legs) | 152 | 15-25 | 3 | No Rest |
| Shoulders –Bent-Over Lateral Raise | 220 | 8-10 | 3 | 45 seconds |

# Weeks 5 & 6

| DAY 3 | | | | WEDNESDAY/SATURDAY |
|---|---|---|---|---|
| **EXERCISE** | **PAGE NO.** | **REPS** | **SETS** | **REST** |
| **GIANT SET # 1** | | | | |
| Lower Abs-Lying Leg Raise | 296 | 15-25 | 4 | No Rest |
| Upper Abs-Crunch | 284 | 15-25 | 4 | No Rest |

**Note**: Continue until all four sets of each exercise have been done. Don't worry if you are not able to perform all of the recommended reps the first few times that you perform this abdominal workout. As you get used to this rigorous workout, your body will adapt and get stronger.

**AEROBIC ACTIVITY**

25 minutes of fast walking, stationary bike, or any other type of aerobic activity that you like at your target heart rate.

Please refer to www.BodySculptingBible.com for updated workouts and additional cardio routines.

# Advanced 14-Day Body Sculpting Workout #1
# Weeks 1 & 2

---

**SPECIAL INSTRUCTIONS FOR WEEKS 1 & 2**

Use modified compound supersets. Perform modified compound supersets by performing the first exercise, resting for the prescribed rest period, performing the second exercise, resting the prescribed rest period, and going back to the first one. Continue in this manner until you have performed all of the prescribed number of sets. Then continue with the next modified compound superset. You will repeat Day 1 on Monday and Thursday, Day 2 on Tuesday and Friday, and Day 3 on Wednesday and Saturday.

---

| DAY 1 | | | | MONDAY/THURSDAY |
|---|---|---|---|---|
| **EXERCISE** | **PAGE NO.** | **REPS** | **SETS** | **REST** |
| **MODIFIED COMPOUND SUPERSET # 1** | | | | |
| Back—Dumbbell One-Arm Row (alternate with Two-Arm Row on the next workout) | 170 | 12-15 | 3 | 90 seconds |
| Chest—Incline Dumbbell Press (alternate with Incline Dumbbell Press; palms facing each other) | 196 | 12-15 | 3 | 90 seconds |
| **MODIFIED COMPOUND SUPERSET # 2** | | | | |
| Back—Dumbbell Pullover (alternate with Low-Pulley Row) | 186 | 12-15 | 3 | 90 seconds |
| Chest—Chest Dip (alternate with Push Up) | 204 | 12-15 | 3 | 90 seconds |
| **MODIFIED COMPOUND SUPERSET # 3** | | | | |
| Back—Wide-Grip Pull-Up (or Pull-Down) to Front (alternate with Neutral Grip Pull-Up or Pull-Down) | 174 | 12-15 | 3 | 90 seconds |
| Chest—Incline Dumbbell Fly (alternate with Incline Cable Crossover) | 202 | 12-15 | 3 | 90 seconds |
| **MODIFIED COMPOUND SUPERSET # 4** | | | | |
| Rear Delts—Bent-Over Lateral Raise (alternate with Seated Rear Delt Machine) | 220 | 12-15 | 3 | 90 seconds |
| Calves—Seated Machine Calf Raise (alternate with Donkey Calf Raise) | 154 | 15-25 | 3 | 90 seconds |

# Advanced 14-Day Body Sculpting Workout #1

## Weeks 1 & 2

| DAY 2 | | | | TUESDAY/ FRIDAY |
|---|---|---|---|---|
| **EXERCISE** | **PAGE NO.** | **REPS** | **SETS** | **REST** |
| **MODIFIED COMPOUND SUPERSET # 1** | | | | |
| Biceps—Dumbbell Curl (alternate with Incline Dumbbell Curl) | 262 | 12-15 | 3 | 90 seconds |
| Triceps—Lying Dumbbell Extension (alternate with Triceps Push-Down) | 242 | 12-15 | 3 | 90 seconds |
| **MODIFIED COMPOUND SUPERSET # 2** | | | | |
| Biceps—Concentration Curl (alternate with Hammer Curl) | 270 | 12-15 | 3 | 90 seconds |
| Triceps—Triceps Kickback (alternate with Overhead Dumbbell Extension) | 256 | 12-15 | 3 | 90 seconds |
| **MODIFIED COMPOUND SUPERSET # 3** | | | | |
| Biceps—Reverse Curl (alternate with Preacher Curl) | 276 | 12-15 | 3 | 90 seconds |
| Triceps—Triceps Dip (alternate with Close-Grip Dumbbell Press | 246 | 12-15 | 3 | 90 seconds |
| **MODIFIED COMPOUND SUPERSET # 4** | | | | |
| Shoulders—Dumbbell Shoulder Press (alternate with Military Press) | 216 | 12-15 | 3 | 90 seconds |
| Shoulders—Dumbbell Upright Row (alternate with Dumbbell Lateral Raise) | 226 | 12-15 | 3 | 90 seconds |

# Advanced 14-Day Body Sculpting Workout #1
# Weeks 1 & 2

| DAY 3 | | | | WEDNESDAY/ SATURDAY |
|---|---|---|---|---|
| **EXERCISE** | **PAGE NO.** | **REPS** | **SETS** | **REST** |
| **MODIFIED COMPOUND SUPERSET # 1** | | | | |
| Thighs—Barbell Squat (alternate with Ballet Squat) | 120 | 12-15 | 3 | 90 seconds |
| Hamstrings—Lying Leg Curl (alternate with Dumbbell Lunge) | 138 | 12-15 | 3 | 90 seconds |
| **MODIFIED COMPOUND SUPERSET # 2** | | | | |
| Thighs—Hack Squat (alternate with Leg Extension) | 128 | 12-15 | 3 | 90 seconds |
| Hamstrings—Stiff-Legged Deadlift (alternate with Seated Leg Curl) | 144 | 12-15 | 3 | 90 seconds |
| **MODIFIED COMPOUND SUPERSET # 3** | | | | |
| Thighs—Leg Press (alternate with Dumbbell Squat) | 134 | 12-15 | 3 | 90 seconds |
| Hamstrings—Standing Leg Curl (alternate with Lying Leg Curl) | 142 | 12-15 | 3 | 90 seconds |
| **MODIFIED COMPOUND SUPERSET # 4** | | | | |
| Calves—Calf Press (alternate with Two-Legged Barbell Calf Raise) | 158 | 15-25 | 3 | 90 seconds |
| Calves—Standing Calf Raise (one-leg) (alternate with Standing Calf Raise, two legs) | 152 | 15-25 | 3 | 90 seconds |

# Cardio and Abs Advanced Workout #1
## Weeks 1 & 2

To be performed from Monday through Saturday first thing in the morning on an empty stomach or right after the workout.

---

**SPECIAL INSTRUCTIONS FOR WEEKS 1 & 2**

Use modified compound supersets. Perform modified compound supersets by performing the first exercise, resting for the prescribed rest period, performing the second exercise, resting the prescribed rest period, and going back to the first one. Continue in this manner until you have performed all of the prescribed number of sets. Then continue with the next modified compound superset.

---

## WEEKS 1 & 2

| EXERCISE | PAGE NO. | REPS | SETS | REST |
|---|---|---|---|---|
| **MODIFIED COMPOUND SUPERSET # 1** | | | | |
| Lower Abs—Lying Leg Raise | 296 | 15-25 | 3 | 90 seconds |
| Upper Abs—Crunch | 284 | 15-25 | 3 | 90 seconds |
| **MODIFIED COMPOUND SUPERSET # 2** | | | | |
| Lower Abs—Knee-In | 294 | 15-25 | 3 | 90 seconds |
| Upper Abs—Bicycle Crunch | 286 | 15-25 | 3 | 90 seconds |

---

**AEROBIC ACTIVITY**

20 minutes of fast walking, stationary bike, or any other type of aerobic activity that you like at your target heart rate.

---

Please refer to www.BodySculptingBible.com for updated workouts and additional cardio routines.

# Advanced 14-Day Body Sculpting Workout #1
# Weeks 3 & 4

### SPECIAL INSTRUCTIONS FOR WEEKS 3 & 4

Use supersets. Perform supersets by pairing exercises with no rest period in between. Only rest after the two exercises have been performed consecutively. Repeat for the prescribed number of sets and then move on to the next pair of exercises. You will repeat Day 1 on Monday and Thursday, Day 2 on Tuesday and Friday, and Day 3 on Wednesday and Saturday.

| DAY 1 | | | | MONDAY/THURSDAY |
|---|---|---|---|---|
| **EXERCISE** | **PAGE NO.** | **REPS** | **SETS** | **REST** |
| **SUPERSET # 1** | | | | |
| Back—Dumbbell One-Arm Row (alternate with Two-Arm Row on the next workout) | 170 | 10-12 | 4 | No Rest |
| Chest—Incline Dumbbell Press (alternate with Incline Dumbbell Press; palms facing you) | 196 | 10-12 | 4 | 60 seconds |
| **SUPERSET # 2** | | | | |
| Back—Dumbbell Pullover (alternate with Low-Pulley Row) | 186 | 10-12 | 4 | No Rest |
| Chest—Chest Dip (alternate with Push-Up) | 204 | 10-12 | 4 | 60 seconds |
| **SUPERSET # 3** | | | | |
| Back—Wide-Grip Pull-Up (or Pull-Down) to Front (alternate with Neutral Grip Pull-Up or Pull-Down) | 174 | 10-12 | 3 | No Rest |
| Chest—Incline Dumbbell Fly (alternate with Incline Cable Crossover) | 202 | 10-12 | 3 | 60 seconds |
| **SUPERSET # 4** | | | | |
| Rear Delts—Bent-Over Lateral Raise (alternate with Seated Rear Delt Machine) | 220 | 10-12 | 3 | No Rest |
| Calves—Seated Machine Calf Raise (alternate with Donkey Calf Raise) | 154 | 15-25 | 3 | 60 seconds |

# Advanced 14-Day Body Sculpting Workout #1
## Weeks 3 & 4

| DAY 2 | | | | TUESDAY/FRIDAY |
|---|---|---|---|---|
| **EXERCISE** | **PAGE NO.** | **REPS** | **SETS** | **REST** |
| **SUPERSET # 1** | | | | |
| Biceps—Dumbbell Curl (alternate with Incline Dumbbell Curl) | 262 | 10-12 | 4 | No Rest |
| Triceps—Lying Dumbbell Extension (alternate with Triceps Pushdown) | 242 | 10-12 | 4 | 60 seconds |
| **SUPERSET # 2** | | | | |
| Biceps—Concentration Curl (alternate with Hammer Curl) | 270 | 10-12 | 4 | No Rest |
| Triceps—Triceps Kickback (alternate with Overhead Dumbbell Extension) | 256 | 10-12 | 4 | 60 seconds |
| **SUPERSET # 3** | | | | |
| Biceps—Reverse Curl (alternate with Preacher Curl) | 276 | 10-12 | 3 | No Rest |
| Triceps—Triceps Dip (alternate with Close-Grip Dumbbell Press) | 246 | 10-12 | 3 | 60 seconds |
| **SUPERSET # 4** | | | | |
| Shoulders—Dumbbell Shoulder Press (alternate with Military Press) | 216 | 10-12 | 3 | No Rest |
| Shoulders—Dumbbell Upright Row (alternate with Dumbbell Lateral Raise) | 226 | 10-12 | 3 | 60 seconds |

# Advanced 14-Day Body Sculpting Workout #1
# Weeks 3 & 4

| DAY 3 | | | | WEDNESDAY/SATURDAY |
|---|---|---|---|---|
| **EXERCISE** | **PAGE NO.** | **REPS** | **SETS** | **REST** |
| **SUPERSET # 1** | | | | |
| Thighs—Barbell Squat (alternate with Ballet Squat) | 120 | 10-12 | 4 | No Rest |
| Hamstrings—Lying Leg Curl (alternate with Dumbbell Lunge) | 138 | 10-12 | 4 | 60 seconds |
| **SUPERSET # 2** | | | | |
| Thighs—Hack Squat (alternate with Leg Extension) | 128 | 10-12 | 4 | No Rest |
| Hamstrings—Stiff-Legged Deadlift (alternate with Seated Leg Curl) | 144 | 10-12 | 4 | 60 seconds |
| **SUPERSET # 3** | | | | |
| Thighs—Leg Press (alternate with Dumbbell Squat) | 134 | 10-12 | 3 | No Rest |
| Hamstrings—Standing Leg Curl (alternate with Lying Leg Curl) | 142 | 10-12 | 3 | 60 seconds |
| **SUPERSET # 4** | | | | |
| Calves—Calf Press (alternate with Standing Calf Raise (two-leg) | 158 | 15-25 | 3 | No Rest |
| Calves—Standing Calf Raise (one-leg) (alternate with Standing Calf Raise, two legs) | 152 | 15-25 | 3 | 60 seconds |

# Cardio and Abs Advanced Workout #1
## Weeks 3 & 4

To be performed from Monday through Saturday first thing in the morning on an empty stomach or right after the workout.

---

**SPECIAL INSTRUCTIONS FOR WEEKS 3 & 4**

Use supersets. Perform supersets by pairing exercises with no rest period in between. Only rest after the two exercises have been performed consecutively. Repeat for the prescribed number of sets and then move on to the next pair of exercises.

---

## WEEKS 3 & 4

| EXERCISE | PAGE NO. | REPS | SETS | REST |
|---|---|---|---|---|
| **SUPERSET # 1** | | | | |
| Lower Abs—Lying Leg Raise | 296 | 15-25 | 4 | No Rest |
| Upper Abs—Crunch | 284 | 15-25 | 4 | 60 seconds |
| **MODIFIED COMPOUND SUPERSET # 2** | | | | |
| Lower Abs—Knee-In | 294 | 15-25 | 3 | No Rest |
| Upper Abs—Bicycle Crunch | 286 | 15-25 | 3 | 60 seconds |

---

**AEROBIC ACTIVITY**

30 minutes of fast walking, stationary bike, or any other type of aerobic activity that you like at the target heart rate.

---

Please refer to www.BodySculptingBible.com for updated workouts and additional cardio routines.

# Advanced 14-Day Body Sculpting Workout #1
## Weeks 5 & 6

**SPECIAL INSTRUCTIONS FOR WEEKS 5 & 6**

Use giant sets. Perform giant sets by performing four exercises with no rest period in between. Only rest after the four exercises have been performed consecutively. Repeat for the prescribed number of sets and then move on to the second group of exercises. You will repeat Day 1 on Monday and Thursday, Day 2 on Tuesday and Friday, and Day 3 on Wednesday and Saturday.

| DAY 1 | | | | MONDAY/THURSDAY |
|---|---|---|---|---|
| EXERCISE | PAGE NO. | REPS | SETS | REST |
| **GIANT SET #1** | | | | |
| Back—Dumbell One-Arm Row (alternate with Two-Arm Row) | 170 | 8-10 | 4 | No Rest |
| Chest—Incline Dumbbell Press (alternate with Incline Dumbbell Press; palms facing you) | 196 | 8-10 | 4 | No Rest |
| Back—Dumbbell Pullover (alternate with Low-Pulley Row) | 186 | 8-10 | 4 | No Rest |
| Chest—Chest Dip (alternate with Push-Up) | 204 | 8-10 | 4 | 60 seconds |
| **GIANT SET # 2** | | | | |
| Back—Wide-Grip Pull-Up (or Pull-Down) to Front (alternate with Neutral Grip Pull-Up or Pull-Down) | 174 | 8-10 | 4 | No Rest |
| Chest—Incline Dumbbell Fly (alternate with Incline Cable Crossover) | 202 | 8-10 | 4 | No Rest |
| Rear Delts—Bent-Over Lateral Raise (alternate with Seated Rear-Delt Machine) | 220 | 8-10 | 4 | No Rest |
| Calves—Seated Machine Calf Raise (alternate with Donkey Calf Raise) | 154 | 15-25 | 4 | 60 seconds |

# Advanced 14-Day Body Sculpting Workout #1
## Weeks 5 & 6

| DAY 2 | | | | TUESDAY/FRIDAY |
|---|---|---|---|---|
| **EXERCISE** | **PAGE NO.** | **REPS** | **SETS** | **REST** |
| **GIANT SET # 1** | | | | |
| Biceps—Dumbbell Curl (alternate with Incline Dumbbell Curl) | 262 | 8-10 | 4 | No Rest |
| Triceps—Lying Dumbbell Extension (alternate with Triceps Pushdown) | 242 | 8-10 | 4 | No Rest |
| Biceps—Concentration Curl (alternate with Hammer Curl) | 270 | 8-10 | 4 | No Rest |
| Triceps—Triceps Kickback (alternate with Overhead Dumbbell Extension) | 256 | 8-10 | 4 | 60 seconds |
| **GIANT SET # 2** | | | | |
| Biceps—Reverse Curl (alternate with Preacher Curl) | 276 | 8-10 | 4 | No Rest |
| Triceps—Triceps Dip (alternate with Close-Grip Dumbbell Press) | 246 | 8-10 | 4 | No Rest |
| Shoulders—Dumbbell Upright Row (alternate with Dumbbell Lateral Raise) | 226 | 8-10 | 4 | No Rest |
| Shoulders—Dumbbell Shoulder Press (alternate with Military Press) | 216 | 8-10 | 4 | 60 seconds |

# Advanced 14-Day Body Sculpting Workout #1
# Weeks 5 & 6

| DAY 3 | | | | WEDNESDAY/SATURDAY |
|---|---|---|---|---|
| **EXERCISE** | **PAGE NO.** | **REPS** | **SETS** | **REST** |
| **GIANT SET # 1** | | | | |
| Thighs—Barbell Squat (alternate with Ballet Squat) | 120 | 8-10 | 4 | No Rest |
| Hamstrings—Lying Leg Curl (alternate with Dumbbell Lunge) | 138 | 8-10 | 4 | No Rest |
| Thighs—Hack Squat (alternate with Leg Extension) | 128 | 8-10 | 4 | No Rest |
| Hamstrings—Standing Leg Curl (alternate with Lying Leg Curl) | 142 | 8-10 | 4 | 60 seconds |
| **GIANT SET # 2** | | | | |
| Thighs—Leg Press (alternate with Dumbbell Squat) | 134 | 8-10 | 4 | No Rest |
| Hamstrings—Stiff-Legged Deadlift (alternate with Seated Leg Curl) | 144 | 8-10 | 4 | No Rest |
| Calves—Calf Press (alternate with Two Legged Barbell Calf Raise)152 | 158 | 15-25 | 4 | No Rest |
| Calves—Standing Calf Raise (one-leg) (alternate with Standing Calf Raise, two legs) | 152 | 15-25 | 4 | 60 seconds |

# Cardio and Abs Advanced Workout #1
## Weeks 5 & 6

To be performed from Monday through Saturday first thing in the morning on an empty stomach or right after the workout.

---

**SPECIAL INSTRUCTIONS FOR WEEKS 5 & 6**

Use giant sets. Perform giant sets by performing four exercises with no rest period in between. Only rest after the four exercises have been performed consecutively. Repeat for the prescribed number of sets and then move on to the second group of exercises.

---

## WEEKS 5 & 6

| EXERCISE | PAGE NO. | REPS | SETS | REST |
|---|---|---|---|---|
| GIANT SET # 1 | | | | |
| Lower Abs—Lying Leg Raise | 296 | 15-25 | 4 | No Rest |
| Upper Abs—Crunch | 284 | 15-25 | 4 | No Rest |
| Lower Abs—Knee-In | 294 | 15-25 | 4 | No Rest |
| Upper Abs—Bicycle Crunch | 286 | 15-25 | 4 | 60 seconds |

---

**AEROBIC ACTIVITY**

40 minutes of fast walking, stationary bike, or any other type of aerobic activity that you like at your target heart rate.

---

Please refer to www.BodySculptingBible.com for updated workouts and additional cardio routines.

# Advanced 14-Day Body Sculpting Workout #2
# Weeks 1 & 2

---

**SPECIAL INSTRUCTIONS FOR WEEKS 1 & 2**

Use modified compound supersets. Perform modified compound supersets by performing the first exercise, resting for the prescribed rest period, performing the second exercise, resting the prescribed rest period and going back to the first one. Continue in this manner until you have performed all of the prescribed number of sets. Then continue with the next modified compound superset.You will repeat Day 1 on Monday and Thursday, Day 2 on Tuesday and Friday, and Day 3 on Wednesday and Saturday.

---

| DAY 1 | | | | MONDAY/ THURSDAY |
|---|---|---|---|---|
| **EXERCISE** | **PAGE NO.** | **REPS** | **SETS** | **REST** |
| **MODIFIED COMPOUND SUPERSET # 1** | | | | |
| Back—Two-Arm Row (alternate with Bent-Over Barbell Row on the next workout) | 172 | 12-15 | 3 | 90 seconds |
| Chest—Incline Dumbbell Press (alternate with Incline Dumbbell Press; palms facing each other) | 196 | 12-15 | 3 | 90 seconds |
| **MODIFIED COMPOUND SUPERSET # 2** | | | | |
| Back—Bent-Arm Pullover (alternate with Neutral-Grip Pull-Up) | 186 | 12-15 | 3 | 90 seconds |
| Chest—Chest Dip (alternate with Flat Dumbbell Press) | 204 | 12-15 | 3 | 90 seconds |
| **MODIFIED COMPOUND SUPERSET # 3** | | | | |
| Back—Wide-Grip Pull-Down to Front (alternate with Close-Grip Pull-Down) | 174 | 12-15 | 3 | 90 seconds |
| Chest—Incline Dumbbell Fly (alternate with Incline Cable Crossover) | 202 | 12-15 | 3 | 90 seconds |
| **MODIFIED COMPOUND SUPERSET # 4** | | | | |
| Rear Delts—Seated Rear Delt Machine (alternate with Bent-Arm Bent-Over Row) | 234 | 12-15 | 3 | 90 seconds |
| Calves—Seated Machine Calf Raise (alternate with Tibia Raise) | 154 | 15-25 | 3 | 90 seconds |

# Advanced 14-Day Body Sculpting Workout #2
## Weeks 1 & 2

| DAY 2 | | | | TUESDAY/FRIDAY |
|---|---|---|---|---|
| **EXERCISE** | **PAGE NO.** | **REPS** | **SETS** | **REST** |
| **MODIFIED COMPOUND SUPERSET # 1** | | | | |
| Biceps—High Cable Curl (alternate with Concentration Curl) | 280 | 12-15 | 3 | 90 seconds |
| Triceps—Triceps Pushdown (with Rope) (alternate with Fixed Bar Bodyweight Triceps Extension) | 254 | 12-15 | 3 | 90 seconds |
| **MODIFIED COMPOUND SUPERSET # 2** | | | | |
| Biceps—Hammer Curl (alternate with Reverse Curl) | 274 | 12-15 | 3 | 90 seconds |
| Triceps—E-Z Curl Bar Close-Grip Press (alternate with Overhead Dumbbell Triceps Extension) | 250 | 12-15 | 3 | 90 seconds |
| **MODIFIED COMPOUND SUPERSET # 3** | | | | |
| Biceps—Standing E-Z Bar Curl (alternate with One-Arm Preacher Curl) | 272 | 12-15 | 3 | 90 seconds |
| Triceps—Bench Dip (alternate with Close-Grip Dumbbell Press) | 248 | 12-15 | 3 | 90 seconds |
| **MODIFIED COMPOUND SUPERSET # 4** | | | | |
| Shoulders—Bent-Over Lateral Raise on Incline Bench (alternate with Two-Arm Cable Lateral Raise) | 230 | 12-15 | 3 | 90 seconds |
| Shoulders—Front Raise (alternate with Dumbbell Shoulder Press) | 224 | 12-15 | 3 | 90 seconds |

# Advanced 14-Day Body Sculpting Workout #2
# Weeks 1 & 2

| DAY 3 | | | | WEDNESDAY/SATURDAY |
|---|---|---|---|---|
| **EXERCISE** | **PAGE NO.** | **REPS** | **SETS** | **REST** |
| **MODIFIED COMPOUND SUPERSET # 1** | | | | |
| Thighs—Hack Squat (alternate with Leg Extension) | 128 | 12-15 | 3 | 90 seconds |
| Hamstrings—Stiff-Legged Deadlift (alternate with Dumbbell Lunge (pressing with heels)) | 144 | 12-15 | 3 | 90 seconds |
| **MODIFIED COMPOUND SUPERSET # 2** | | | | |
| Thighs—Front Squat (alternate with Ballet Squat) | 130 | 12-15 | 3 | 90 seconds |
| Hamstrings—Lying Leg Curl (alternate with Seated Leg Curl) | 138 | 12-15 | 3 | 90 seconds |
| **MODIFIED COMPOUND SUPERSET # 3** | | | | |
| Thighs—Leg Press (alternate with Barbell Squat) | 134 | 12-15 | 3 | 90 seconds |
| Hamstrings—Standing Leg Curl (alternate with Step-Up) | 142 | 12-15 | 3 | 90 seconds |
| **MODIFIED COMPOUND SUPERSET # 4** | | | | |
| Calves—Calf Press (alternate with Standing Calf Raise) | 158 | 15-25 | 3 | 90 seconds |
| Calves—Standing Calf Raises (one-leg) (alternate with Seated Machine Calf Raise) | 152 | 15-25 | 3 | 90 seconds |

# Cardio and Abs Advanced Workout #2
## Weeks 1 & 2

To be performed from Monday through Saturday first thing in the morning on an empty stomach or right after the workout.

### SPECIAL INSTRUCTIONS FOR WEEKS 1 & 2

Use modified compound supersets. Perform modified compound supersets by performing the first exercise, resting for the prescribed rest period, performing the second exercise, resting the prescribed rest period and going back to the first one. Continue in this manner until you have performed all of the prescribed number of sets. Then continue with the next modified compound superset.

## WEEKS 1 & 2

| EXERCISE | PAGE NO. | REPS | SETS | REST |
|---|---|---|---|---|
| **MODIFIED COMPOUND SUPERSET # 1** | | | | |
| Lower Abs—Lying Leg Raise | 296 | 15-25 | 3 | 90 seconds |
| Upper Abs—Trunk Curl and Crunch | 288 | 15-25 | 3 | 90 seconds |
| **MODIFIED COMPOUND SUPERSET # 2** | | | | |
| Lower Abs—Knee-In | 294 | 15-25 | 3 | 90 seconds |
| Upper Abs—Incline Board Partial Sit-Up | 300 | 15-25 | 3 | 90 seconds |

## AEROBIC ACTIVITY

20 minutes of fast walking, stationary bike, or any other type of aerobic activity that you like at your target heart rate.

Please refer to www.BodySculptingBible.com for updated workouts and additional cardio routines.

# Advanced 14-Day Body Sculpting Workout #2
## Weeks 3 & 4

**SPECIAL INSTRUCTIONS FOR WEEKS 3 & 4**

Use supersets. Perform supersets by pairing exercises with no rest period in between. Only rest after the two exercises have been performed consecutively. Repeat for the prescribed number of sets and then move on to the next pair of exercises. You will repeat Day 1 on Monday and Thursday, Day 2 on Tuesday and Friday, and Day 3 on Wednesday and Saturday.

| DAY 1 | | | | MONDAY/THURSDAY |
|---|---|---|---|---|
| **EXERCISE** | **PAGE NO.** | **REPS** | **SETS** | **REST** |
| **SUPERSET # 1** | | | | |
| Back—Wide-Grip Pull-Up to Front (alternate with Close-Grip Pull-Down) | 174 | 10-12 | 4 | No Rest |
| Chest—Incline Dumbbell Fly (alternate with Incline Cable Crossover) | 202 | 10-12 | 4 | 60 seconds |
| **SUPERSET # 2** | | | | |
| Back—Close-Grip Pull-Up (alternate with Wide-Grip Pull-Down) | 176 | 10-12 | 4 | No Rest |
| Chest—Incline Dumbbell Press; palms facing you (alternate with Chest Dip) | 196 | 10-12 | 4 | 60 seconds |
| **SUPERSET # 3** | | | | |
| Back—Seated Low-Pulley Row (alternate with Bent-Over Barbell Row) | 184 | 10-12 | 3 | No Rest |
| Chest—Flat Dumbbell Press (alternate with Incline Dumbbell Press) | 198 | 10-12 | 3 | 60 seconds |
| **SUPERSET # 4** | | | | |
| Rear Delts—Seated Rear-Delt Machine (alternate with Bent-Over Lateral Raise) | 234 | 10-12 | 3 | No Rest |
| Calves—Tibia Raise (alternate with Donkey Calf Raise) | 160 | 15-25 | 3 | 60 seconds |

# Advanced 14-Day Body Sculpting Workout #2
## Weeks 3 & 4

| DAY 2 | | | | TUESDAY/FRIDAY |
|---|---|---|---|---|
| EXERCISE | PAGE NO. | REPS | SETS | REST |
| **SUPERSET # 1** | | | | |
| Biceps—Dumbbell Curl (alternate with Barbell Curl) | 262 | 10-12 | 4 | No Rest |
| Triceps—Overhead Dumbbell Extension (alternate with Triceps Kickback) | 240 | 10-12 | 4 | 60 seconds |
| **SUPERSET # 2** | | | | |
| Biceps—E-Z Reverse Preacher Curl (alternate with Hammer Curl) | 268 | 10-12 | 4 | No Rest |
| Triceps—Fixed Bar Bodyweight Triceps Extension (alternate with Lying E-Z Bar Extension) | 258 | 10-12 | 4 | 60 seconds |
| **SUPERSET # 3** | | | | |
| Biceps—Reverse Curl (alternate with Preacher Curl) | 276 | 10-12 | 3 | No Rest |
| Triceps—Bench Dip (alternate with Close-Grip Dumbbell Press) | 248 | 10-12 | 3 | 60 seconds |
| **SUPERSET # 4** | | | | |
| Shoulders—Dumbbell Upright Row (alternate with Bent-Over Lateral Raise on Incline Bench) | 226 | 10-12 | 3 | 60 seconds |
| Shoulders—Rotator Cuff (alternate with Military Press) | 236 | 10-12 | 3 | No Rest |

# Advanced 14-Day Body Sculpting Workout #2
## Weeks 3 & 4

| DAY 3 | | | | WEDNESDAY/SATURDAY |
|---|---|---|---|---|
| **EXERCISE** | **PAGE NO.** | **REPS** | **SETS** | **REST** |
| **SUPERSET # 1** | | | | |
| Thighs—Barbell Squat (alternate with Ballet Squat) | 120 | 10-12 | 4 | No Rest |
| Hamstrings—Lying Leg Curl (alternate with Hamstring Leg Press) | 138 | 10-12 | 4 | 60 seconds |
| **SUPERSET # 2** | | | | |
| Thighs—Hack Squat (alternate with Leg Extension) | 128 | 10-12 | 4 | No Rest |
| Hamstrings—Stiff-Legged Deadlift (alternate with Seated Leg Curl) | 144 | 10-12 | 4 | 60 seconds |
| **SUPERSET # 3** | | | | |
| Thighs—Leg Press (alternate with Sissy Squat) | 134 | 10-12 | 3 | No Rest |
| Hamstrings—Standing Leg Curl (alternate with Lying Leg Curl) | 142 | 10-12 | 3 | 60 seconds |
| **SUPERSET # 4** | | | | |
| Calves—Calf Press (alternate with Standing Calf Raises (Two-Legged Barbell) | 158 | 15-25 | 3 | No Rest |
| Calves—Standing Calf Raise (one-leg) (alternate with Standing Calf Raise, two legs) | 152 | 15-25 | 3 | 60 seconds |

# Cardio and Abs Advanced Workout #2
## Weeks 3 & 4

To be performed from Monday through Saturday first thing in the morning on an empty stomach or right after the workout.

### SPECIAL INSTRUCTIONS FOR WEEKS 3 & 4

Use supersets. Perform supersets by pairing exercises with no rest period in between. Only rest after the two exercises have been performed consecutively. Repeat for the prescribed number of sets and then move on to the next pair of exercises.

## WEEKS 3 & 4

| EXERCISE | PAGE NO. | REPS | SETS | REST |
|---|---|---|---|---|
| **SUPERSET # 1** | | | | |
| Lower Abs—V-Up | 292 | 15-25 | 4 | No Rest |
| Upper Abs—Crunch | 284 | 15-25 | 4 | 60 seconds |
| **SUPERSET # 2** | | | | |
| Lower Abs—Reverse Crunch with the Ball | 298 | 15-25 | 3 | No Rest |
| Upper Abs—Bicycle Crunch | 286 | 15-25 | 3 | 60 seconds |

### AEROBIC ACTIVITY

30 minutes of fast walking, stationary bike, or any other type of aerobic activity that you like at the target heart rate.

Please refer to www.BodySculptingBible.com for updated workouts and additional cardio routines.

# Advanced 14-Day Body Sculpting Workout #2
## Weeks 5 & 6

---

### SPECIAL INSTRUCTIONS FOR WEEKS 5 & 6

Use giant sets. Perform giant sets by performing four exercises with no rest period in between. Only rest after the four exercises have been performed consecutively. Repeat for the prescribed number of sets and then move on to the second group of exercises. You will repeat Day 1 on Monday and Thursday, Day 2 on Tuesday and Friday, and Day 3 on Wednesday and Saturday.

---

| DAY 1 | | | | MONDAY/THURSDAY |
|---|---|---|---|---|
| **EXERCISE** | **PAGE NO.** | **REPS** | **SETS** | **REST** |
| **GIANT SET # 1** | | | | |
| Back—Wide-Grip Pull-Up to Front (alternate with Close-Grip Pull-Up on the next workout) | 174 | 8-10 | 4 | No Rest |
| Chest—Incline Barbell Press (alternate with Incline Dumbbell Press) | 196 | 8-10 | 4 | No Rest |
| Back—Dumbbell One-Arm Row (alternate with Bent-Over Barbell Row) | 170 | 8-10 | 4 | No Rest |
| Chest—Flat Dumbbell Press (alternate with Chest Dip) | 198 | 8-10 | 4 | 60 seconds |
| **GIANT SET # 2** | | | | |
| Back—Wide-Grip Pull-Up to Front (alternate with Bent-Knee Deadlift) | 174 | 8-10 | 4 | No Rest |
| Chest—Incline Cable Crossover (alternate with Standing Cable Crossover) | 206 | 8-10 | 4 | No Rest |
| Rear Delts—Seated Rear Delt Row (alternate with Seated Rear-Delt Machine) | 234 | 8-10 | 4 | No Rest |
| Calves—Calf Press (alternate with Tibia Raise) | 158 | 15-25 | 4 | 60 seconds |

# Advanced 14-Day Body Sculpting Workout #2
## Weeks 5 & 6

| DAY 2 | | | | TUESDAY/FRIDAY |
|---|---|---|---|---|
| **EXERCISE** | **PAGE NO.** | **REPS** | **SETS** | **REST** |
| **GIANT SET # 1** | | | | |
| Biceps—E-Z Preacher Curl (alternate with Neutral-Grip Chin-Up) | 268 | 8-10 | 4 | No Rest |
| Triceps—Triceps Dip (alternate with E-Z Curl Bar Close-Grip Press) | 246 | 8-10 | 4 | No Rest |
| Biceps—Close-Grip Chin-Up (alternate with Incline Curl) | 176 | 8-10 | 4 | No Rest |
| Triceps—Close-Grip Dumbbell Press (alternate with Overhead Dumbbell Extension) | 252 | 8-10 | 4 | 60 seconds |
| **GIANT SET # 2** | | | | |
| Biceps—Reverse Curl (alternate with Incline Hammer Curl) | 276 | 8-10 | 4 | No Rest |
| Triceps—Triceps Pushdown (with rope) (alternate with Triceps Pushdown) | 254 | 8-10 | 4 | No Rest |
| Shoulders—Dumbbell Lateral Raise (alternate with Dumbbell Upright Row) | 218 | 8-10 | 4 | No Rest |
| Shoulders—Dumbbell Shoulder Press (alternate with Military Press) | 216 | 8-10 | 4 | 60 seconds |

# Advanced 14-Day Body Sculpting Workout #2
# Weeks 5 & 6

| DAY 3 | | | | WEDNESDAY/SATURDAY |
|---|---|---|---|---|
| **EXERCISE** | **PAGE NO.** | **REPS** | **SETS** | **REST** |
| **GIANT SET # 1** | | | | |
| Thighs—Barbell Squat (alternate with Ballet Squat) | 120 | 8-10 | 4 | No Rest |
| Hamstrings—Lying Leg Curl (alternate with Dumbbell Lunge pressing with heels) | 138 | 8-10 | 4 | No Rest |
| Thighs—Leg Press (alternate with Leg Extension) | 134 | 8-10 | 4 | No Rest |
| Hamstrings—Standing Leg Curl (alternate with Glute-Ham Raise) | 142 | 8-10 | 4 | 60 seconds |
| **GIANT SET # 2** | | | | |
| Thighs—Front Squat (alternate with Hack Squat) | 130 | 8-10 | 4 | No Rest |
| Hamstrings—Stiff-Legged Deadlift (alternate with Seated Leg Curl) | 144 | 8-10 | 4 | No Rest |
| Calves—Calf Press (alternate with Standing Calf Raise (Two-Legged Barbell)) | 158 | 15-25 | 4 | No Rest |
| Calves—Standing Calf Raise (One-Legged Dumbbell) (alternate with Standing Calf Raise, two legs) | 152 | 15-25 | 4 | 60 seconds |

# Cardio and Abs Advanced Workout #2
# Weeks 5 & 6

To be performed from Monday through Saturday first thing in the morning on an empty stomach or right after the workout.

### SPECIAL INSTRUCTIONS FOR WEEKS 5 & 6

Use giant sets. Perform giant sets by performing four exercises with no rest period in between. Only rest after the four exercises have been performed consecutively. Repeat for the prescribed number of sets and then move on to the second group of exercises.

## WEEKS 5 & 6

| EXERCISE | PAGE NO. | REPS | SETS | REST |
|---|---|---|---|---|
| **GIANT SET # 1** | | | | |
| Lower Abs—Hanging Leg Raise | 296 | 15-25 | 4 | No Rest |
| Upper Abs—Crunch on the Ball | 284 | 15-25 | 4 | No Rest |
| Lower Abs—Crunch/Pelvic Lift Combination | 298 | 15-25 | 4 | No Rest |
| Upper Abs—Ab-Bench Crunch | 302 | 15-25 | 4 | 60 seconds |

### AEROBIC ACTIVITY

40 minutes of fast walking, stationary bike, or any other type of aerobic activity that you like at your target heart rate.

Please refer to www.BodySculptingBible.com for updated workouts and additional cardio routines.

## WHAT TO DO AFTER WEEK 6
## OF THE ADVANCED WORKOUT

After week six, you can start over at week one but exchange the recommended exercises with similar ones. Don't be afraid to experiment! Also, if you want to gain additional muscle mass, then feel free to reduce the amount of repetitions in the following manner:

Weeks 1-2: 10-12 reps
Weeks 3-4: 8-10 reps
Weeks 5-6: 6-8 reps

Also, reduce the cardiovascular/abs component of the workout to three days a week instead of six. All other aspects of the program remain the same.

# 14-Day Body Sculpting Mass Workout

---

**SPECIAL INSTRUCTIONS FOR WEEKS 1 & 2**

Use modified compound supersets. Perform these sets by completing the first set of the first exercise, resting for the prescribed rest period, performing the first set of the second exercise, resting the prescribed rest period, and then doing the second set of the first exercise. Continue in this manner until you have completed all of the prescribed number of sets for each exercise. Then move on to the next modified compound superset.

---

| DAY 1 | | | | MONDAY/THURSDAY |
|---|---|---|---|---|
| **EXERCISE** | **PAGE NO.** | **REPS** | **SETS** | **REST** |
| **MODIFIED COMPOUND SUPERSET # 1** | | | | |
| Back—Dumbbell One-Arm Row | 170 | 10-12 | 3 | 90 seconds |
| Chest—Incline Dumbbell Press | 196 | 10-12 | 3 | 90 seconds |
| **MODIFIED COMPOUND SUPERSET # 2** | | | | |
| Back—Wide-Grip Pull-Up to Front | 174 | 10-12 | 2 | 90 seconds |
| Chest—Chest Dip | 204 | 10-12 | 2 | 90 seconds |
| **MODIFIED COMPOUND SUPERSET # 3** | | | | |
| Biceps—Standing E-Z Bar Curl | 272 | 10-12 | 3 | 90 seconds |
| Triceps—Lying E-Z Bar Extension | 244 | 10-12 | 3 | 90 seconds |
| **MODIFIED COMPOUND SUPERSET # 4** | | | | |
| Biceps—Hammer Curl | 274 | 10-12 | 2 | 90 seconds |
| Triceps—Overhead Dumbbell Extension | 240 | 10-12 | 2 | 90 seconds |

# Weeks 1 & 2

| DAY 2 | | | | TUESDAY/FRIDAY |
|---|---|---|---|---|
| **EXERCISE** | **PAGE NO.** | **REPS** | **SETS** | **REST** |
| **MODIFIED COMPOUND SUPERSET # 1** | | | | |
| Thighs—Leg Press | 134 | 10-12 | 3 | 90 seconds |
| Hamstrings—Seated Leg Curl | 140 | 10-12 | 3 | 90 seconds |
| **MODIFIED COMPOUND SUPERSET # 2** | | | | |
| Thighs—Dumbbell Lunge | 132 | 10-12 | 2 | 90 seconds |
| Hamstrings—Stiff-Legged Deadlift | 144 | 10-12 | 2 | 90 seconds |
| **MODIFIED COMPOUND SUPERSET # 3** | | | | |
| Calves—Standing Calf Raise (one leg) | 152 | 12-15 | 3 | 90 seconds |
| Shoulders—Dumbbell Shoulder Press | 216 | 10-12 | 3 | 90 seconds |
| **MODIFIED COMPOUND SUPERSET # 4** | | | | |
| Calves—Standing Calf Raise (two legs) | 152 | 12-15 | 2 | 90 seconds |
| Shoulders—Bent-Over Lateral Raise | 220 | 10-12 | 2 | 90 seconds |

| DAY 3 | | | | WEDNESDAY/SATURDAY |
|---|---|---|---|---|
| **EXERCISE** | **PAGE NO.** | **REPS** | **SETS** | **REST** |
| **MODIFIED COMPOUND SUPERSET # 1** | | | | |
| Lower Abs—Lying Leg Raise | 296 | 10-12 | 3 | 90 seconds |
| Upper Abs—Crunch | 284 | 10-12 | 2 | 90 seconds |

| AEROBIC ACTIVITY |
|---|
| 20 minutes of fast walking, stationary bike, or any other type of aerobic activity that you prefer at the target heart rate. |

Please refer to www.BodySculptingBible.com for updated workouts and additional cardio routines.

# 14-Day Body Sculpting Mass Workout

### SPECIAL INSTRUCTIONS FOR WEEKS 3 & 4

Use supersets. Perform these sets by pairing exercises with no rest period in between. Rest only after the two exercises have been performed consecutively. Repeat this routine for the prescribed number of sets before moving on to the next pair of exercises. You will repeat Day 1 on Monday and Thursday, Day 2 on Tuesday and Friday, and Day 3 on Wednesday and Saturday.

| DAY 1 | | | | MONDAY/THURSDAY |
|---|---|---|---|---|
| **EXERCISE** | **PAGE NO.** | **REPS** | **SETS** | **REST** |
| **SUPERSET # 1** | | | | |
| Back—Close-Grip Pull-Up | 176 | 8-10 | 4 | No Rest |
| Chest—Flat Dumbbell Press | 198 | 8-10 | 4 | 60 seconds |
| **SUPERSET # 2** | | | | |
| Back—Bent-Over Barbell Row | 166 | 8-10 | 3 | No Rest |
| Chest—Flat Dumbbell Fly | 200 | 8-10 | 3 | 60 seconds |
| **SUPERSET # 3** | | | | |
| Biceps—Incline Dumbbell Curl | 264 | 8-10 | 4 | No Rest |
| Triceps—Close-Grip Dumbbell Press | 252 | 8-10 | 4 | 60 seconds |
| **SUPERSET # 4** | | | | |
| Biceps—Reverse Curl | 276 | 8-10 | 3 | No Rest |
| Triceps—Triceps Pushdown | 254 | 8-10 | 3 | 60 seconds |

# Weeks 3 & 4

| DAY 2 | | | | TUESDAY/FRIDAY |
|---|---|---|---|---|
| **EXERCISE** | **PAGE NO.** | **REPS** | **SETS** | **REST** |
| **SUPERSET # 1** | | | | |
| Thighs—Close Stance Barbell Squat | 120 | 8-10 | 4 | No Rest |
| Hamstrings—Lying Leg Curl | 138 | 8-10 | 4 | 60 seconds |
| **SUPERSET # 2** | | | | |
| Thighs—Leg Extension | 136 | 8-10 | 3 | No Rest |
| Hamstrings—Leg Press | 134 | 8-10 | 3 | 60 seconds |
| **SUPERSET # 3** | | | | |
| Calves—Standing Calf Raise | 152 | 12-15 | 4 | No Rest |
| Shoulders—Dumbbell Upright Row | 226 | 8-10 | 4 | 60 seconds |
| **SUPERSET # 4** | | | | |
| Calves—Seated Machine Calf Raise | 154 | 12-15 | 3 | No Rest |
| Shoulders—Bent-Over Lateral Raise | 220 | 8-10 | 3 | 60 seconds |

| DAY 3 | | | | WEDNESDAY/SATURDAY |
|---|---|---|---|---|
| **EXERCISE** | **PAGE NO.** | **REPS** | **SETS** | **REST** |
| **SUPERSET # 1** | | | | |
| Lower Abs—Leg Raise | 296 | 10-12 | 4 | No Rest |
| Upper Abs—Crunch | 284 | 10-12 | 3 | 60 seconds |

**AEROBIC ACTIVITY**

25 minutes of fast walking, stationary bike, or any other type of aerobic activity that you prefer at your target heart rate.

Please refer to www.BodySculptingBible.com for updated workouts and additional cardio routines.

# 14-Day Body Sculpting Mass Workout

**SPECIAL INSTRUCTIONS FOR WEEKS 5 & 6**

Use giant sets. Perform these sets by doing four exercises with no rest periods in between. Rest only after the four exercises have been performed consecutively. Repeat for the prescribed number of sets before moving on to the next group of exercises. You will repeat Day 1 on Monday and Thursday, Day 2 on Tuesday and Friday, and Day 3 on Wednesday and Saturday.

| DAY 1 | | | | MONDAY/THURSDAY |
|---|---|---|---|---|
| EXERCISE | PAGE NO. | REPS | SETS | REST |
| **GIANT SET # 1** | | | | |
| Back—Close-Grip Pull-Down | 182 | 6-8 | 4 | No Rest |
| Chest—Incline Dumbbell Press | 196 | 6-8 | 4 | No Rest |
| Back—Dumbbell One-Arm Row | 170 | 6-8 | 4 | No Rest |
| Chest—Flat Dumbbell Press | 198 | 6-8 | 4 | 60 seconds |
| **GIANT SET # 2** | | | | |
| Biceps—One-Arm Preacher Curl | 266 | 8-10 | 4 | No Rest |
| Triceps—Triceps Dip | 246 | 8-10 | 4 | No Rest |
| Biceps—Reverse Curl | 276 | 8-10 | 4 | No Rest |
| Triceps—E-Z Curl Bar Close-Grip Press | 250 | 8-10 | 4 | 60 seconds |

| DAY 2 | | | | TUESDAY/FRIDAY |
|---|---|---|---|---|
| **EXERCISE** | **PAGE NO.** | **REPS** | **SETS** | **REST** |
| **GIANT SET # 1** | | | | |
| Thighs—Barbell Squat | 120 | 6-8 | 4 | No Rest |
| Hamstrings—Barbell Lunge | 132 | 6-8 | 4 | No Rest |
| Thighs—Ballet Squat | 124 | 6-8 | 4 | No Rest |
| Hamstrings—Barbell Stiff-Legged Deadlift | 144 | 6-8 | 4 | 60 seconds |
| **GIANT SET # 2** | | | | |
| Calves—Calf Press | 158 | 6-8 | 4 | No Rest |
| Shoulders—Military Press | 222 | 6-8 | 4 | No Rest |
| Calves—Donkey Calf Raise | 156 | 6-8 | 4 | No Rest |
| Shoulders—Seated Rear Delt Machine | 234 | 6-8 | 4 | 60 seconds |

| DAY 3 | | | | WEDNESDAY/SATURDAY |
|---|---|---|---|---|
| **EXERCISE** | **PAGE NO.** | **REPS** | **SETS** | **REST** |
| **GIANT SET # 1** | | | | |
| Lower Abs—Lying Leg Raise | 296 | 10-12 | 4 | No Rest |
| Upper Abs—Crunch | 284 | 10-12 | 4 | No Rest |

**Note:** Continue until you complete all four sets of each exercise. Don't worry if the first few times that you perform this abdominal workout you are not able to perform all of the recommended reps. As you get used to this rigorous workout, your body will adapt and become stronger.

**AEROBIC ACTIVITY**

30 minutes of fast walking, stationary bike, or any other type of aerobic activity that you prefer at your target heart rate.

Please refer to www.BodySculptingBible.com for updated workouts and additional cardio routines.

# 14-Day Bodyweight Body Sculpting Workout

---

**SPECIAL INSTRUCTIONS FOR WEEKS 1 & 2**

Use modified compound supersets. Perform modified compound supersets by performing the first exercise, resting for the prescribed rest period, performing the second exercise, resting the prescribed rest period, and going back to the first exercise. Continue in this manner until you have performed all of the prescribed number of sets. Then continue with the next modified compound superset. You will repeat Day 1 on Monday and Thursday, Day 2 on Tuesday and Friday, and Day 3 on Wednesday and Saturday.

---

## DAY 1 — MONDAY/THURSDAY

| EXERCISE | PAGE NO. | REPS | SETS | REST |
|---|---|---|---|---|
| **MODIFIED COMPOUND SUPERSET # 1** | | | | |
| Back—Wide-Grip Pull-Up to Front | 174 | As many as possible | 2 | 60 seconds |
| Chest—Push-Up (feet on raised surface) | 210 | As many as possible | 2 | 60 seconds |
| | | | | |
| **MODIFIED COMPOUND SUPERSET # 2** | | | | |
| Back—Close-Grip Pull-Up | 176 | As many as possible | 2 | 60 seconds |
| Chest—Push-Up (feet on floor) | 210 | As many as possible | 2 | 60 seconds |
| | | | | |
| **MODIFIED COMPOUND SUPERSET # 3** | | | | |
| Biceps—Close-Grip Pull-Up (emphasize biceps) | 176 | As many as possible | 2 | 60 seconds |
| Triceps—Bench Dip | 248 | As many as possible | 2 | 60 seconds |
| | | | | |
| **MODIFIED COMPOUND SUPERSET # 4** | | | | |
| Biceps—Neutral Grip Chin-Up (emphasize biceps) | 278 | As many as possible | 2 | 60 seconds |
| Chest— Push-Up (narrow hand-width) | 210 | As many as possible | 2 | 60 seconds |

# Weeks 1 & 2

## DAY 2 | TUESDAY/FRIDAY

| EXERCISE | PAGE NO. | REPS | SETS | REST |
|---|---|---|---|---|
| **MODIFIED COMPOUND SUPERSET # 1** | | | | |
| Thighs—Dumbbell Lunge (bodyweight only; one leg at a time; press with toes) | 132 | As many as possible | 2 | 60 seconds |
| Hamstrings— Dumbbell Lunge (bodyweight only; press with heels; alternate with legs in a walking motion) | 132 | As many as possible | 2 | 60 seconds |
| **MODIFIED COMPOUND SUPERSET # 2** | | | | |
| Thighs—Sissy Squat | 126 | As many as possible | 2 | 60 seconds |
| Hamstrings— Dumbbell Lunge (bodyweight only; press with heels; alternate with legs in a walking motion) | 132 | As many as possible | 2 | 60 seconds |
| **MODIFIED COMPOUND SUPERSET # 3** | | | | |
| Calves—Standing Calf Raise (one leg) | 152 | As many as possible | 2 | 60 seconds |
| Calves—Standing Calf Raise (two legs) | 152 | As many as possible | 2 | 60 seconds |
| **MODIFIED COMPOUND SUPERSET # 4** | | | | |
| Abs—Lying Leg Raise | 296 | As many as possible | 2 | 60 seconds |
| Abs—Crunch | 284 | As many as possible | 2 | 60 seconds |

## DAY 3 | WEDNESDAY/SATURDAY

**AEROBIC ACTIVITY**

20 minutes of fast walking, stationary bike, or any other type of aerobic activity that you like at the target heart rate.

Please refer to www.BodySculptingBible.com for updated workouts and additional cardio routines.

# 14-Day Bodyweight Body Sculpting Workout

<table>
<tr><td>SPECIAL INSTRUCTIONS FOR WEEKS 3 & 4<br>Use supersets. Perform supersets by pairing exercises with no rest in between. Only rest after the two exercises have been performed consecutively. Repeat for the prescribed number of sets and then move on to the next pair of exercises. You will repeat Day 1 on Monday and Thursday, Day 2 on Tuesday and Friday, and Day 3 on Wednesday and Saturday.</td></tr>
</table>

| DAY 1 | | | | MONDAY/THURSDAY |
|---|---|---|---|---|
| **EXERCISE** | **PAGE NO.** | **REPS** | **SETS** | **REST** |
| **SUPERSET #1** | | | | |
| Back—Wide-Grip Pull-Up to Front | 174 | As many as possible | 3 | No Rest |
| Chest—Push-Up (feet on raised surface) | 210 | As many as possible | 3 | 60 seconds |
| **SUPERSET #2** | | | | |
| Back—Close-Grip Pull-Up | 176 | As many as possible | 3 | No Rest |
| Chest—Push-Up (feet on floor) | 210 | As many as possible | 3 | 60 seconds |
| **SUPERSET #3** | | | | |
| Biceps—Close-Grip Pull-Up (emphasize biceps) | 176 | As many as possible | 3 | No Rest |
| Triceps—Bench Dip | 248 | As many as possible | 3 | 60 seconds |
| **SUPERSET #4** | | | | |
| Biceps—Neutral Grip Chin-Up (emphasize biceps) | 278 | As many as possible | 3 | No Rest |
| Chest— Push-Up (narrow hand-width) | 210 | As many as possible | 3 | 60 seconds |

# Weeks 3 & 4

| DAY 2 | | | | TUESDAY/FRIDAY |
|---|---|---|---|---|
| **EXERCISE** | **PAGE NO.** | **REPS** | **SETS** | **REST** |
| **SUPERSET # 1** | | | | |
| Thighs—Dumbbell Lunge (bodyweight only; one leg at a time; press with toes) | 132 | As many as possible | 3 | No Rest |
| Hamstrings— Dumbbell Lunge (bodyweight only; press with heels; alternate with legs in a walking motion) | 132 | As many as possible | 3 | 60 seconds |
| **SUPERSET # 2** | | | | |
| Thighs—Sissy Squat | 126 | As many as possible | 3 | No Rest |
| Hamstrings— Dumbbell Lunge (bodyweight only; press with heels; alternate with legs in a walking motion) | 132 | As many as possible | 3 | 60 seconds |
| **SUPERSET # 3** | | | | |
| Calves—Standing Calf Raise (one leg) | 152 | As many as possible | 3 | No Rest |
| Calves—Standing Calf Raise (two legs) | 152 | As many as possible | 3 | 60 seconds |
| **SUPERSET # 4** | | | | |
| Abs—Lying Leg Raise | 296 | As many as possible | 3 | No Rest |
| Abs—Crunch | 284 | As many as possible | 3 | 60 seconds |

| DAY 3 | WEDNESDAY/SATURDAY |
|---|---|
| **AEROBIC ACTIVITY** | |
| 30 minutes of fast walking, stationary bike, or any other type of aerobic activity that you like at the target heart rate. | |

Please refer to www.BodySculptingBible.com for updated workouts and additional cardio routines.

# 14-Day Bodyweight Body Sculpting Workout

| SPECIAL INSTRUCTIONS FOR WEEKS 5 & 6 |
|---|
| Use giant sets. Perform giant sets by performing four exercises with no rest in between. Only rest after the four exercises have been performed consecutively. Repeat for the prescribed number of sets and then move on to the second group of exercises. You will repeat Day 1 on Monday and Thursday, Day 2 on Tuesday and Friday, and Day 3 on Wednesday and Saturday. |

| DAY 1 | | | | MONDAY/THURSDAY |
|---|---|---|---|---|
| **EXERCISE** | **PAGE NO.** | **REPS** | **SETS** | **REST** |
| **GIANT SET #1** | | | | |
| Back—Wide-Grip Pull-Up to Front | 174 | As many as possible | 4 | No Rest |
| Chest—Push-Up (feet on raised surface) | 210 | As many as possible | 4 | No Rest |
| Back—Close-Grip Pull-Up | 176 | As many as possible | 4 | No Rest |
| Chest—Push-Up (feet on floor) | 210 | As many as possible | 4 | 60 seconds |
| | | | | |
| **GIANT SET # 2** | | | | |
| Biceps—Close-Grip Pull-Up (emphasize biceps) | 176 | As many as possible | 4 | No Rest |
| Triceps—Bench Dip | 248 | As many as possible | 4 | No Rest |
| Biceps—Neutral Grip Chin-Up (emphasize biceps) | 278 | As many as possible | 4 | No Rest |
| Chest—Push-Up (narrow hand-width) | 210 | As many as possible | 4 | 60 seconds |

| DAY 2 | | | | TUESDAY/FRIDAY |
|---|---|---|---|---|
| **EXERCISE** | **PAGE NO.** | **REPS** | **SETS** | **REST** |
| **GIANT SET # 1** | | | | |
| Thighs—Dumbbell Lunge<br>(bodyweight only; one leg at a time; press with toes) | 132 | As many as possible | 4 | No Rest |
| Hamstrings— Dumbbell Lunge<br>(bodyweight only; press with heels;<br>alternate with legs in a walking motion) | 132 | As many as possible | 4 | No Rest |
| Thighs—Sissy Squat | 126 | As many as possible | 4 | No Rest |
| Hamstrings— Dumbbell Lunge (bodyweight only;<br>press with heels; alternate with legs in<br>a walking motion) | 132 | As many as possible | 4 | 60 seconds |
| **GIANT SET # 2** | | | | |
| Calves—Standing Calf Raise (one leg) | 152 | As many as possible | 4 | No Rest |
| Calves—Standing Calf Raise (two legs) | 152 | As many as possible | 4 | No Rest |
| Abs—Lying Leg Raise | 296 | As many as possible | 4 | No Rest |
| Abs—Crunch | 284 | As many as possible | 4 | 60 seconds |

| DAY 3 | WEDNESDAY/SATURDAY |
|---|---|
| **AEROBIC ACTIVITY** | |
| 40 minutes of fast walking, stationary bike, or any other type of aerobic activity that you like at the target heart rate. | |

Please refer to www.BodySculptingBible.com for updated workouts and additional cardio routines.

# Appendix A
## Glossary

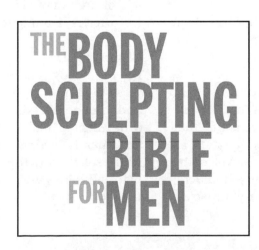

**Aerobic Exercise:** Constant moderate intensity work that uses oxygen at a rate in which the cardio respiratory system can replenish oxygen in the working muscles. Examples of such activity are stationary bike riding or walking. It is a good activity for fat loss when done in the right amounts but highly catabolic if done in excess.

**Anaerobic Exercise:** Exercise in which oxygen is used more quickly than the body is able to replenish it inside the working muscle. Weight training is an example of such an activity. It is highly anabolic in nature but also highly catabolic if done in excess.

**Anabolic State:** Favorable state in the body created by a combination of good training, nutrition, and rest that leads to favorable changes in body composition.

**Anabolic Steroids:** Synthetic (man-made) hormones that simulate the effects of the male hormone testosterone.

**Anti-catabolic Properties:** Properties provided by certain nutrients that protect the muscle mass in the body from being broken down.

**Anti-lypolitic Properties:** Properties provided by certain nutrients that prevent the body from turning calories into fat.

**Antioxidant Properties:** Properties provided by certain nutrients that protect the body from disease.

**Basic Exercises:** Exercise movement that involves a large number of muscles in the body. They are generally multi-joint movements that target the larger muscles of the body (such as chest, back, and thighs) but also involve the smaller muscles as well (such as shoulders, arms, calves, and abs) as auxiliary muscles.

Examples of such movements are chin-ups, pull-ups, dips, bench presses, squats, and lunges.

**Bulk Minerals:** Minerals which the body needs in great quantities (in the order of grams) such as calcium, magnesium, potassium, sodium, and phosphorus.

**Carbohydrates:** Macronutrient used by the body as its main source of energy. Carbohydrates are divided into complex carbs and simple carbs. The complex carbs give you sustained energy ("timed release") while the simple carbs give you immediate energy. This macronutrient can be found in rice (complex, starchy), pasta (complex, starchy), breads (complex, starchy), fruits (simple), sugars (simple), fruit juices (simple), dairy products (simple), and vegetables (complex, fibrous).

**Catabolic State:** Unfavorable state in the body created by a combination of too much training, lack of good nutrition and lack of rest that leads to muscle loss and fat accumulation.

**Cortisol:** Catabolic hormone secreted by the adrenal glands in situations of stress (both physical and mental), lack of calories/nutrients and lack of sleep. This hormone is associated with loss of muscle mass, loss of strength, and fat accumulation. An excess of it over long periods of time may also contribute to hardening of the arteries, leading to heart disease.

**Diuretics:** Drugs used to remove excess water from the body. There are two versions: the drug version (can only be prescribed by a physician), and the herbal version. Excessive use of the drug version has as side effects muscle cramps and harsh arrhythmia. The herbal version, while safer than the drug version, can lead to potassium loss and excessive use puts stress on the kidneys.

**Dumbbell:** A short-handled barbell 10-12 inches long that can be carried in one hand. Dumbbells allow flexibility in the execution of a movement and full range of motion.

**Endorphins:** Hormones that make us feel good and happy. The production of these hormones is stimulated by exercise.

**Essential Fatty Acids (EFAs):** Fats that have anti-catabolic, anti-lypolitic, and antioxidant properties. These fats affect good cholesterol in a positive way. In addition, these fats aid in the muscle-building, fat-loss process. The Omega 3 Fatty Acids found in fats such as fish oils and flaxseed oil are a good source of EFAs.

**Estrogen:** Female hormone that regulates and sustains female sexual development and reproductive function. An excess of this hormone appears to be related to heart disease and cancer. In addition, when this hormone is in excess, it causes fat gain and water retention. Estrogen deficits, on the other hand, cause memory problems, trouble finding words, inability to pay attention, mood swings, and irritability. Exercise reduces the risk of these diseases and conditions by helping to balance the levels of this hormone.

**Exercise Volume:** The amount of work performed in an exercise session defined by the product resulting from the amount of weight lifted, multiplied by the number of sets and multiplied by the number of repetitions. For example, if you had a workout that consisted of 10 sets of dumbbell curls, and for each set you used 30 pounds and performed 10 repetitions, then your biceps routine volume equals 10 x 10 x 30=3000 pounds. Too much volume leads to overtraining.

**Fats:** Macronutrient needed by the body in order to manufacture hormones and sustain cell metabolism. All the cells in the body have some fat in them. Hormones are manufactured from fats. Also, fats lubricate your joints. If you eliminate the fat from your diet, your hormonal production will go down and a whole array of chemical reactions will be interrupted. There are three types of fats: saturated, polyunsaturated, and monounsaturated.

**Fat-Soluble Vitamins:** Vitamins stored in fat that if taken in excessive amounts will become toxic. They include vitamins A, D, E, and K.

**Giant Set:** Giant sets are four exercises done one after the other with no rest in between sets. Again, there are two ways to implement this. You can either use four exercises for the same muscle group or perform two pairs of opposing muscle group exercises. For the purposes of this manual, whenever we do giant sets, we will perform two pairs of opposing muscle group exercises with no rest. The exception is when we do abs in which we will alternate between lower abs and upper abs.

**Growth Hormone:** Hormone secreted by the pituitary gland that aids in fat loss and muscle building.

**Hormones:** Fats similar to, and usually synthesized from, cholesterol, starting with Acetyl-CoA, moving through squalene, lanosterol, cholesterol, and, in the gonads and adrenal cortex, a number of steroid hormones. Because they stimulate cell growth, either by changing the internal structure or increasing the rate of proliferation, they are often called anabolic steroids.

**Hypertrophy:** Scientific term for describing an increase in muscle mass and strength caused by the stimulation of the muscles.

**Intensity:** Intensity has two definitions in the weight-training world. (1) Relative term that indicates the level of effort exerted during the performance of an exercise. (2) In strength training circles, intensity refers to the amount of weight used on a specific exercise.

**Insulin:** Hormone secreted by the pancreas responsible for carbohydrate metabolism. This hormone determines if carbohydrates are to be used for energy, storage inside the muscle cells as glycogen, or converting and storing the carbohydrates as fats when they are found in excess in the bloodstream.

**Isolation Exercises:** Exercise movements that are generally single jointed and serve to isolate a single area of the body. Examples of such are dumbbell flys, concentration curls, triceps kickbacks, leg extensions, and leg curls.

**Lactic Acid:** By-product created by a lack of oxygen flow to the working muscles. Lactic acid is created by anaerobic activities such as weight training exercises. It is believed that its presence causes a surge in growth hormone levels.

**Macronutrient:** One of the three major nutrients that the body needs for survival. These nutrients are carbohydrates, proteins, and fats.

**Metabolism:** The rate at which the body utilizes calories and nutrients in order to sustain its daily activities.

**Minerals:** Minerals are inorganic compounds (not produced by animals or vegetables) whose main function is to assure that your brain receives the correct signals from the body, as well as to ensure balance of fluids, make muscular contractions possible and allow energy production, as well as building muscle and bones. There are two types of minerals: bulk and trace minerals.

**Modified Compound Superset:** In a modified compound set, you pair exercises for opposing muscle groups or for opposing muscle movements (e.g. Push vs. Pull). First you perform one exercise, rest the recommended amount of seconds and then perform the second exercise (for instance, first do biceps, rest, then do triceps). You then rest the prescribed amount of time again and go back to the first exercise. Using this technique of pairing exercises in a modified superset fashion not only saves time and keeps the body warm, but allows for faster recovery of the nervous system between sets. This will allow the person to lift heavier weights than possible if he just stayed idle for 2-3 minutes waiting to recover.

**Monounsaturated Fats:** Fats that have a positive effect on good cholesterol levels. These fats are usually high in essential fatty acids and may have antioxidant properties. Sources of these fats are fish oils, virgin olive oil, canola oil, and flaxseed oil.

**Muscle Failure:** Point during the exercise at which it becomes impossible to perform another repetition in good form. This point is reached due to the lack of oxygen reaching the working muscles and the increased levels of lactic acid.

**Overtraining:** Condition caused by an excess of volume in a training routine that leads to muscle loss, strength loss, and fat accumulation. Symptoms include depression, insomnia, lethargy, and lack of energy.

**Polyunsaturated Fats:** Fats that do not have an affect on cholesterol levels. Most of the fats in vegetable oils, such as corn, cottonseed, safflower, soybean, and sunflower oil are polyunsaturated.

**Protein:** Every tissue in your body is made from protein (i.e. muscle, hair, skin, nails).

Proteins are the building blocks of muscle tissue. This macronutrient can be found in poultry, meats, and dairy products.

**Repetitions:** The amount of times you perform an exercise. For instance, pretend that you are performing a bench press. You pick up the bar, lower it, pause, and lift it up. That action of executing the movement for one time counts for one repetition. If you perform that same movement a second time, then that is your second repetition, and so on.

**Rest Interval:** The amount of time a person rests between sets. For instance, a rest interval of 60 seconds means that after you finish your first set, you will remain idle for 60 seconds before going on to the next set.

**Saturated Fats:** Saturated fats are associated with heart disease and high cholesterol levels. They are found to a large extent in products of animal origin. However, some vegetable fats are altered in a way that increases the amount of saturated fats in them by a chemical process known as hydrogenation. Hydrogenated vegetable oils are generally found in packaged foods. In addition, coconut oil, palm oil, and palm kernel oil, which are also frequently used in packaged foods and non-dairy creamers are also highly saturated.

**Sets:** A set is a collection of repetitions that culminates in the muscle reaching muscular failure.

**Supersets:** A superset is a combination of one exercise performed right after the other with no rest in between. There are two ways to implement a superset. The first way is to do two exercises for the same muscle group at once; for example dumbbell curls immediately followed by concentration curls. The drawback to this technique is that you will not be as strong as you usually are on the second exercise. The second and best way to superset is by pairing exercises of opposing muscle groups or different muscle movements such as back and chest, thighs and hamstrings, biceps and triceps, shoulders and calves, upper abs and lower abs. When pairing antagonistic exercises, there is no drop of strength once your cardiovascular system is well conditioned.

**Trace Minerals:** Minerals which are needed by the body in minute amounts, usually in the order of micrograms, such as chromium, copper, cobalt, silicon, selenium, iron, and zinc.

**Testosterone:** Hormone responsible for increasing muscle size. Even though this hormone is predominantly present in males, it is also present in women to a lesser degree. It is believed that this hormone also aids in fat loss to a lesser degree.

**Vitamins:** Vitamins are organic compounds (produced by both animals and vegetables) whose function is to enhance the actions of proteins that cause chemical reactions such as muscle building, fat burning and energy production. There are two types of vitamins: fat - soluble and water-soluble.

**Water Soluble Vitamins:** Vitamins that are not stored in the body, such as B-Complex vitamins and vitamin C. Therefore, they need to be taken on a frequent basis.

# Table of Food Values

**B**

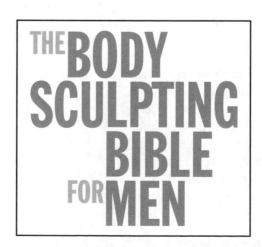

# Nutrition Chart and Glycemic Index

| STARCHY CARBOHYDRATES | | | |
|---|---|---|---|
| Eat with all 5-6 meals throughout the day. Around 50-54 grams of carbohydrates per serving. 1 serving per meal. | | | |
| **FOOD ITEM** | **SERVING SIZE (MEASURE DRY)** | **GLYCEMIC INDEX** | **DESIRABLE** |
| Old Fashioned Oats | 1 cup dry | Low | Highly |
| Cream of Rice | 1/2 cup dry | High | Good After Workout Only |
| Cream of Wheat | 8 tablespoons dry | Medium | Good |
| Baked Potatoes | 8 ounce cooked | Medium | Good |
| Sweet Potatoes | 8 ounce cooked | Medium | Good |
| Rice (Brown Whole Grain) | 1 cup cooked | Medium | Good |
| White Rice | 1 cup cooked | High | Good After Workout Only |
| Spaghetti | 8 oz cooked | Low | Good in GI but too many carbs for a small serving. |
| Whole wheat flour bread | 4 slices | High | Not a great choice but ok in moderation. |
| Corn | 1-1/2 cup | Medium | Good |
| Peas | 2 cups | Medium | Good |
| Low GI=1-55 Medium GI=56-69 High GI=70-100 | | | |

## SIMPLE CARBOHYDRATES

If you must, eat 1 serving with Breakfast and 1 after workout as even though they are low to medium in GI, too many simple sugars from fruits in the diet throughout the day can prevent fat loss. If your post workout meal is breakfast, then just consume 1 serving per day of fruits.

Around 20 grams of carbohydrates per serving. If breakfast is the post workout meal: 1 serving per day with post work-out meal. If post workout meal is not breakfast: 1 serving with breakfast and 1 serving with post workout meal.

| FOOD ITEM | SERVING SIZE | GLYCEMIC INDEX | DESIRABLE |
|---|---|---|---|
| Apples | 1 | Low | Good |
| Oranges | 1 | Low | Good |
| Grapefruit | 1 | Low | Good |
| Cherries | 14 | Low | Good |
| Pears | 2/3 | Low | Good |
| Bananas | 2/3 | Medium | After Workout Only |
| Lemons | 2 | Low | Good |
| Cantaloupe | 1/2 melon | High | After Workout Only |
| Strawberries | 2 cups | 1 cup | Good |
| Apricots | 6 | Medium | After Workout Only |
| Grapes | 1 cup | Low | Good |
| Mango | 2/3 cup | Medium | After Workout Only |
| Papaya | 1 cup | Medium | After Workout Only |

Low GI=1-55 Medium GI=56-69 High GI=70-100Low GI=1-55 Medium GI=56-69 High GI=70-100

## FIBROUS CARBOHYDRATES

Eat at least 1 serving with lunch and 1 serving with dinner though more can be consumed if desired; consider these free foods as they do not get absorbed.

Around 10 grams of carbohydrates per serving. At least 1 serving at lunch and 1 serving at dinner.

| FOOD ITEM | SERVING SIZE (MEASURE COOKED) | GLYCEMIC INDEX | DESIRABLE |
|---|---|---|---|
| Broccoli | 1 cup | Low | Good |
| Green Beans | 1 cup | Low | Good |
| Asparagus | 12 spears or 1 cup | Low | Good |
| Lettuce | 1 head raw | Low | Good |
| Tomatoes | 2 cups chopped | Low | Good |
| Green Peppers (chopped) | 1-1/2 cup raw | Low | Good |
| Onions | 1/2 cup | Low | Good |
| Mushrooms | 1 cup | Low | Good |
| Cucumber sliced | 3 cups | Low | Good |
| Cauliflower | 2 cups | Low | Good |
| Spinach | 4 cups | Low | Good |
| Cabbage | 2 cups | Low | Good |
| Carrots | 1/2 cup sliced | High | After Workout |

Low GI=1-55 Medium GI=56-69 High GI=70-100

## PROTEINS

Eat with all 5-6 meals throughout the day. Around 40-46 grams of protein per serving. 1 serving per meal.

| FOOD ITEM | SERVING SIZE (MEASURE COOKED) | GLYCEMIC INDEX | DESIRABLE |
|---|---|---|---|
| Chicken breast (skinless) | 6 ounces | Low | Good |
| Turkey | 6 ounces | Low | Good |
| Veal | 6 ounces | Low | Good |
| Top Sirloin | 6 ounces | Low | Good |
| Tuna | 6 ounces | Low | Good |
| Wild Alaskan Salmon | 6 ounces | Low | Good |
| Egg Whites (in carton) | 2 cups | Low | Good |
| Whey Protein | 2 scoops | Low | Good |
| Orange Roughy | 6 ounces | Low | Good |

## GOOD FATS

Around 10 grams of fats per serving. 1 serving at lunch, dinner, and any other meal except post workout meal.

| FOOD ITEM | SERVING SIZE | GLYCEMIC INDEX | DESIRABLE |
|---|---|---|---|
| Fish Oils | 2 teaspoons | Low | Good |
| Flax Oils | 2 teaspoons | Low | Good |
| Extra Virgin Olive Oil | 2 teaspoons | Low | Good |
| Natural Peanut Butter | 4 teaspoons | Low | Good |

All fats are low in glycemic index and by combining a carbohydrate with a protein the combined glycemic index of the whole meal goes down. The fats included here were selected due to their high essential fatty acids content and their health properties.

NOTES: Avoid cooking with flax oil as the heat degrades the oil. Bake and broil instead of frying. Also, if eating salmon, eliminate 2 servings of good fats as salmon is high on EFAs.

The complete list of the glycemic index and glycemic load for 750 foods can be found in the article "International tables of glycemic index and glycemic load values: 2002," by Kaye Foster-Powell, Susanna H.A. Holt, and Janette C. Brand-Miller in the July 2002 American Journal of Clinical Nutrition, Vol. 62, pages 5–56. <http://www.ajcn.org/cgi/content/full/76/1/5>

## NOTES:

- While the foods above contain trace amounts of other macronutrients (for example, skinless chicken breasts contain 2.5 to 5 grams of fat), for the purposes of our calculations, we will assume that these food contain only the macronutrient under which they are listed.

- Always try to use natural foods. Avoid using canned or pre-prepared types of foods as they usually contain too much fats, sodium, and carbs.

- Stay within plus or minus 10 grams of the recommended amount of carbs and proteins. For fats, stay within +/- 5 grams.

- Always choose low-fat protein sources. If you eat really low-fat meals, don't worry about incurring into a fat deficiency since the supplements program takes care of the need for essential fatty acids. Besides, there are trace amounts of fats even in the low-fat protein sources that we choose.

- If you choose to include skim milk in your diet, remember that it not only has protein (8 to 9 grams for every 8 ounces of milk) but also simple carbs (12 to 13 grams for every 8 ounces of milk). Therefore, count milk as both. Note that since the carbs in milk are simple carbs, this food item should only be used in the post workout meal. However, if due to schedule you need to include more protein shakes throughout the day, and the carbs that you will rely on are those found in skim milk, ensure that you add a teaspoon of flaxseed oil to it as the oil will slow down the release of the simple carbs into the blood stream. Guys interested in competing should however eliminate any dairy products from the diet as these products tend to make you retain water and the lactose in them make it harder to get to the desired low body fat percentage required for contest condition. In addition, whole-wheat products should also be minimized during this phase as they may contain pytho-estrogens that would make it harder to lose fat.

- Try to include fibrous carbs in at least two meals.

- Post-workout meal should contain high glycemic carbs combined with fast released proteins such as whey protein isolate. Fats and fibers should be eliminated from this meal.

- If you use flaxseed oil as your Essential Fatty Acids supplement, remember to count itas fat grams. Each teaspoon contains approximately 5 grams of good fats.

- If you use fish oil capsules as your Essential Fatty Acids supplement, count each capsule as 1 gram of good fats.

- Remember that carbohydrates have 4 calories per gram. Therefore, a 6-ounce banana has 27 grams of carbs x 4 = 108 calories.

- Remember that protein has 4 calories per gram. Therefore, a 3.5-ounce chicken breast has 35 grams of protein x 4 = 140 calories.

- Remember that fat has 9 calories per gram. Therefore, a teaspoon of flaxseed oil has 5 grams of fat x 9 = 45 calories.

Now that you know your approved list of foods, simply use the following guidelines to create your meal plan.

## WEEKS 1-2: CALORIES: LOW (Approximately 2400 calories)

Around 250 grams of carbohydrates (mostly complex with simple carbs being saved for after the workout)

Around 250 grams of protein

Around 40 grams of fats

### MEAL #1 (7:30 AM) BREAKFAST (POST-WORKOUT)

Choose 1 serving of Proteins
Choose 1 serving of Starchy Carbs
Optionally, you may choose to add 1 serving of Simple Carbs in the form of Fruit, if you can't live without them.

### MEAL #2 (10:30 AM) MORNING BREAK SNACK

Choose 1 serving of Proteins
Choose 1 serving of Starchy Carbs
Choose 1 serving of Good Fats

### MEAL #3 (1:30 PM) LUNCH TIME

Choose 1 serving of Proteins
Choose 1 serving of Starchy Carbs
Choose 1 serving of Fibrous Carbs
Choose 1 serving of Good Fats

### MEAL #4 (3:30 PM) AFTERNOON BREAK SNACK

Choose 1 serving of Proteins
Choose 1 serving of Starchy Carbs

### MEAL #5 (6:30 PM) DINNER

Choose 1-1/2 serving of Proteins
Choose 1/2 serving of Starchy Carbs
Choose 1 serving of Fibrous Carbs
Choose 1 serving of Good Fats

## WEEKS 3-4 CALORIES: HIGH (Approximately 2800 calories)

310 grams of carbohydrates (mostly complex with simple carbs being saved for after the workout)

310 grams of protein

40 grams of fats

### MEAL #1 (7:30 AM) BREAKFAST (POST-WORKOUT)

Choose 1 serving of Proteins
Choose 1 serving of Starchy Carbs
Optionally, you may choose to add 1 serving of Simple Carbs in the form of Fruit, if you can't live without them.

### MEAL #2 (10:30 AM) MORNING BREAK SNACK

Choose 1 serving of Proteins
Choose 1 serving of Starchy Carbs

### MEAL #3 (1:30 PM) LUNCH TIME

Choose 1 serving of Proteins
Choose 1 serving of Starchy Carbs
Choose 1 serving of Fibrous Carbs
Choose 1 serving of Good Fats

### MEAL #4 (3:30 PM) AFTERNOON BREAK SNACK

Choose 1 serving of Proteins
Choose 1 serving of Starchy Carbs

### MEAL #5 (6:30 PM) DINNER

Choose 1-1/2 serving of Proteins
Choose 1 serving of Starchy Carbs
Choose 1 serving of Fibrous Carbs
Choose 1 serving of Good Fats

### MEAL #6 (8:30 PM) LATE SNACK

Choose 1-1/2 serving of Proteins
Choose 1/2 serving of Starchy Carbs
Choose 1 serving of Fibrous Carbs
Choose 1 serving of Good Fats

For sample diets that use these exact measurements, please see Appendix C.

# Appendix C
## Sample Diets

**C**

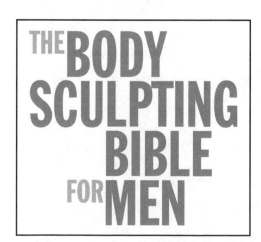

THE **BODY**
**SCULPTING**
**BIBLE**
FOR **MEN**

These diets were created using the Appendix B menu charts. These diets are samples of what you can eat on a daily basis. Remember that you don't have to be stuck to just what is written here. You can vary your daily plan by using the food tables from Appendix B in conjunction with the daily menus. Also remember that these diets are samples of the normal Body Sculpting Bible diet program. For the advanced carb cycling program, follow the recommendations on that section of the Nutrition chapter.

## WEEKS 1-2: CALORIES:LOW (Approximately 2400 calories)

Around 250 grams of carbohydrates (mostly complex with simple carbs being saved for after the workout)

Around 250 grams of protein

Around 40 grams of fats

### MEAL #1 (7:30 AM) BREAKFAST (POST-WORKOUT)

Choose 1 serving of Proteins
Choose 1 serving of Starchy Carbs
Optionally, you may choose to add 1 serving of Simple Carbs in the form of Fruit, if you can't live without them.

### MEAL #2 (10:30 AM) MORNING BREAK SNACK

Choose 1 serving of Proteins
Choose 1 serving of Starchy Carbs
Choose 1 serving of Good Fats

### MEAL #3 (1:30 PM) LUNCH TIME

Choose 1 serving of Proteins
Choose 1 serving of Starchy Carbs
Choose 1 serving of Fibrous Carbs
Choose 1 serving of Good Fats

### MEAL #4 (3:30 PM) AFTERNOON BREAK SNACK

Choose 1 serving of Proteins
Choose 1 serving of Starchy Carbs

### MEAL #5 (6:30 PM) DINNER

Choose 1-1/2 serving of Proteins
Choose 1/2 serving of Starchy Carbs
Choose 1 serving of Fibrous Carbs
Choose 1 serving of Good Fats

## WEEKS 3-4 CALORIES: HIGH (Approximately 2800 calories)

310 grams of carbohydrates (mostly complex with simple carbs being saved for after the workout)

310 grams of protein

40 grams of fats

### MEAL #1 (7:30 AM) BREAKFAST (POST-WORKOUT)

Choose 1 serving of Proteins
Choose 1 serving of Starchy Carbs
Optionally, you may choose to add 1 serving of Simple Carbs in the form of Fruit, if you can't live without them.

### MEAL #2 (10:30 AM) MORNING BREAK SNACK

Choose 1 serving of Proteins
Choose 1 serving of Starchy Carbs

### MEAL #3 (1:30 PM) LUNCH TIME

Choose 1 serving of Proteins
Choose 1 serving of Starchy Carbs
Choose 1 serving of Fibrous Carbs
Choose 1 serving of Good Fats

### MEAL #4 (3:30 PM) AFTERNOON BREAK SNACK

Choose 1 serving of Proteins
Choose 1 serving of Starchy Carbs

### MEAL #5 (6:30 PM) DINNER

Choose 1-1/2 serving of Proteins
Choose 1 serving of Starchy Carbs
Choose 1 serving of Fibrous Carbs
Choose 1 serving of Good Fats

### MEAL #6 (8:30 PM) LATE SNACK

Choose 1-1/2 serving of Proteins
Choose 1/2 serving of Starchy Carbs
Choose 1 serving of Fibrous Carbs
Choose 1 serving of Good Fats

## SAMPLE 14-DAY LOW-CALORIE MILK-FREE DIET
(THIS DIET IS GOOD FOR THOSE WHO WANT TO ELIMINATE MILK PRODUCTS FROM THEIR PROGRAM.)

| MEAL # | FOOD | SERVING SIZE |
|---|---|---|
| MEAL 1<br>BREAKFAST<br>(POST-WORKOUT)<br>7:30 AM | WHEY PROTEIN<br><br>BANANA<br>CREAM OF RICE | 2 SCOOPS<br><br>2/3 BANANA<br>1/2 CUP DRY |
| MEAL 2<br>10:30 AM | WHEY PROTEIN<br>OLD-FASHIONED OATS<br>FLAXSEED OIL | 2 SCOOPS<br>1 CUP (MEASURED DRY)<br>1 TABLESPOON |
| MEAL 3<br>1:30 PM | BROWN RICE<br>GREEN BEANS<br>CHICKEN BREAST<br>EXTRA-VIRGIN OLIVE OIL | 1 CUP COOKED<br>1 CUP<br>6 OUNCES<br>1 TABLESPOON |
| MEAL 4<br>3:30 PM | WHEY PROTEIN<br>OLD-FASHIONED OATS | 2 SCOOPS<br>1 CUP (MEASURED DRY) |
| MEAL 5<br>6:30 PM | WILD ALASKAN SALMON<br>SWEET POTATOES<br>BROCCOLI | 9 OUNCES<br>4 OUNCES COOKED<br>1 CUP |

## SAMPLE 14-DAY HIGH-CALORIE MILK-FREE DIET

(THIS DIET IS GOOD FOR THOSE WHO WANT TO ELIMINATE MILK PRODUCTS FROM THEIR PROGRAM.)

| MEAL # | FOOD | SERVING SIZE |
|---|---|---|
| MEAL 1<br>BREAKFAST<br>(POST-WORKOUT)<br>7:30 AM | WHEY PROTEIN<br><br>BANANA<br>CREAM OF RICE | 2 SCOOPS<br><br>2/3 BANANA<br>1/2 CUP DRY |
| MEAL 2<br>10:30 AM | WHEY PROTEIN<br>OLD-FASHIONED OATS<br>FLAXSEED OIL | 2 SCOOPS<br>1 CUP (MEASURED DRY)<br>1 TABLESPOON |
| MEAL 3<br>1:30 PM | BROWN RICE<br>GREEN BEANS<br>CHICKEN BREAST<br>EXTRA-VIRGIN OLIVE OIL | 1 CUP COOKED<br>1 CUP<br>6 OUNCES<br>1 TABLESPOON |
| MEAL 4<br>3:30 PM | WHEY PROTEIN<br>OLD-FASHIONED OATS | 2 SCOOPS<br>1 CUP (MEASURED DRY) |
| MEAL 5<br>6:30 PM | WILD ALASKAN SALMON<br>SWEET POTATOES<br>BROCCOLI | 9 OUNCES<br>4 OUNCES COOKED<br>1 CUP |
| MEAL 6<br>8:30 PM | ORANGE ROUGHY<br>BAKED POTATOES<br>ASPARAGUS<br>FLAXSEED OIL | 9 OUNCES<br>4 OUNCES COOKED<br>1 CUP<br>1 TABLESPOON |

# SAMPLE 14-DAY LOW-CALORIE DIET WITH MILK PRODUCTS

| MEAL # | FOOD | SERVING SIZE |
|---|---|---|
| MEAL 1<br>BREAKFAST<br>(POST-WORKOUT)<br>7:30 AM | WHEY PROTEIN<br>SKIM MILK<br>CREAM OF RICE | 1 SCOOP<br>16 OUNCES<br>1/2 CUP DRY |
| MEAL 2<br>10:30 AM | WHEY PROTEIN<br>OLD-FASHIONED OATS<br>SKIM MILK<br>FLAXSEED OIL | 1 SCOOP<br>1/2 CUP (MEASURED DRY)<br>16 OUNCES<br>1 TABLESPOON |
| MEAL 3<br>1:30 PM | BROWN RICE<br>GREEN BEANS<br>CHICKEN BREAST<br>EXTRA-VIRGIN OLIVE OIL | 1 CUP COOKED<br>1 CUP<br>6 OUNCES<br>1 TABLESPOON |
| MEAL 4<br>3:30 PM | WHEY PROTEIN<br>OLD-FASHIONED OATS | 2 SCOOPS<br>1 CUP (MEASURED DRY) |
| MEAL 5<br>6:30 PM | WILD ALASKAN SALMON<br>SWEET POTATOES<br>BROCCOLI | 9 OUNCES<br>4 OUNCES COOKED<br>1 CUP |

## SAMPLE 14-DAY HIGH-CALORIE DIET WITH MILK PRODUCTS

| MEAL # | FOOD | SERVING SIZE |
|---|---|---|
| MEAL 1<br>BREAKFAST<br>(POST-WORKOUT)<br>7:30 AM | WHEY PROTEIN<br>SKIM MILK<br>CREAM OF RICE | 1 SCOOP<br>16 OUNCES<br>1/2 CUP DRY |
| MEAL 2<br>10:30 AM | WHEY PROTEIN<br>OLD-FASHIONED OATS<br>SKIM MILK<br>FLAXSEED OIL | 1 SCOOP<br>1/2 CUP (MEASURED DRY)<br>16 OUNCES<br>1 TABLESPOON |
| MEAL 3<br>1:30 PM | BROWN RICE<br>GREEN BEANS<br>CHICKEN BREAST<br>EXTRA-VIRGIN OLIVE OIL | 1 CUP COOKED<br>1 CUP<br>6 OUNCES<br>1 TABLESPOON |
| MEAL 4<br>3:30 PM | WHEY PROTEIN<br>OLD-FASHIONED OATS | 2 SCOOPS<br>1 CUP (MEASURED DRY) |
| MEAL 5<br>6:30 PM | WILD ALASKAN SALMON<br>SWEET POTATOES<br>BROCCOLI | 9 OUNCES<br>4 OUNCES COOKED<br>1 CUP |
| MEAL 6<br>8:30 PM | ORANGE ROUGHY<br>BAKED POTATOES<br>ASPARAGUS<br>FLAXSEED OIL | 9 OUNCES<br>4 OUNCES COOKED<br>1 CUP<br>1 TABLESPOON |

# SAMPLE 14-DAY LOW-CALORIE OVO-LACTO VEGETARIAN DIET

| MEAL # | FOOD | SERVING SIZE |
|---|---|---|
| MEAL 1 BREAKFAST (POST-WORKOUT) 7:30 AM | WHEY PROTEIN SKIM MILK CREAM OF RICE | 1 SCOOP 16 OUNCES 1/2 CUP DRY |
| MEAL 2 10:30 AM | WHEY PROTEIN OLD-FASHIONED OATS SKIM MILK FLAXSEED OIL | 1 SCOOP 1/2 CUP (MEASURED DRY) 16 OUNCES 1 TABLESPOON |
| MEAL 3 1:30 PM | BROWN RICE GREEN BEANS EGG WHITES EXTRA-VIRGIN OLIVE OIL | 1 CUP COOKED 1 CUP 2 CUPS 1 TABLESPOON |
| MEAL 4 3:30 PM | WHEY PROTEIN OLD-FASHIONED OATS | 2 SCOOPS 1 CUP (MEASURED DRY) |
| MEAL 5 6:30 PM | EGG WHITES SWEET POTATOES BROCCOLI | 2 CUPS 4 OUNCES COOKED 1 CUP |

## SAMPLE 14-DAY HIGH-CALORIE OVO-LACTO VEGETARIAN DIET

| MEAL # | FOOD | SERVING SIZE |
|--------|------|--------------|
| MEAL 1<br>BREAKFAST<br>(POST-WORKOUT)<br>7:30 AM | WHEY PROTEIN<br>SKIM MILK<br>CREAM OF RICE | 1 SCOOP<br>16 OUNCES<br>1/2 CUP DRY |
| MEAL 2<br>10:30 AM | WHEY PROTEIN<br>OLD-FASHIONED OATS<br>SKIM MILK<br>FLAXSEED OIL | 1 SCOOP<br>1/2 CUP (MEASURED DRY)<br>16 OUNCES<br>1 TABLESPOON |
| MEAL 3<br>1:30 PM | BROWN RICE<br>GREEN BEANS<br>EGG WHITES<br>EXTRA-VIRGIN OLIVE OIL | 1 CUP COOKED<br>1 CUP<br>2 CUPS<br>1 TABLESPOON |
| MEAL 4<br>3:30 PM | WHEY PROTEIN<br>OLD-FASHIONED OATS | 2 SCOOPS<br>1 CUP (MEASURED DRY) |
| MEAL 5<br>6:30 PM | EGG WHITES<br>SWEET POTATOES<br>BROCCOLI | 2 CUPS<br>4 OUNCES COOKED<br>1 CUP |
| MEAL 6<br>8:30 PM | EGG WHITES<br>BAKED POTATOES<br>ASPARAGUS<br>FLAXSEED OIL | 2 CUPS<br>4 OUNCES COOKED<br>1 CUP<br>1 TABLESPOON |

# Appendix D
## Workout Journal

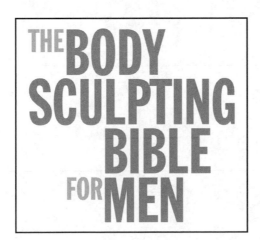

THE BODY SCULPTING BIBLE FOR MEN

# BREAK-IN ROUTINE #1

## Daily Workout Journal

Week ◯ Day ◯

| Exercise Main (Alternate) | | Set 1 Reps | Weight | Set 2 Reps | Weight | Set 3 Reps | Weight | Set 4 Reps | Weight | Set 5 Reps | Weight |
|---|---|---|---|---|---|---|---|---|---|---|---|
| **Group 1** | | | | | | | | | | | |
| | | | | | | | | | | | |
| | | | | | | | | | | | |
| **Group 2** | | | | | | | | | | | |
| | | | | | | | | | | | |
| | | | | | | | | | | | |
| **Group 3** | | | | | | | | | | | |
| | | | | | | | | | | | |
| | | | | | | | | | | | |
| **Group 4** | | | | | | | | | | | |
| | | | | | | | | | | | |
| | | | | | | | | | | | |
| **Abs** | | | | | | | | | | | |
| | | | | | | | | | | | |
| | | | | | | | | | | | |

**Cardio**

**Cardio Activity:**     **Notes:**

**Average Heart Rate:**

**Duration:**

# BREAK-IN ROUTINE #2

## Daily Workout Journal
**Week** ⬤ **Day** ⬤

| Exercise<br>Main (Alternate) | | Set 1 Reps | Set 1 Weight | Set 2 Reps | Set 2 Weight | Set 3 Reps | Set 3 Weight | Set 4 Reps | Set 4 Weight | Set 5 Reps | Set 5 Weight |
|---|---|---|---|---|---|---|---|---|---|---|---|
| **Group 1** | | | | | | | | | | | |
| **Group 2** | | | | | | | | | | | |
| **Group 3** | | | | | | | | | | | |
| **Group 4** | | | | | | | | | | | |
| **Abs** | | | | | | | | | | | |

**Cardio**

**Cardio Activity:**

**Average Heart Rate:**

**Duration:**

**Notes:**

# 14-DAY BODY SCULPTING WORKOUT #1

## Daily Workout Journal     Week ⬤ Day ⬤

| Exercise<br>Main (Alternate) | Set 1<br>Reps / Weight | Set 2<br>Reps / Weight | Set 3<br>Reps / Weight | Set 4<br>Reps / Weight | Set 5<br>Reps / Weight |
|---|---|---|---|---|---|
| **Group 1** | | | | | |
| **Group 2** | | | | | |
| **Group 3** | | | | | |
| **Group 4** | | | | | |
| **Abs** | | | | | |

**Cardio**

Cardio Activity:

Average Heart Rate:

Duration:

**Notes:**

# 14-DAY BODY SCULPTING WORKOUT #2

## Daily Workout Journal    Week ⚪ Day ⚪

| Exercise Main (Alternate) | Set 1 Reps | Set 1 Weight | Set 2 Reps | Set 2 Weight | Set 3 Reps | Set 3 Weight | Set 4 Reps | Set 4 Weight | Set 5 Reps | Set 5 Weight |
|---|---|---|---|---|---|---|---|---|---|---|
| **Group 1** | | | | | | | | | | |
| | | | | | | | | | | |
| | | | | | | | | | | |
| | | | | | | | | | | |
| **Group 2** | | | | | | | | | | |
| | | | | | | | | | | |
| | | | | | | | | | | |
| | | | | | | | | | | |
| **Group 3** | | | | | | | | | | |
| | | | | | | | | | | |
| | | | | | | | | | | |
| | | | | | | | | | | |
| **Group 4** | | | | | | | | | | |
| | | | | | | | | | | |
| | | | | | | | | | | |
| | | | | | | | | | | |
| **Abs** | | | | | | | | | | |
| | | | | | | | | | | |
| | | | | | | | | | | |
| | | | | | | | | | | |

**Cardio**

Cardio Activity:

Average Heart Rate:

Duration:

**Notes:**

# 14-DAY BODY SCULPTING WORKOUT # 3

## Daily Workout Journal       Week ⬤ Day ⬤

| Exercise Main (Alternate) | | Set 1 Reps | Set 1 Weight | Set 2 Reps | Set 2 Weight | Set 3 Reps | Set 3 Weight | Set 4 Reps | Set 4 Weight | Set 5 Reps | Set 5 Weight |
|---|---|---|---|---|---|---|---|---|---|---|---|
| **Group 1** | | | | | | | | | | | |
| | | | | | | | | | | | |
| | | | | | | | | | | | |
| | | | | | | | | | | | |
| **Group 2** | | | | | | | | | | | |
| | | | | | | | | | | | |
| | | | | | | | | | | | |
| | | | | | | | | | | | |
| **Group 3** | | | | | | | | | | | |
| | | | | | | | | | | | |
| | | | | | | | | | | | |
| | | | | | | | | | | | |
| **Group 4** | | | | | | | | | | | |
| | | | | | | | | | | | |
| | | | | | | | | | | | |
| | | | | | | | | | | | |
| **Abs** | | | | | | | | | | | |
| | | | | | | | | | | | |
| | | | | | | | | | | | |
| | | | | | | | | | | | |

**Cardio**

Cardio Activity:

Average Heart Rate:

Duration:

Notes:

# 14-DAY RAPID BODY SCULPTING WORKOUT #1

## Daily Workout Journal  Week ⬤ Day ⬤

| Exercise Main (Alternate) | | Set 1 Reps | Set 1 Weight | Set 2 Reps | Set 2 Weight | Set 3 Reps | Set 3 Weight | Set 4 Reps | Set 4 Weight | Set 5 Reps | Set 5 Weight |
|---|---|---|---|---|---|---|---|---|---|---|---|
| **Group 1** | | | | | | | | | | | |
| | | | | | | | | | | | |
| | | | | | | | | | | | |
| | | | | | | | | | | | |
| **Group 2** | | | | | | | | | | | |
| | | | | | | | | | | | |
| | | | | | | | | | | | |
| | | | | | | | | | | | |
| **Group 3** | | | | | | | | | | | |
| | | | | | | | | | | | |
| | | | | | | | | | | | |
| | | | | | | | | | | | |
| **Group 4** | | | | | | | | | | | |
| | | | | | | | | | | | |
| | | | | | | | | | | | |
| | | | | | | | | | | | |
| **Abs** | | | | | | | | | | | |
| | | | | | | | | | | | |
| | | | | | | | | | | | |

**Cardio**

Cardio Activity:     Notes:

Average Heart Rate:

Duration:

# 14-DAY RAPID BODY SCULPTING WORKOUT #2

## Daily Workout Journal          Week ◯ Day ◯

| Exercise Main (Alternate) | Set 1 Reps | Set 1 Weight | Set 2 Reps | Set 2 Weight | Set 3 Reps | Set 3 Weight | Set 4 Reps | Set 4 Weight | Set 5 Reps | Set 5 Weight |
|---|---|---|---|---|---|---|---|---|---|---|
| **Group 1** | | | | | | | | | | |
| | | | | | | | | | | |
| | | | | | | | | | | |
| **Group 2** | | | | | | | | | | |
| | | | | | | | | | | |
| | | | | | | | | | | |
| **Group 3** | | | | | | | | | | |
| | | | | | | | | | | |
| | | | | | | | | | | |
| **Group 4** | | | | | | | | | | |
| | | | | | | | | | | |
| | | | | | | | | | | |
| **Abs** | | | | | | | | | | |
| | | | | | | | | | | |
| | | | | | | | | | | |

**Cardio**

Cardio Activity:                    Notes:

Average Heart Rate:

Duration:

# ADVANCED 14-DAY BODY SCULPTING WORKOUT #1

## Daily Workout Journal    Week ◯ Day ◯

| | Exercise Main (Alternate) | Rest | Set 1 Reps | Set 1 Weight | Set 2 Reps | Set 2 Weight | Set 3 Reps | Set 3 Weight | Set 4 Reps | Set 4 Weight | Set 5 Reps | Set 5 Weight | |
|---|---|---|---|---|---|---|---|---|---|---|---|---|---|
| Group 1 | | | | | | | | | | | | | Group 1 |
| | | | | | | | | | | | | | |
| | | | | | | | | | | | | | |
| Group 2 | | | | | | | | | | | | | Group 2 |
| | | | | | | | | | | | | | |
| | | | | | | | | | | | | | |
| Group 3 | | | | | | | | | | | | | Group 3 |
| | | | | | | | | | | | | | |
| | | | | | | | | | | | | | |
| Group 4 | | | | | | | | | | | | | Group 4 |
| | | | | | | | | | | | | | |
| | | | | | | | | | | | | | |
| Abs | | | | | | | | | | | | | Abs |
| | | | | | | | | | | | | | |
| | | | | | | | | | | | | | |

**Cardio**

Cardio Activity: _____  Notes: _____

Average Heart Rate: _____

Duration: _____

**Notes**

# ADVANCED 14-DAY BODY SCULPTING WORKOUT #2

## Daily Workout Journal   Week ⬤ Day ⬤

| | Exercise Main (Alternate) | Rest | Set 1 Reps | Set 1 Weight | Set 2 Reps | Set 2 Weight | Set 3 Reps | Set 3 Weight | Set 4 Reps | Set 4 Weight | Set 5 Reps | Set 5 Weight | |
|---|---|---|---|---|---|---|---|---|---|---|---|---|---|
| **Group 1** | | | | | | | | | | | | | **Group 1** |
| **Group 2** | | | | | | | | | | | | | **Group 2** |
| **Group 3** | | | | | | | | | | | | | **Group 3** |
| **Group 4** | | | | | | | | | | | | | **Group 4** |
| **Abs** | | | | | | | | | | | | | **Abs** |

| **Cardio** | **Cardio Activity:** | **Notes:** | **Notes** |
|---|---|---|---|
| | **Average Heart Rate:** | | |
| | **Duration:** | | |

# 14-DAY BODY SCULPTING MASS WORKOUT

## Daily Workout Journal    Week ◯ Day ◯

| | Exercise<br>Main (Alternate) | Rest | Set 1<br>Reps / Weight | Set 2<br>Reps / Weight | Set 3<br>Reps / Weight | Set 4<br>Reps / Weight | Set 5<br>Reps / Weight | |
|---|---|---|---|---|---|---|---|---|
| **Group 1** | | | | | | | | **Group 1** |
| **Group 2** | | | | | | | | **Group 2** |
| **Group 3** | | | | | | | | **Group 3** |
| **Group 4** | | | | | | | | **Group 4** |
| **Abs** | | | | | | | | **Abs** |

**Cardio**

Cardio Activity:          Notes:

Average Heart Rate:

Duration:

**Notes**

# 14-DAY BODYWEIGHT BODY SCULPTING WORKOUT

## Daily Workout Journal — Week ⚪ Day ⚪

| | Exercise Main (Alternate) | Rest | Set 1 Reps | Set 1 Weight | Set 2 Reps | Set 2 Weight | Set 3 Reps | Set 3 Weight | Set 4 Reps | Set 4 Weight | Set 5 Reps | Set 5 Weight | |
|---|---|---|---|---|---|---|---|---|---|---|---|---|---|
| Group 1 | | | | | | | | | | | | | Group 1 |
| Group 2 | | | | | | | | | | | | | Group 2 |
| Group 3 | | | | | | | | | | | | | Group 3 |
| Group 4 | | | | | | | | | | | | | Group 4 |
| Abs | | | | | | | | | | | | | Abs |

**Cardio**

Cardio Activity:

Average Heart Rate:

Duration:

**Notes:**

# Appendix E
# Nutrition Journal

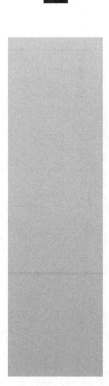

E

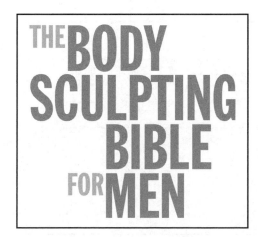

# Daily Nutrition Journal

Week ⬤ Day ◯

| | Food | Serving Size | Calories | Carbs (grams) | Protein (grams) | Fat (grams) |
|---|---|---|---|---|---|---|
| Meal 1 | | | | | | |
| Meal 2 | | | | | | |
| Meal 3 | | | | | | |
| Meal 4 | | | | | | |
| Meal 5 | | | | | | |
| Meal 6 | | | | | | |
| **Total** | | | | | | |

# Appendix F
## Tracking Your Progress

**F**

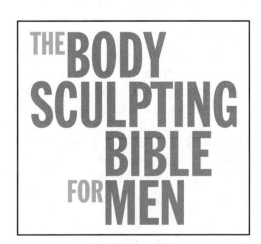

THE **BODY SCULPTING BIBLE** FOR **MEN**

The only way to know if your program is working or not is by tracking your progress. A simple way to do this is by using the following formulas excerpted from the book *Hardcore Bodybuilding: A Scientific Approach,* written by strength training authority Frederick C. Hatfield, Ph.D. Dr. Hatfield, better known as Dr. Squat, is the co-founding Director of Sports and Fitness Sciences for the prestigious International Sports Sciences Association (ISSA). As a three-time winner of the World Championships of Powerlifting, Dr. Hatfield not only is well versed on weight training theory, but on its application as well.

## FOR MEN:

Before you use the formulas, there are two measurements that are required:
**Measurement 1:** Bodyweight
**Measurement 2:** Waist Girth (measured at the umbilicus)

## PROCEDURE:

1) Multiply your bodyweight by 1.082. Add the result to 94.42. Once your calculation is complete, save the number. ➜ (Bodyweight x 1.082) + 94.42=Result 1

2) Multiply your waist girth by 4.15. Once you get this result, subtract it from the number obtained in step 1 (ie: Step 1 result-Step 2 result). The result obtained after the subtraction is done is your lean bodyweight (your weight if you had no fat in your body at all).

   ➜ Result 1—(Waist Girth x 4.15)= Lean Body Weight

3) Finally, subtract your lean bodyweight from your total bodyweight (Total weight-Lean Bodyweight). Once you get the result, multiply that number by 100. Once you get the result divide it by your total bodyweight. This final result is your percentage of body fat.
   ➜ ((Total Bodyweight—Lean Bodyweight) x 100) divided by (Your Body Weight) = Your Percentage of Body Fat.

## EXAMPLE:

I weigh 190 and I have a 30.5 inch waist. Therefore, step 1 is (190 x 1.082) + 94.42 = 300. Step 2 says that my lean body weight equals 300-(30.5 x 4.15)=173.425. Finally, Step 3 says that my body fat percentage is ((190-173.425) x 100) divided by 190= 8.72%.

**Notes:** The formulas above are approximations. The goal here is to have a point of reference from which to work. I recommend that you measure your body fat every three weeks. If you see a pattern where you are gaining muscle and losing fat, then you know your program is on track. If not, examine which part of your program is not optimal. Assuming that you are following the recommended training routines, then the only things that could be going wrong are either you are not getting enough rest at night, or more likely that you are not following the nutrition plan properly. You will also want to take your body fat measurements and can do so by purchasing a pair of body fat calipers. This will be a very good indicator of how much fat you are losing, much better than the mistaken theory of "weight" being the method of calculating improvements.

# Appendix G
## Grocery Shopping List

G

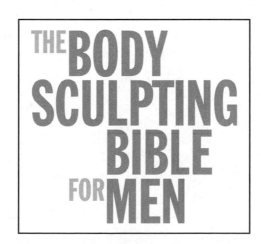

**Note:** Eat a meal prior to going grocery shopping to ensure that you don't buy junk foods. Another strategy is to do your grocery shopping on Sundays, when you are allowed to eat whatever you want for one meal.

Obviously, you do not need to purchase all of the items on this grocery list. We provide it as a reminder of the types of foods that your shopping list should include.

## CARBOHYDRATES

Brown rice
Chickpeas
Cream of rice
Yams (sweet potatoes)
Whole-wheat bread
Plain oatmeal (old fashion, not instant)
Corn
Baking potato
Lentils
Pita bread
Lentils
Grits
Fruits
Fresh green vegetables

## PROTEINS

Chicken breasts (avoid deli meats; they
    are high in sodium and low in protein)
Turkey breasts (avoid deli meats; they are
    high in sodium and low in protein)
Water-packed Tuna
White fish
Eggs
Halibut
Cod
Round steak
Top sirloin

## FATS
Flaxseed Oil

## SUPPLEMENTS

Vitamin and mineral formula
Vitamin C
Chromium picolinate
Fish oil capsules (if you don't use
    flaxseed oil)
Meal replacement powders
Whey protein powders
Protein bars
Creatine
Glutamine

## DAIRY

Skim Milk

## MISCELLANEOUS ITEMS

Garlic powder (for flavoring)
Onion powder (for flavoring)
Balsamic vinegar
Crystal light
Any sugar-free and salt-free seasoning

(Photocopy these pages for your own personal use)

# Appendix H
# Body Hair Free

**H**

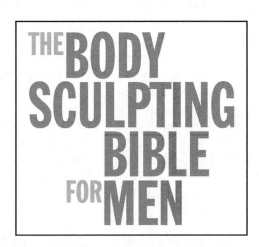

## ELIMINATING BODY HAIR

This particular section is dedicated to a topic that many men either don't think about or, because of the "masculinity" thing, believe they shouldn't think about. The topic we're talking about is body hair and whether or not you should shave it or, at least, trim it. Now, I understand that there are men and women out there who like and even love body hair. For all of you that do in fact enjoy the hairy side of life, this is not a plea to change your personal preference. It is merely a "How To" guide created to help those who would like to make a change.

When I was a young man, I never thought about shaving my body hair. The reasons for this were simple. First, I really didn't have much hair to begin with and second, I was fat! Speaking for myself and for many heavy people, the last thing a heavy person wants to do is reveal their naked body. Whether it is with the help of the clothes we wear or the body hair we accumulate over time, we would much rather try and hide from what we aren't comfortable with showing.

Over the years I began working out and, as a result, began depleting my body fat while simultaneously building lean muscle mass. I knew I was losing fat because my fat calipers indicated so. I knew I was gaining muscle because the tape measure showed an increase in my measurements. That made me feel great but whenever I took off my shirt, I didn't look as good as I thought I would. This pushed me towards working even harder than ever but to no avail, I still wasn't pleased. I got to the point where I became obsessed with working out and ended up pushing too hard. In fact, I pushed so hard that I began physically injuring myself. Furthermore, it didn't even help with my appearance.

One day, at the age of 18, I bought a copy of a fitness magazine called MuscleMag. I discovered that these guys looked amazing and not one of them had body hair! That's how I wanted to look. Without the body hair, you could clearly see all of the hard work these guys put in to working out. I began to think. What if I shaved? Will it look right on me? I concluded that it just wouldn't look right on me. With that thought, I didn't shave for the next three years.

When I finally did decide to shave, I did so with a disposable razor and shaving cream. I was merely experimenting so I started with my chest only. At first, I really didn't like it. I looked and felt like a little kid. About two weeks later, I decided to shave my stomach.

Believe me when I tell you that it looks much better when both are shaved, rather than having a bare chest and a hairy stomach.

All of a sudden I could see my abs and, although I knew I had great abs there somewhere, I could finally see a six-pack! It was like they had just suddenly appeared. I looked at my chest again and noticed that I had these muscle striations and deep cuts in my chest region. All I could think was: "Where the heck did these come from?" At that point, the shocking realization was that, for the three years prior to me shaving, this same body existed. Wow, I actually had really looked like this for about three years! Can you believe that? For three years I could have taken off my shirt at the beach and had people admiring my body. I could have felt confident and who knows how much further I could have come during that time.

I've told this story to many people since my discovery and many of them felt that this story was perhaps exaggerated. The suggestion that I suddenly noticed that I had this nice body seemed far-fetched. I posed this question to them and to you now: why do you think all of those fitness or supplement companies are so successful when running those "before and after" pictorial fitness contests? I'm sure you've seen them before. They are before and after picture campaigns where the featured men are all plump, pasty, and hairy in their before pictures. In these men's after pictures though, did you happen to notice that they are all tanned up in addition to being hairless? Of course, you must give credit where credit is due and admit that some of these men have made some very admirable changes to their physiques. While this is true for some, the majority of these pictures depict improvements made possible with the help of suntan lotions and a razor.

Why do you think these companies would have their male contestants shave and go tanning before they took their after pictures? Let's be honest, many of you have been complimented when you've gotten a tan. When we're tan, we often get compliments regarding our "nice color" or our seemingly "thinner frame". A tan obviously makes us LOOK much better than when we're pale. A tan can help us look more vibrant, more toned, and yes, even more muscular. The companies that hold these fitness contests are smart to make these powerful improvements to their contestants' physiques.

The point here is that you can also help improve your physical appearance when you are tan. If you are concerned about your health regarding overexposure to the sun, there are many new and safe tanning methods including, but not limited to, self-tanning lotions.

Do some research and explore the many options available to you.

As far as eliminating body hair is concerned, there are many options from which you can choose. The first method we will speak of is the traditional method of shaving with a razor. Trying out this particular method should be based on how sensitive your skin is to shaving. If you have a history of skin problems or a tendency to getting skin irritations when you shave your face, you should probably avoid this option. I personally have sensitive skin and do not prefer this method of body hair elimination. Shaving with a razor can also greatly increase

your chances of getting ingrown hairs. In addition to these potential problems, shaving with a razor can be time consuming. If you do decide to go with this method, go slow and apply some type of skin conditioning cream on your shaved body parts when you've finished.

The second method of shaving, and my personal favorite, is trimming the body hair with a hair buzzer. I recommend a hair buzzer that has a built in hair length mechanism, which will allow you to quickly and easily increase or decrease the amount of hair you would like to buzz away. Keep in mind that the best results will appear when you buzz in the opposite direction that the hair is growing in. Even if your goal is not to get a close buzz, shaving in the opposite direction of hair growth will allow you to achieve an even buzz cut. As you're buzzing away the hair, you might notice that the hair accumulates in the hair length mechanism and razor heads. Be aware that this can inhibit the buzzer from cutting evenly and can cause the buzzer head to yank hair from the root. This can be painful so make sure to hold the buzzer upside down and clean out the hair every so often. You can complete your entire body very quickly using this method of hair elimination and usually without any chance of skin irritation. Just remember that there is no need to push the buzzer abrasively along the skin. You might have to go over some areas more than once or twice but remember to use light, even strokes.

The third method of body hair elimination, and one you must be careful in trying out, is the hair removal lotions. I can't stress to you enough how careful you must be when using this method, as misuse or even slight carelessness can cause bad irritations and even burns. You must pay attention to the amount of time you're suppose to leave the lotion on. If you leave it on for a longer period of time than recommended, you risk being burned. Usually, these lotions call for dabbing large amounts of the lotion over the body while avoiding sensitive areas. Usually, they indicate to only leave the lotion on for fifteen minutes. You then get a damp washcloth and wipe the hair right off your body. You might be recommended to apply a skin conditioning lotion when complete. To make you understand how careful you must be with these lotions, I will tell you about my experience with a hair removal lotion. I did exactly what the lotions instructions indicated. I tested the lotion on my chest and tried to make sure that I avoided my nipples. When the recommended fifteen minutes were up, I immediately grabbed a damp washcloth and wiped the hair from my chest. It was working but I did start to experience some burning sensations in my chest area. Remember, fifteen minutes was the maximum time I was allowed to leave the lotion on for. I was in a race to wipe off the lotion and must have accidentally gotten some on my nipples. Now, in that moment I truly did not realize just how serious it could be getting even a trace of that lotion on my nipple area. The next day I had a blister on my nipple and some bad irritation on the skin of my chest. Still, I went to the gym and, when I started to sweat, OH MY GOSH!  My chest and nipples burned so bad that I can't even describe it. Two days later, I had a fairly large scab on my left nipple. As you can see, even after carefully following the directions, you can still run into problems with these products. You must be very careful not to take the cautions lightly. Please pay close attention to the directions and monitor your application of the lotions at all times.

The fourth method, and one that I refuse to ever try again, is waxing. It is by far the most painful method I know for eliminating body hair. I've heard all the different claims stating how this and that waxing system is a pain free means to removing unwanted body hair. Well, apparently the people making those claims have not tried waxing themselves or perhaps their pain receptors in their body were numb when they did try it. Regardless, waxing, my friends, is painful. But hey, if you can handle the pain, go for it!  If you can withstand the pain of waxing, it will provide you with one of the smoothest results you will get from all of the body hair removal methods we've mentioned so far.

The last two methods we will mention are for you to research yourself. They are the Electrolysis method and Laser hair removal methods. Both can be expensive and require a medical doctor or licensed technician to perform. Either ask your dermatologist to refer you to a practitioner or look in the phone book for a list of local offices.

As you can see, you have many options to choose from when it comes to body hair elimination. If I were to make a suggestion, I would suggest that you first try the buzzer method since it is the most mild of the methods.

I should point something out to you before you get too excited about removing your body hair. If this is the first time you've ever started working out and wish to shave because you think you'll look much better than you do now, please don't mislead yourself. If it's simply a matter of removing the hair because you really don't like it, then by all means do so. However, don't do it expecting to look like someone who has been working out for a long time. Too many people have strong expectations of what they should look like and can easily get discouraged when they don't see what they thought they would see. You need to be thick-skinned and face the fact that you need to work out, eat well and pay your dues in order to look the way you want. When you do begin to work hard and pay attention to all of the variables that help to create a healthy and fit lifestyle, it would not be surprising to see that your results end up being much better than even those high expectations of what you originally thought you'd look like.

If I were you and were just starting out with the fitness lifestyle, I would not shave my body hair right now. I would set a goal for myself and look forward to seeing those goals met. When you're ready, you'll know the right time to eliminate that body hair and when you do, WOW! You'll be amazed at yourself. Think of it as an unveiling ceremony.

Yeah it might seem a little corny, but you'll be the only one laughing.

# Appendix I
## Body Sculpting Under Special Circumstances

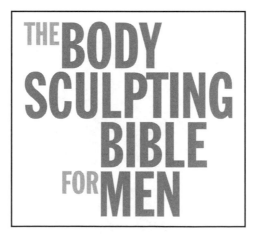

## BODY SCULPTING FOR OLDER MEN

During the past several years, many point to the many benefits and safety of weight training exercise for aging adults. Among these benefits are the usual benefits of reduced cholesterol, reduced blood pressure, reduced resting pulse rate, increased levels of muscle mass, increased levels of bone density, and decreased levels of body fat. In addition to those benefits, weight training for older men offers the following:

- Improved digestion
- Improved blood glucose levels
- Reduced discomfort caused by arthritis
- Reduced lower back pain
- Increased mobility (due to an increase in muscle strength)
- Reduced possibility of a fall due to loss of balance caused by loose joints and weak leg muscles

In order for older men to get all of the benefits that strength training has to offer the following guidelines must be followed:

**First and foremost, consult with your doctor and/or physical therapist before you start any exercise program.** Depending on your present condition, you may or may not need someone to supervise you during your weight training session. If you have been physically active all your life, you should have no problems going full bore into a weight training routine. If you have never been very physically active and you suffer from ailments like loss of balance, then supervision will be required.

**Educate yourself on how to perform the exercises correctly!** Read the exercise description section in this book as many times as necessary. Study the illustrations and practice the movement mentally. It is crucial that exercise form is followed in order to avoid injury.

**Ensure that you follow the nutritional guidelines of our Nutrition Chapter.** Many senior citizens in this country are malnourished, as their appetites have decreased over the years. Also, certain medications cause a loss of appetite as well. Force yourself to follow our nutrition guidelines and we guarantee that you won't be malnourished. Remember that in order to get the maximum effect from training, the diet has to be in order. Being malnourished leads to a loss of muscle mass (the body is using such mass as fuel) and a resulting loss of strength and bone density (which leads to brittle bones).

You have two choices for the exercise program. If you have always been physically active and you are in good health, go ahead and start with our Break-In Routine and progress to the 14-Day Body Sculpting Workout. If on the other hand, you suffer from ailments like loss of balance and have perhaps limited mobility, use the following program that is composed of machines:

## DAY 1

- Leg Extensions
- Seated Leg Curls
- Leg Press
- Calf Press
- Lower Back Machine
- Abdominal Machine

**DAY 2**

- Pulldown to Front
- Close-Grip Pulldown
- Overhead Press Machine
- Rear-Delt Machine
- Biceps Curl Machine
- Triceps Extension Machine

## HOW TO PROGRESS

- Follow the same structure of the 14-Day Body Sculpting Workout.
- Use weights on Mon/Wed/Fri alternating between Day 1 and 2.
- Do cardio on Tue/Thu/ Saturday.
- Sundays are for complete rest.
- Weeks 1-2: Perform 2 sets of 15 to 18 repetitions per exercise. Take 2 seconds to lift the weight and 4 to lower it. Rest 1 minute in between sets. No weight training techniques such as modified compound supersets are to be utilized. Perform one set after the other in straight set fashion.
- Weeks 3-4: Increase to 3 sets of 12 to 15 repetitions. Take 2 seconds to lift the weight and 4 to lower it. Rest 1 minute in between sets. No weight training techniques such as modified compound supersets are to be utilized. Perform one set after the other in straight set fashion.
- Weeks 5-6: Go up to 4 sets of 10-12 repetitions. Take 2 seconds to lift the weight and 4 to lower it. Rest 1 minute in between sets. No weight training techniques such as modified compound supersets are to be utilized. Perform one set after the other in straight set fashion.
- On cardio days, build up to 25 minutes of continuous aerobic exercise performed at 70-75 percent of your maximum heart rate. Start with 5 minutes of aerobics 3 times a week, and add 2 minutes every week to the original 5 minutes. At the end of 10 weeks, you should be able to do 25 minutes of continuous aerobic exercise with no problems. Use Sundays as your complete rest day from diet and exercise. If after a while of using this routine you feel that you are in shape to do the 14-Day Body Sculpting Routine, then by all means do so by using the exercises listed above. If you feel that you are ready to incorporate some free weight exercises as well, then go for it!

## YOUNGSTERS AND WEIGHT TRAINING

At what age a teenage boy can start working out with weights has always been a topic of debate. Some people say that weights should not be touched until after all of the growing is done or else you could affect the growth platelets and stunt your growth. Others say it is okay to start lifting weight at an early age. We have arrived at the following conclusions based on the latest research on this subject.

We believe that youngsters (anybody **less than 12 years old**) are better off doing exercises with just their body weight. The following exercises should compose a youngster's program:

- Running
- Dips
- Push-ups
- Pull-ups
- Chin-ups
- Squats with no weights
- Lunges with no weights
- Calf raises with no weight
- Crunches
- Leg raises

Depending on the age and motivation of the person, anywhere between 2-5 sets of each exercise for the maximum amount of reps possible is sufficient. There should be 30 seconds of rest in between exercises and they should be performed 3 times a week.

An additional 15-20 minutes of running on their rest day is enough exercise for anyone who wishes to start an exercise program before the age of 13.

**13-year-olds** can start working out with weights as long as they're using weights light enough to allow 20-30 reps per set. They should basically follow the same program described above with the same set, repetition, and rest scheme, plus adding the following dumbbell exercises: dumbbell curls, dumbbell overhead triceps extensions, and lateral raises. In addition, dumbbells can also be used to perform lunges, squats and calf raises. The complete program will look like the following:

- Running
- Dips
- Push-ups
- Pull-ups
- Chin-ups
- Lateral raises
- Dumbbell curls
- Dumbbell overhead triceps extensions
- Dumbbell squats
- Dumbbell lunges
- Dumbbell calf raises
- Crunches
- Leg raises

Continue this program for the next three years.

**15-year-olds** can start increasing the weight but should stay within 13-20 reps. For the next two years they should concentrate on perfecting their exercise technique and form. They must make sure to only increase the weight when they can do over 20 repetitions easily. They should not go to absolute muscular failure or use any fancy weight training techniques, since there is still some bone growth and development occurring in their bodies. Remember, strenuous and heavy weighted exercise can interfere with the growth process, so keep it simple!

At this age it is okay to use the 14-Day Body Sculpting routines from this book as long as the 13-20 repetition rule is kept (Weeks 1-2: 18-20 reps are used, weeks 3-4: 16-18, weeks 5-6: 13-15).

**After 18,** you can start going heavier in weight with no problems; by then all of the growth platelets, bones, and joint structures should be fully developed.

## FITNESS WHILE TRAVELING

We always use traveling as an excuse to not get in shape. Getting in shape while traveling is more challenging, but it is certainly possible. Provided that you are determined, the key is planning and preparation. We have taught all of our clients to learn to treat exercise as a way of life. This way, you are innately drawn to exercising even during vacation time. We have gotten some of the best workouts of our lives during vacation and traveling. It is refreshing to go to train in new environments and surroundings, plus a great way to meet people.

Before you go on your next trip, find out if the hotel that you are going to stay in has a fitness facility or at least a set of dumbbells. If not, then find out where the closest fitness facility is and plan to work out there. If, by some twist of fate, there are no fitness facilities in the area (hard to believe), then try to do the youngsters weight training routine which consists of dips, push-ups, pull-ups, chin-ups, squats with no weights, lunges with no weights, calf raises with no weight, crunches and leg raises performed 3 times a week for 5 sets with 30 seconds of rest in between sets of as many reps as possible. Run for 20-30 minutes first thing in the morning on rest days. All you need for this routine is a park with a chin-up bar and parallel bars. If there is no park within the area, then you can still do push-ups, pull-ups, chin-ups, squats with no weights, lunges with no weights, calf raises with no weight, crunches, and leg raises. All you need to carry is a portable chin-up bar that you can place in the hotel room. Once you get back home, you can start doing the 14-Day Body Sculpting Workout as laid out with the only exception being that you should start it on Week 3, since you have already done high repetition, light weight work.

With diet, you will need to get creative. Follow the rules from the section on eating out. Also, carry with you protein bars so that you are prepared with all of the required meals for the day. Missing meals too often guarantees failure with this program.

As you can see, even though it will take more effort to get in shape if you travel, it is not impossible. If you are determined enough to change your body, then nothing is impossible!

## TRAINING WHILE YOU ARE SICK

Nothing can bring progress to a halt more than when you are sick. We are often asked the question, should I train while I am sick? The answer to that question really depends on what you mean by sick. Is it a cold? The flu? Allergies? Most people confuse the common cold for the flu. However, these are different types of illnesses. The flu is caused by viruses known as Influenza A or Influenza B, while the common cold is caused by viruses called coronaviruses and rhinoviruses. There are over 200 different types of coronaviruses and rhinoviruses. If one of them hits you, your immune system builds a lifelong immunity to it (therefore, the same virus

will never hit you twice). However, you have the rest of the viruses that have not yet affected you to worry about; and there are enough to last a lifetime.

The flu, as you may have already found out by experience, is much more severe as it is usually accompanied by an array of body aches and fever. Therefore, your body's immune system is taxed much more by the flu than by the common cold. At this time, training would not only be detrimental to muscle growth, but it would also be very detrimental to your health as well. Remember that while training can help us gain muscle, lose fat, and feel good and energetic, it is still a catabolic activity. The body needs to be in good health in order to go from the catabolic state caused by the exercise to an anabolic state of recuperation and muscle growth. So if you have the flu, your body is already fighting a catabolic state caused by the Influenza virus. In this case, weight training would only add more catabolism, which in turn would negatively affect the efficacy of the immune system against the virus, causing you to get sicker. Therefore, absolutely no training if you have the flu. Instead, concentrate on very good nutrition and on drinking large amounts of fluids (water and electrolyte replacement drinks like Gatorade in order to prevent dehydration). Once the flu completely runs its course, you can slowly start up the 14-Day Body Sculpting Workout on week 1 starting with light weights. Don't push yourself too hard during this first week. The next week you'll repeat week 1 again, but pushing yourself closer to muscular failure. By the second week of the program you should be back on track.

If it is the common cold that is hitting you and the particular virus is mild (you know that it is mild when your symptoms are just a runny nose and slight coughing), you may get away with training as long as you stop the sets short of reaching muscular failure and you decrease the weight poundages by 25 percent (divide the weights that you usually use by 4 and that will give you the amount of weight that you need to take off the bar) in order to prevent you from pushing too hard. Again, if the cold virus is causing you to feel run down, achy, with a sore throat and headaches, it would be best to stop training all together, until the symptoms subside. If this is the case, just follow the exercise program start-up recommendations described above for after the flu. Remember that we do not want to make it any harder for the immune system to fight the virus by introducing more catabolic activity, so intense training is out during that time.

If your ailment is something other than the common cold or the flu, consult your doctor.

Now that we have seen how a flu or a cold can throw a wrench into your progress, let's see how we can prevent these buggers from affecting us during the flu season or during any other season for that matter.

While it is still unknown why the cold and flu season generally comes during the winter months, it is known that you have to let the virus into your system in order for it to affect you. Therefore, it is only logical that we implement a two-fold prevention approach:

**Prevent the virus from infiltrating your system.** Keeping in mind that cold viruses spread by human contact, that they get into your system through the mouth, eyes and nose, and that they can remain active for up to three hours, you can accomplish this by doing the following:

• Keep your hands away from your face
• Wash your hands with anti bacterial soap frequently throughout the day (especially as soon as you finish your workout at the gym).

**Maintain immune system operation at peak efficiency levels at all times.** Remembering that excessive exercise, a bad diet, and losing sleep are all catabolic activities, do the following:

• Avoid overtraining by using the principles advocated in this book.
• Maintain a balanced diet as described in the nutrition chapter and avoid processed foods that contain high levels of saturated fats, refined flours or sugar since these types of foods lower the immune system function.
• Get a healthy dose of sleep a day (anywhere from 7 to 9 hours depending on your individual requirements).

So remember, stay healthy by following the tips above, and if you get sick, then "don't beat a tired horse" as former Mr. Olympia Lee Haney used to say. Rest until you get better! If you don't you will end up more seriously ill and this will take you out of the gym for a longer period of time.

# Appendix J
## Anatomy Charts

J

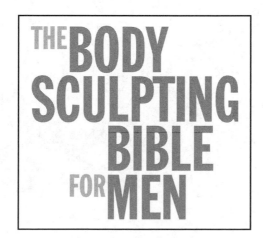
THE **BODY SCULPTING BIBLE** FOR **MEN**

# MALE MUSCULAR AND SKELETAL ANATOMY

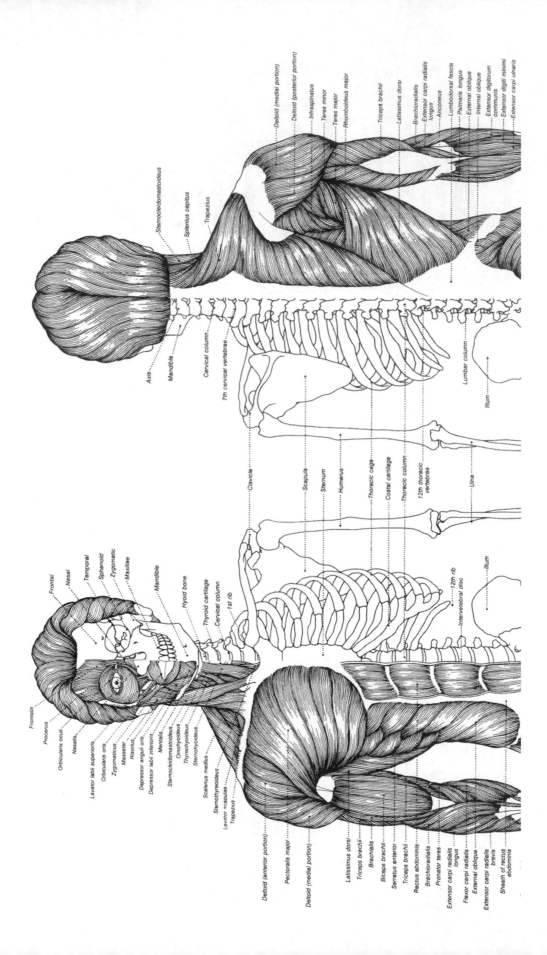

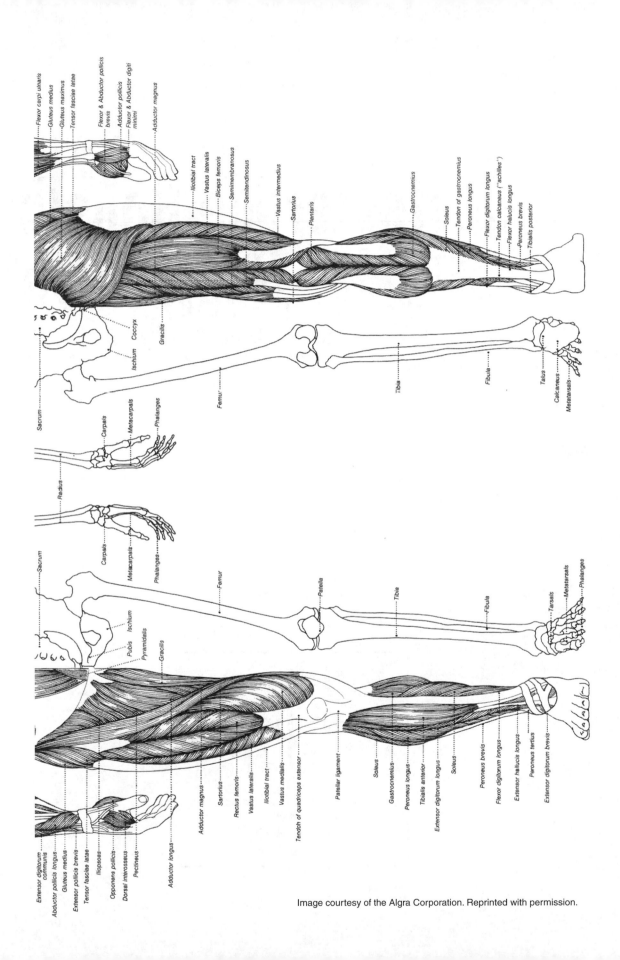

Image courtesy of the Algra Corporation. Reprinted with permission.

# Testosterone Boosting Supplements

**K**

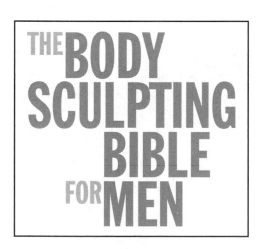

THE **BODY**
**SCULPTING**
**BIBLE**
FOR **MEN**

These are the types of supplements that you can take if you plan to compete, if you have the budget to try them, and only if you are older than 25 when the hormonal production begins to decline (except when noted otherwise).

Teenagers should stay away from any supplement that has an effect on hormonal levels as there is no need to upset a teen's delicate hormonal balance. Teenagers produce the equivalent of a 300 mg shot of testosterone per week anyway, so there is no need to attempt to increase the production of testosterone in a system that is already producing at peak levels.

The usefulness of some of these supplements is still under debate by some of the experts in the field, but in my opinion as a competitive athlete, I have seen an edge by using them. Also, I would like to mention that by increasing your hormonal levels you may experience some acne and slightly increased aggression. Finally, if you have a propensity for male pattern baldness and/or an increased prostate you should monitor these things if you still decide to use some of these products.

# TESTOSTERONE

As most of you fellow lifters know, testosterone is the male hormone responsible for the development of the male sex and reproduction organs. It also promotes male characteristics such as a deep voice, facial hair, increased levels of muscle mass, sex drive, aggressiveness, and confidence. Men's testicles produce this hormone in large quantities while female's ovaries produce some of it in very small quantities.

Low levels of this hormone create metabolic issues that have immediate and long-term consequences for the person suffering from a deficiency.

## MALADIES OF LOW TESTOSTERONE LEVELS

Needless to say low levels of testosterone can cause a male to first and foremost lose his sex drive. Depending on how low your levels are impotence may become an issue down the road. Also energy levels will plummet as well as muscle mass and strength. Even if you are giving it all you got in the gym and following your diet, you may find that getting a good pump at the gym is hard, and also that gaining muscle is becoming a very hard task to accomplish. Worst of all, fat loss seems harder than ever as well.

If you suffer from low testosterone your mood may also take a dive and you may often feel depressed. In addition to the above, the following are also maladies of low testosterone levels:

- Increased insulin resistance (which makes it hard to lose body fat as insulin levels will increase in the body due to the fact that the cells are not accepting this hormone efficiently; this can of course lead to diabetes).
- Constant fatigue and reduced zest for life.
- Reduced mental capacity.

## AGE FOR DECLINE

At what age does this decline start happening? The time at which this decline in levels begins is still much debated amongst experts but recent research seems to indicate that it can begin as early as 25-30 years old. My advice to you is that if your sex drive is low, then you should have your levels checked because this is the most common symptom of low testosterone.

Below are the normal values for testosterone levels:

- Normal range of total testosterone is between 300 - 1200 nanograms per deciliters (ng/dl)
- Normal ranges for free testosterone (the actual active testosterone that your body can use) are: 8.7 - 25 picograms per milliliters (pg/ml).

Needless to say the closer to the upper level you are in both ranges the better.

## TOP NATURAL SUPPLEMENTS THAT CAN HELP BOOST TESTOSTERONE LEVELS (NOT RECOMMENDED FOR TEENAGERS)

Once you find that your levels of testosterone are beginning to decline, there are several supplements that one can use in order to keep them optimized naturally. Please remember that for the most part only if you are older than 25 years old, when the hormonal production may begin to decline, should you start considering the use of these supplements.

## ZMA

A scientifically designed anabolic mineral formula. This formula consists of Zinc Monomethionine Aspartate, Magnesium Aspartate, and vitamin B-6. This all-natural product has been clinically proven to significantly increase anabolic hormone levels and muscle strength in trained athletes. Hard-training athletes typically deplete the body from these essential minerals.

Studies have shown that supplementing with 30mg of Zinc and 450mg of Magnesium per day can elevate testosterone levels up to 30%! I take 2 caps in the evening time.

**Note:** Due to the fact that ZMA consists of two minerals and a vitamin B, teenagers can safely use this product.

## QNT USA TESTEK

This is another pro-hormone free testosterone booster that naturally increases growth hormone and testosterone levels through different pathways than the ZMA and HumanoGrowth. In addition, Testek has ingredients that help to increase focus and memory, regulate your mood, and increase your recovery capacity at the gym.

## FLAVONE COMPLEX

The testosterone increase in this product is accomplished via a flavone complex that causes a reduction in estrogen. By reducing estrogen levels, the body begins to manufacture more testosterone.

## ALPHA GPC

An acetylcholine precursor that increases growth factors by inhibiting somatostatin, which is the growth hormone-inhibiting hormone. As you inhibit somatostatin, you increase GH levels dramatically by 333%. As a matter of fact, in a study performed at the Center for Applied Health Sciences, subjects consuming Alpha GPC prior to resistance exercise increased their peak anabolic growth factors by 333%.

## PHOSPHATIDYLSERINE (PS)

Naturally-occurring phospholipid, which research has shown can speed up recovery, prevent muscle soreness and, more importantly, reduce the cortisol response to intense exercise. This improves the testosterone/cortisol ratio by as much as 184%, which ultimately results in a more anabolic environment.

## DHT REDUCTION COMPLEX

Finally, Testek protects the user against the increased DHT production caused by increased testosterone levels via the use of flavones and lycopene. In addition, Testek's combination of ingredients promotes good mood and increased concentration and focus at the gym.

**How to Use:** Take 1 serving (4 capsules) 1-2 times daily with water. Use one serving in the morning and/or early evening. Use for approximately 6-8 weeks, then cycle off for 2 weeks.

## LABRADA NUTRITION'S HUMANOGROWTH

This testosterone booster is composed of two ingredients that help to increase testosterone and growth hormone levels, lower cortisol, improve mood, and maximize recovery as well as protein synthesis (ability of the body to turn the protein you eat into muscle).

## HUMANOFORT

A patented standardized embryo extract from Europe that has been shown to boost testosterone and growth hormone levels while reducing cortisol. It is rich in various growth factors that are good for hormonal production and general health as well. It even helps to improve the quality of your sleep!

## LEAN MUSCLE ACCELERATOR (LMA)

A purified plasma protein that improves pro-

tein efficiency by up to 31% and promotes a positive nitrogen balance by up to 20%. In simple terms, this all means that you convert more of the protein that you eat into muscle. In addition, this plasma protein also helps your body to burn more fat (instead of muscle tissue) for fuel during periods of dieting.

**How to Use:** Take 4 capsules of Humano-Growth prior to sleep. There is no need to cycle off this product.

## FINAL THOUGHTS ON TESTOSTERONE BOOSTING SUPPLEMENTATION

If you are an over 25-year-old trainee whose testosterone levels have already begun to decline and who wishes to increase them naturally, then you may want to try some of these supplements. There is no need to take all of these at the same time. You could get great benefit from doing 6 weeks of one, 6 weeks of another and so on. But if you have the finances to use them all, I have found no adverse effects from doing so.

# Addendum
## Exercise Technique and Why Some Exercises Give You Better Results

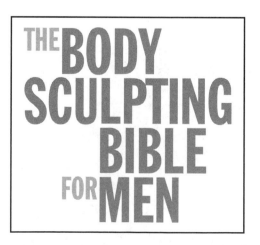

THE **BODY SCULPTING BIBLE** FOR **MEN**

## PROPER EXERCISE TECHNIQUE

Learning proper exercise technique is the backbone of every fitness program. If you train improperly you will not stimulate the intended muscle, and will risk major injury as well as receiving little or no results. When you learn to use proper exercise technique you will receive twice the results in half the time, guaranteed! We see people in the gym day in and day out who have no idea how to properly train their muscles. Some of them are professional bodybuilders, some are professional athletes, and some are even certified fitness trainers. Unfortunately, the ones who really suffer the most are people like you who rely on these role models for wisdom and guidance. We will show you the proper exercise technique to use for optimal results. Just remember to utilize your newfound knowledge. Like the old saying, "Feed a man a fish and he'll eat for a day, teach a man to fish and he'll eat for a lifetime." We expect the same of you. We don't want you to read this book once and forget everything you've learned. We want you to learn and utilize that knowledge to achieve astounding results.

Applying proper exercise form and technique is without doubt the most important component of any fitness program. Without it, many setbacks will occur. First, the musculature you intend to exercise will not be stimulated as efficiently as possible. Exercise should not be focused around just lifting barbells and weights. It shouldn't just be about how much you can lift. Optimum fitness is about the quality of exercise, the quality of your form and how you maintain that form, especially during heavier lifting. Proper exercise technique coupled with the Zone-Tone principle that we presented in **Chapter 1** will bring you the most astonishing results with the minimum amount of sets. Why? Because as we

have already discussed, one properly executed set is equivalent to five sets of "just going through the motions" type of exercise. *It comes down to this; if you want to get the most out of your workout, keep the intensity high without sacrificing proper form.* Neglecting to focus on proper form quickly leads to no results, while practicing perfect proper form equals incredible results quickly!

## WHICH EXERCISES ARE THE BEST FOR FAST RESULTS?

In weight training, there are a variety of exercises that one can choose from to sculpt the body of your dreams. Results in bodybuilding or body sculpting are generally measured in body composition changes; increased muscle mass or tone, depending on the goal, along with decreases in body fat. The speed at which such changes are acquired depends on the training protocol used, the nutrition plan followed and the amount of rest that the trainee gets. In order for a training protocol to work at peak efficiency, not only must it be periodized or cycled but it also must include exercises that give you the most stimulation in the minimum amount of time.

Different exercises provide different levels of stimulation. Exercises like leg extensions, while excellent for sculpting the lower part of the quadriceps, produce less of a stimulating effect than an exercise like the squat. The efficacy of an exercise really depends on the exercise's ability to involve the maximum amount of muscle fibers and also on its ability to provide a neuromuscular stimulation (NMS). Neuromuscular stimulation is of crucial importance as it is the nervous system that ultimately sends a signal to the brain requesting to start the muscle growth process. How do we determine what the stimulation factor of each exercise is?

## THE NMS CLASSES

In order to rate what the NMS of each exercise is, we borrowed the Class rating system used for classifying the speed of DSL systems (the technology used to achieve high speed connections to the Internet through your phone line) and tailored it to fit our purpose. In this system a Class 1 technology has lower speeds than a Class 2 technology. Therefore, in our exercise rating system composed of four classes, a Class 1 exercise yields the lowest NMS (this class is composed of variable resistance machine type exercises) while a Class 4 exercise yields the highest NMS and is therefore the hardest but most stimulating one. In each class, we may also have subclasses such as Class 1a and Class 1b. A Class 1a exercise will yield less NMS than a Class 1b.

Class 1a exercises are composed of isolation (one joint) exercises performed in variable resistance machines (such as Nautilus) where the whole movement of the exercise is controlled. These type of exercises provide the least amount of stimulation as stabilizer muscles do not need to get involved since the machine takes care of the stabilization process. An example of such an exercise would be the machine curl.

Class 1b exercises are compound (multi-joint) movements performed in a variable resistance machine. An example of such movement would be the incline bench press performed in a Hammer Strength machine. Since the movement is a compound one, more muscles get involved and therefore the neuromuscular stimulation is higher than that offered by a machine curl. However, the fact that the machine takes care of the stabilization issues limits the growth offered by the exercise.

Class 2a exercises are composed of isolation (one joint) exercises performed with non-variable resistance machines. An example of such exercise would be the leg extension exercise performed in one of those leg extensions attachments that come with the benches that are sold for home gyms. These attachments lack the pulleys and the cams that would make the exercise a variable resistance exercise. Therefore, the muscles need to get more involved in the movement, providing better stimulation.

Class 2b exercises are composed of basic (multi-joint) exercises performed with non-variable resistance machines. An example of such would be the bench press unit that is attached to the Universal type of machines or a leg press machine that contains no pulleys or cams that would make the exercise easier. Since there are no pulleys or cams to make the exercise easier as you lift the weight, the NMS is higher.

Class 3a exercises are isolation (one joint) exercises performed with free weights. An example of such exercise would be a concentration curl performed with a dumbbell. It is still not very clear whether a multi joint exercise performed on a machine offers the same amount or better NMS than the one offered by a free weight isolation exercise. However, for the purposes of this discussion, we will assume that the free weight isolation exercise provides more stimulation as stabilizer muscles come into play (especially if you do the exercise standing up).

Class 3b exercises are multi-jointed basic exercises performed with barbell free weights.

Class 3c exercises are multi-jointed basic exercises performed with dumbbell free weights. The barbell exercises provide less NMS as the movement is more restrained as opposed to dumbbells where the weights can go in all directions unless all of your stabilizer muscles jump in and constrain the movement. Because of this, dumbbells provide the highest NMS in this category.

Finally, Class 4 exercises are free weight exercises where your body moves through space. In other words, any exercise where your torso is the one moving, such as squats, deadlifts, pull-ups, close grip chins, pushups, lunges, and dips, will provide the most stimulation possible and therefore, the fastest results. Haven't you seen at the gym how many people do great amounts of weights in a pulldown machine but have trouble doing pull-ups? The reason for this is that in order for you to perform these type of exercises you need to be capable of not only carrying the added resistance but also involving your bodyweight as well. Therefore, many muscles are called into play in order to perform this feat. Performing dips, chinups, squats and deadlifts you are really hitting every single muscle in your body! These exercises not only give you fast results, but they also create functional strength; in other words strength that can be used for your daily activities. If you are great at performing pull-ups and you go to perform a pulldown you'll see how easy the task of performing a pulldown is. As a matter of fact, depending on your pull-up strength, you might be able to lift the whole stack in most pulldown machines. However, the reverse is not true. While you may be very good at performing pulldowns you may not be able to perform many pull-ups as the strength gained in the pulldown exercise is not as transferable as the one gained in a pull-up. Again, the reason for this phenomenon is NMS.

## CONCLUSION

Now that you know what exercises are the ones that give you the most bang for your buck, my recommendations are as follows:
- If you follow the normal *14-Day Body Sculpting Workout*, stick to Class 3 and 4 region exercises.

- If you follow the *Advanced 14-Day Body Sculpting Workout* you can get away with having 1/3 of your routine composed of lower class (Classes 2 and below) exercises.

Remember, convincing your body to grow and develop muscle is not an easy task. However it becomes an impossible one if you choose exercises that do not provide a significant NMS effect. Therefore, always choose exercises from the higher classes in order to show your body that you mean business.

# Resources

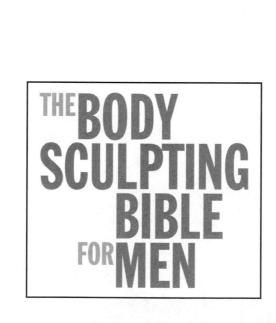

**www.bodysculptingbible.com**
The official page of the *Body Sculpting Bibles*. Pass through here and have access to tons of free resources!

**www.facebook.com/bodysculptingbibles**
The official Facebook page of the *Body Sculpting Bibles*. Come and interact with the Body Sculpting Bible online Facebook community and motivate each other.

**www.fitnessbusinesscoach.com**
A site for all health and fitness professionals looking to achieve their highest level of success and wealth. James Villepigue will now help you sculpt your business wealthy. When you visit the site, in the contact box, write "BSB" for a one-hour complimentary coaching session with James.

**www.hugorivera.net**
Hugo Rivera's personal site. Great information on all aspects of bodybuilding, body sculpting, and how to live a healthy lifestyle

**www.losefatandgainmuscle.com**
If you're looking for a companion resource that will truly help you lose fat and gain muscle, this is the website that people visit to achieve it!

## TRAINING REFERENCES

Bompa, T.O. (1983). Theory and Methodology of Training—The Key to Athletic Performance. Kendall/Hunt Publishing; Dubuque, Ia.

Bompa, Tudor O., Cornacchia, Lorenzo J., (1998). Serious Strength Training, Human Kinetics Publishers.

Bompa, Tudor O., (1990). Periodization of strength: the most effective methodology of strength training, National Strength and Conditioning Association Journal, 12(5), 49-52.

Bompa, Tudor O. Periodization of strength: the new wave in strength training. Toronto, ON: Veritas Publishing Inc., pg. 28, 1993.

Chernyak, A.V., Karimov, E.S. Butinchinov, Z.T. (1979). Distribution of Load Volume and Intensity Throughout the Year (Weightlifting). Soviet Sports Review. 14(2): 98-101.

Ebbing, C. and P. Clarkson, (1989). Exercise-induced muscle damage and adaptation. Sports Medicine. Vol 7: 207-234.

Edgerton, R.V. (1976), "Neuromuscular adaptation to power and endurance work." Canadian Journal of Applied Sports Sciences, 1:49-58.

Fleck, S.J. Periodized Strength Training: A Critical Review. The Journal of Strength and Conditioning Research, 13 (1) 82-89, 1999.

Fry AC, Kreamer WJ, Stone MH, Koziris LP, Thrush JT, Fleck SJ, (2000). Relationship between serum testosterone, cortisol, and weightlifting performance. Journal of Strength and Conditioning Research, 14(13): 338-343.

Fry, R.W., R Morton, and D. Keast. (1991), "Overtraining in athletics." Sports Medicine, 2(1):32-65.

Gilliam, G.M. (1981). Effects of Frequency of Weight Training on Muscle Strength Training. Journal of Sports Medicine. 21: 432-436.

Goldberg, A.L., J.D.Etlinger,D.F.Goldspink, and C.Jablecki.(1975), "Mechanism of work-induced hypertrophy of skeletal muscles." Medicine and Science in Sports and Exercise, 7:185-198.

Hakkinen, K. (1989), "Neuromuscular and hormonal adaptations during strength and power training." A Review of Sports Medicine Physical Fitness, 29(1):9-26.

Hakkinen KA, Pskarinen A, Alen M, Kau hanen H, Komi PV (1987). Relationships between training volume, physical performance capacity, and serum hormone concentrations during prolonged training in elite weight lifters. International Journal of Sports Medicine, 8 (suppli): 61-65.

Kuipers, H. and H.A. Keizer. (1988), "Overtraining in Elite Athletes: Review and directions for the future." Sports Medicine, 6:79-92.

McDonagh, M.J.N. and C.T.M. Davis. (1984). Adaptive response of mammalian skeletal muscle to exercise with high loads. European Journal of Applied Physiology. 52:139-155.

Minchenko, V.G. (1989). The Distribution of Training Load Throughout the Yearly Training Cycles of Athletes. Soviet Sports Review. 24(1): 1-6.

Rhea MR, Ball SD, Phillips WT, Burkett LN., A comparison of linear and daily undulating periodized programs with equated volume and intensity for strength. J Strength Cond Res. 2002 May;16(2):250-5.

Starkey, D.B., Pollock, M.L., Ishida, Y., Welsch, M.A., Brechue, W.F., Graves, J.E., Feigenbaum, M.S. (1996). Effect of resistance training volume on strength and muscle thickness, Medicine and Science in Sports and Exercise, 1311-1320.

Terjung R.L. and D.A. Hood. (1986). Biochemical adaptation in skeletal muscle induced by exercise training.

## NUTRITION REFERENCES

Dragan GI, Vasiliu A, Georgescu E. "Effects of increased supply of protein on elite weightlifters." In Milk Proteins 1984: Galesloot TE, Tinbergen BJ, (Eds). Pudoc, Wageningen, The Netherlands Pudoc, 99-103

Ivy, J.L. (1991), "Muscle glycogen synthesis before and after exercise." Sports Medicine, 11:6-19.

Lemon, Peter W.R. (1991), "Protein and amino acid needs of the strength athlete." International Journal of Sports Nutrition, 1:127-390.

Munro, H.N. (1951), "Carbohydrate and fat as factors in protein utilization and metabolism." Physiol. Rev., 31:449-488.

## STEROID REFERENCES

Bahrke, M.S., Yesalis, C. E. 3rd, Wright, J. E. (1996) Psychological and behavioural effects of endogenous testosterone and anabolic-androgenic steroids. An update. Sports Medicine, 22, 367-90

DiPasquale, M.G. (1990), Anabolic Steroid Side Effects-Fact, Fiction and Treatment. Warkworth, Ontario: MGD Press.

Gruber, A.J., Pope, H.G. Jr. (1999) Complusive weight lifting and anabolic drug abuse among women rape victims. Comprehensive Psychiatry, 40, 273-277

Hickson, R.C., Ball, K.L., Falduto M.T. (1989) Adverse effects of anabolic steroids. Med Toxicol Adverse Drug Exp, 4, 254-271

Hughes, T.K. Jr., Rady, P.L., Smith, E.M. (1998) Potential for the effects of anabolic steroid abuse in the immune and neuroendocrine axis. Journal of Neuroimmunol, 83, 162-167

Lamb, D. (1984). Anabolic steroids in athletics: how do they work and how dangerous are they? American Journal of Sports Medicine. 12(1):31-37.

Malarkey, W.B., Strauss, R.H., Leizman, D.J., Liggett, M., Demers, L.M. (1991) Endocrine effects in female weight lifters who self-administer testosterone and anabolic steroids. American Journal of Obstetrics and Gynecology, 165, 1385-1390

Strauss, R.H., Liggett, M.T., Lanese, R.R. (1985) Anabolic steroids use and perceived effects in ten weight-trained women athletes. JAMA, 253, 2871-2873

Wu, F.C. (1997) Endocrine aspects of anabolic steroids. Clinical Chemistry, 43, 1289-1292

## WHEY PROTEIN REFERENCES

Bounous, G. "Dietary whey protein inhibits the development of dimethylhydrazine induced malignancy." Clin. Invest. Medic. (1988), p. 213-217.

Bounous, G., P., Konshaven and P.Gold. "The immuno-enhancing properties of dietary whey protein concentrates," Clin. Invest. Med. 11 (1988), p. 271-278.

Burke, D.G. and P.D. Chilibeck, et al. "The effect of whey protein supplementation with and without creatne monohydrate combined with resistance training on lean tissue mass and muscle strength," Int. Jour. Sport Nutr. Exerc. Metab. 11/3 (2001), p. 349-64.

## CREATINE REFERENCES

Odland, L.M., J.D. MacDougall, et al. "Effect of oral creatine supplementation on muscle [PCr] and short term maximum power output," Med. Sci. Sports Exerc. 29/2 (1997), p.216-9.

Pearson, D.R., D.G. Hamby, et al. "Long-term effects of creatine monohydrate on strength and power," Journal of Strength and Conditioning Research 13/3 (1999), p. 187-192.

## FINAL THOUGHTS

The techniques presented in the sections above combined with the 14-Day Body Sculpting Training and Nutrition Principles, along with the knowledge presented on how to use your mind to improve your results at the gym and in anything else you do in life are what separate the 14-Day Body Sculpting Workout from anything you have ever read.

After reading this book you should have the knowledge necessary to control the way your body looks. Knowledge is power and the power to change the way your body looks will give you a sense of control that will spill over into other areas of your life. Soon you will discover that the discipline you use to re-sculpt your body can be used to accomplish any other goal that you want to reach in life. Now stop wishing and start doing! Go for it!

# About the Authors

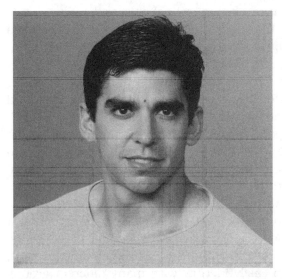

**Hugo A. Rivera** graduated from the University of South Florida with a Bachelor of Science in Engineering and also holds two certifications from ISSA, as a trainer and a specialist in nutrition. Born on December 5, 1974 in Bayamon, Puerto Rico, he was an overweight child and experienced at an early age the insecurity that comes with obesity and the ridicule of those around him. After going anorexic at the age of 13 and losing a total of 70 pounds in less than a year, his concerned parents took him to a nutritionist in an effort to stop the anorexic cycle. This nutritionist mentioned one thing that would change Hugo's outlook on dieting forever: "Eating food will not make you fat; only abusing the quantities of the bad foods will." Hugo decided to kick his anorexia and instead dedicate his life to studying the effects of foods on the human physiology.

By the age of fifteen, Hugo's interest in how food affects the shape and the form of your body naturally led to an interest in exercise, something that led him to become an avid natural bodybuilder.

He discovered early on that there wasn't much realistic or practical bodybuilding/fitness advice and went on to record what did and didn't work for him. After much trial and error, he started finding principles that he noticed worked on any healthy human being. The best part of it all was his discovery of the fact that there was no necessity to stay all day at the gym in order to get results! Upset at the fact that not many people in the industry cared about trainees actually reaching their goals, he decided to create a web site and start conducting personal training during his college years in an effort to spread all of the knowledge that he had acquired.

Twenty years later Hugo holds a Statewide Natural Bodybuilding Title (Mr. Typhoon Bay) and also a 4th Place in the Nationwide NPC Team Universe (the natural bodybuilder's highest and most competitive contest). Hugo is now considered an expert in the industry and he has dedicated much of his time to helping normal people achieve their dream figures by sharing sensible and practical knowledge that he has found over the years to work ever on the most stubborn metabolisms. Hugo has shared his knowledge on his website www.hrfit.net, through various radio interviews and speaking engagements, as well as on several articles published in the numerous magazines and websites all over the world, such as:

- *Muscular Development en Español* Magazine
- *Maximum Fitness* Magazine
- *Physique* Magazine
- *Be Healthy and Beautiful* Magazine
- *Muscle*
- *Natural Muscle* Magazine
- *Olympian Muscle News*
- *SuperOnda*
- Bodybuilding.About.com
- Bodybuilding.com
- DaveDraper.com
- Dolfzine.com
- MidwestChristianBodybuilding.com
- MSNBC.com
- StrengthPlanet.com

Hugo authored and self-published an online bodybuilding manual called *Body Re-Engineering*. In 2001 he commercially published two books called *The Body Sculpting Bible for Men* and *The Body Sculpting Bible for Women* with co-author James Villepigue, an authority in exercise form and the connection between the mind and the muscle. In these books, both authors apply the periodization principles used by pro athletes to workouts geared for people whose main goal is to lose weight and firm up. Both books soon became bestsellers and now there are over eight book extensions on that franchise.

Hugo was selected from thousands of applicants from all over the world to become the new www.Bodybuilding.About.com guide, an About.com website owned by the *New York Times* Company whose goal is to help beginners start a safe and healthy weight-lifting program, choose the right gear for their needs, and offer motivation to help users meet their personal goals.

Finally, Hugo has co-authored nutrition and training programs along with actress, fitness icon, and six-time Ms. Olympia Cory Everson. He has also served as consultant to high schools helping to put together bodybuilding shows and educating the students on the several aspects of bodybuilding competition and the dangers of steroids. Hugo also visits elementary schools and talks to kids about the importance of a solid education coupled with fitness and exercise. Hugo serves as a consultant to nutrition companies designing nutritional formulas and does seminars all over the world on the subjects of training, nutrition and supplementation.

Hugo's knowledge of the human physiology and anatomy (something that he was exposed to from an early age as his grandfather was a medical doctor), combined with his analytical skills developed through his engineering profession, enable him to produce extremely efficient programs that anyone can fit into their schedule. Because he was overweight and then extremely underweight, he can easily identify with many different groups of people-and his history of juggling several jobs allows him to offer practical advice that people who live a hectic lifestyle can follow.

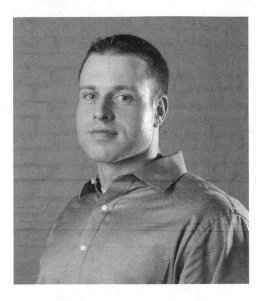

**James Villepigue** has over 20 years of quality certified experience in the health and fitness industry as a nationally certified personal trainer with The American Council on Exercise and The International Sports Science Association. He has received a degree from the New York College of Health Professions and is a massage therapist. James has also attended the accredited and highly acclaimed training school, the Institute for Professional Empowerment Coaching.

The success of the *Body Sculpting Bible* system and his extensive training and coaching experience have propelled James to appearances on national television programs and publication in nationally recognized health and fitness magazines such as:

- *Live with Regis and Kelly*
- *Maury*
- CBS, NBC, FOX, ABC, The WB, and many others
- *Fitness*
- *Women's World*
- *Oxygen*
- *Marie Claire*
- *Cosmopolitan*
- *Muscle-Mag International*

In his own words:

"Fitness training has allowed me to help hundreds of thousands of people throughout the world, of all ages and from all walks of life, to achieve extraordinary results. Besides seeing great changes to their bodies, my clients have additionally received profound changes to all aspects of their lives. This includes being happier, having better relationships, making more money, finding their dream jobs, and achieving all their dreams.

"I've overcome many obstacles in my own life and even most recently, have been dealing with the most challenging obstacle of my life—the tragic death of my beloved father, James Robsam Villepigue. This has been the greatest test for me and my family's very courageous ability to move forward in the wake of chaos. The love that I hold for my dad has empowered me to continue on my wonderful journey of success. I honor my dad and am able to keep to the path I set for myself.

"For those of you who are new to the *Body Sculpting Bible* series, I grew up a skinny kid, who suddenly became very overweight around the age of 14. I was bullied and teased, all the while dreaming for a slim, muscled physique. Unfortunately, in an attempt to lose weight quickly, I became bulimic. I managed to get very thin, but very sick. One's not worth the other, trust me!

"I soon discovered the importance of a clean and healthy lifestyle, comprised of healthy eating, fitness, meditation, and major self-discovery. Fitness gave me the confidence I needed to stand-up for myself and conquer all obstacles in my way. I am so thankful for my discovery of a healthy and fit lifestyle and only wish that everyone could experience it for themselves."

Believe and achieve!

James Villepigue